Acute Topics in Anti-Doping

Medicine and Sport Science

Vol. 62

Series Editors

Dennis J. Caine Georgetown, TX
Andrew P. Hills Brisbane, QLD
Timothy Noakes Cape Town

Acute Topics in Anti-Doping

Volume Editors

Olivier Rabin Montreal, QC
Yannis Pitsiladis Eastbourne

15 figures, 8 in color, and 9 tables, 1 in color, 2017

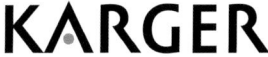

Basel · Freiburg · Paris · London · New York · Chennai · New Delhi ·
Bangkok · Beijing · Shanghai · Tokyo · Kuala Lumpur · Singapore · Sydney

Medicine and Sport Science

Founded 1968 by E. Jokl, Lexington, KY

Honorary Series Editors: J. Borms, Brussels; M. Hebbelinck, Brussels

Olivier Rabin, PhD
Senior Executive Director, Sciences and International Partnerships
World Anti-Doping Agency (WADA)
Stock Exchange Tower
800 Place Victoria, Suite 1700
Montreal, QC H4Z 1B7 (Canada)

Yannis Pitsiladis, MMedSci, PhD, FACSM
Professor of Sport and Exercise Science
University of Brighton
Welkin House
30 Carlisle Road
Eastbourne BN20 7SN (UK)

Library of Congress Cataloging-in-Publication Data

Names: Rabin, Olivier, editor. | Pitsiladis, Yannis, 1967- editor.
Title: Acute topics in anti-doping / volume editors, Olivier Rabin, Yannis Pitsiladis.
Other titles: Medicine and sport science ; v. 62. 0254-5020
Description: Basel, New York : Karger, [2017] | Series: Medicine and sport science, ISSN 0254-5020 ; vol. 62 | Includes bibliographical references and index.
Identifiers: LCCN 2017018114| ISBN 9783318060430 (hard cover : alk. paper) | ISBN 9783318060447 (e-ISBN)
Subjects: | MESH: Doping in Sports--prevention & control | Doping in Sports--legislation & jurisprudence
Classification: LCC RC1230 | NLM QT 262 | DDC 362.29/088796--dc23 LC record available at https://lccn.loc.gov/2017018114

Bibliographic Indices. This publication is listed in bibliographic services, including Current Contents® and Index Medicus.

Disclaimer. The statements, opinions and data contained in this publication are solely those of the individual authors and contributors and not of the publisher and the editor(s). The appearance of advertisements in the book is not a warranty, endorsement, or approval of the products or services advertised or of their effectiveness, quality or safety. The publisher and the editor(s) disclaim responsibility for any injury to persons or property resulting from any ideas, methods, instructions or products referred to in the content or advertisements.

Drug Dosage. The authors and the publisher have exerted every effort to ensure that drug selection and dosage set forth in this text are in accord with current recommendations and practice at the time of publication. However, in view of ongoing research, changes in government regulations, and the constant flow of information relating to drug therapy and drug reactions, the reader is urged to check the package insert for each drug for any change in indications and dosage and for added warnings and precautions. This is particularly important when the recommended agent is a new and/or infrequently employed drug.

All rights reserved. No part of this publication may be translated into other languages, reproduced or utilized in any form or by any means electronic or mechanical, including photocopying, recording, microcopying, or by any information storage and retrieval system, without permission in writing from the publisher.

© Copyright 2017 by S. Karger AG, P.O. Box, CH–4009 Basel (Switzerland)
www.karger.com
Printed in Germany on acid-free and non-aging paper (ISO 9706)
ISSN 0254–5020
e-ISSN 1662–2812
ISBN 978–3–318–06043–0
e-ISBN 978–3–318–06044–7

Contents

VII Preface
Reedie, C. (Glasgow)

1 Brief History of Anti-Doping
Ljungqvist, A. (Stockholm)

Regulatory and Legal Issues

11 The Development of the World Anti-Doping Code
Young, R. (Colorado Springs, CO)

22 Is the Fight against Doping in Sport a Legal Minefield like Any Other?
Haas, U. (Zurich)

34 How Will the Legal and Sport Environment Influence a Future Code?
Niggli, O. (Montreal, QC)

The Anti-Doping Science

39 Structure and Development of the List of Prohibited Substances and Methods
Kinahan, A. (Montreal, QC/Ennis); Budgett, R. (Montreal, QC/London);
Mazzoni, I. (Montreal, QC/Dublin)

55 Therapeutic Use Exemptions
Gerrard, D. (Montreal, QC); Pipe, A. (Ottawa, ON)

68 Challenges in Modern Anti-Doping Analytical Science
Ayotte, C. (Laval, QC); Miller, J. (Glasgow); Thevis, M. (Cologne)

77 Achievements and Challenges in Anti-Doping Research
Bowers, L.D. (Colorado Springs, CO); Bigard, X. (Paris)

91 Gene and Cell Doping: The New Frontier – Beyond Myth or Reality
Neuberger, E.W.I.; Simon, P. (Mainz)

Next Generation Anti-Doping Approaches

107 The Athlete Biological Passport: How to Personalize Anti-Doping Testing across an Athlete's Career?
Robinson, N. (Epalinges); Sottas, P.-E. (Lausanne); Schumacher, Y.O. (Doha)

119 Next Generation "Omics" Approaches in the "Fight" against Blood Doping
Wang, G. (Eastbourne/Rome); Karanikolou, A.; Verdouka I. (Eastbourne); Friedmann, T. (San Diego, CA); Pitsiladis, Y. (Eastbourne/Rome)

129 Integration of the Forensic Dimension into Anti-Doping Strategies
Marclay, F.; Saugy, M. (Epalinges/Lausanne)

139 How to Develop Intelligence Gathering in Efficient and Practical Anti-Doping Activities
Holz, M. (Lausanne); Robertson, J. (Montreal, QC)

Social and Ethical Dimensions of Anti-Doping

153 Education in Anti-Doping: The Art of Self-Imposed Constraints
Loland, S. (Oslo)

160 Can We Better Integrate the Role of Anti-Doping in Sports and Society? A Psychological Approach to Contemporary Value-Based Prevention
Petróczi, A. (Kingston upon Thames/Sheffield); Norman, P. (Sheffield); Brueckner, S. (Kingston upon Thames/Saarbrücken)

177 Sport, Society, and Anti-Doping Policy: An Ethical Overview
Bloodworth, A.J.; McNamee, M. (Swansea)

186 A Moral Foundation for Anti-Doping: How Far Have We Progressed? Where Are the Limits?
Murray, T.H. (Brewster, MA)

194 Conclusion and Perspectives
Howman, D. (Wellington)

202 Author Index
203 Subject Index

Preface

As we now operate under a revised and stronger version of the World Anti-Doping Code that came into force in January 2015, it is the appropriate time to provide the anti-doping community with an updated view of the approaches being taken to protect the clean athletes all around the world. This publication, edited by Olivier Rabin, the Science Director of the World Anti-Doping Agency (WADA), and Yannis Pitsiladis, a leading researcher, covers a wide range of issues including the revised regulatory framework, anti-doping science, possible future changes in emphasis, and the social and ethical dimensions of anti-doping, all entirely appropriate as we look towards the future.

WADA has become a major investor in anti-doping science and has invested since its inception close to USD 75 million. The opportunity now exists to develop this program further as governments around the world have provided some matching funding to meet the USD 10-million fund created by the International Olympic Committee (IOC). This is an exciting development and will widen the range of opportunities open to the scientific community to develop further new and potentially revolutionary processes necessary to protect sport and its athletes.

Progress of science and its implementation in routine anti-doping activities is pivotal in our strategy to expose doped athletes. That was particularly true at an individual level with the retesting program of samples collected by the IOC during the Beijing and London Olympic Games, which revealed more than a hundred new doping cases. Also, in 2016, the combination of science with intelligence and investigations revealed the proofs of the instituitonalized doping program in Russia.

Contributions to this volume of work come from some of the world leading experts in their fields of work and study and provide a wide-ranging picture of the current situation and future opportunities facing the anti-doping community. This is entirely relevant to the challenges faced and the efforts being made to advance the science and knowledge essential to the important tasks ahead.

I commend this book to the reader and thank all the contributors for their willingness to advance the cause of clean sport.

Sir Craig Reedie
President of WADA

Brief History of Anti-Doping

Arne Ljungqvist

Professor Arne Ljungqvist Anti-Doping Foundation, Stockholm, Sweden

Abstract

The fight against doping in sport as we know it today commenced by the creation of the International Olympic Committee (IOC) Medical Commission in 1961 following the death of a Danish cyclist during the Rome Olympic Games the year before. After a slow start, the fight got under way as from the early 1970s under the leadership of the IOC and of the International Association of Athletics Federations. Despite a lack of understanding and weak support even from the sports community, a series of measures were taken during the 1970s and 1980s which still form cornerstones of today's anti-doping strategy. In addition to information and education campaigns, the most important examples are the introduction of procedural rules for doping controls, the establishment and follow-up of a list of prohibited substances and methods, the accreditation of doping control laboratories, the introduction of in- and out-of-competition testing, rules for therapeutic use exemption, and the introduction of blood sampling. During the 1990s, the anti-doping fight gained increasing support both inside and outside the sport community. In order to harmonize the wide variety of rules that had developed both in sport organizations and at the domestic level and to promote anti-doping activities, the World Anti-Doping Agency (WADA) was jointly created by the Olympic movement and the public authorities in 1999. WADA is today carrying on the fight supported by the universally accepted WADA Code and an International Anti-Doping Convention under UNESCO.

© 2017 S. Karger AG, Basel

Introduction

The Rome Olympic Games took place in the summer of 1960. During the team road race, Knud Enemark Jensen, a Danish cyclist, collapsed and died. Some of his team mates also suffered but recovered. Heat stroke? Possibly. But the athletes had been given some sort of stimulating "cocktail" by a team leader. One report stated that it contained Ronicol, a vasodilator [1], and another that it contained some amphetamine-like substance [2]. It was well known that cyclists often used cocktails of different drugs, but the actual content of the Danish one was never officially confirmed. Probably stimulating/vasodilating drugs and the heat together caused the tragedy.

The Rome Olympic Games were the first Summer Games to be televised live to an international audience. The fact that the death of an Olympian while competing was captured live by millions of spectators around the world was too much to accept for the IOC. Although some leaders like the British IOC member Lord Burghley – the 1928 Olympic champion in 400-m hurdles – had warned already at the IOC Session in Warsaw in 1937 about the practice of drug use in elite sport [3], not much had been done to combat it. Now, something needed to be done. The reputation of Olympic sports, and elite sports in general, was at stake. In 1961, the IOC created a Medical Commission (MC) chaired by the IOC member from New Zealand, Sir Arthur Porritt. The remit of the IOC-MC was to design a strategy to combat the drug use in Olympic sports.

The use of performance-enhancing substances, however, has a long history both in sport and in society in general. For example, various kinds of herbal extracts were used by athletes for the purpose of performance enhancement in the ancient Olympic Games and "Ma Huang" (an extract from the *Ephedra* plant) was used as a stimulating drug by the Chinese emperor and his people 2700 BC [4]. The stimulating substance in Ma Huang was identified in 1924 and given the name "ephedrine", which is today on the list of prohibited substances in sport. A more recent example is the use of amphetamines by soldiers during the 2nd World War.

In today's sports, the use of performance-enhancing substances and methods is forbidden and known as "doping," a term that reportedly appeared for the first time in an English dictionary in 1889. Doping was described as an opium-containing remedy which was used to "dope" horses, the word "dope" stemming from the Boer language in South Africa in which "dope" was an extract with stimulating effects [5].

The creation of the IOC-MC signaled the start of the fight against doping in sport. The MC started from scratch. Little was known about what drugs were being used in sport and the extent of their use. Practically no rules were in place. The International Association of Athletics Federations (IAAF) had been the first sport organization to introduce some general rules prohibiting the use of stimulating drugs in 1928, but there is no report on any testing or enforcement of these rules.

The First Steps (1961–1972)

It took Sir Porritt and his Commission many years to assess the situation and to define a strategy. It was not until the 1967 IOC Session in Tehran that the MC presented a proposal which basically consisted of a list of prohibited substances (sympathomimetic amines, central nervous stimulants, narcotics, antidepressants, and major tranquillizers) and rules for testing for those substances at the Olympic Games [3]. At the Teheran Session, Sir Porritt was succeeded by the Belgian IOC member, Prince Alexandre de Mérode, who enthusiastically embraced this role and came to chair the MC for 35 years.

Because of the tragedy in Rome in 1960, the IOC and the UCI (International Cycling Union) planned for some testing in cycling at the 1964 Tokyo Games, but the attempt failed [3]. Samples were collected at the 1968 Mexico City Games, and the first Olympic doping case was found. A member of the Swedish modern pentathlon team tested positive for alcohol after having consumed some beer, and the team was stripped of its bronze medal.

It was not until the Munich Summer Games in 1972, however, that a comprehensive testing program was introduced. About 7,000 athletes competed and over 2,000 samples were collected and analyzed for different stimulants. At these Games, the 16-year-old gold medalist in 400-m freestyle swimming from USA, Rick DeMont, tested positive for ephedrine, which he had been taking routinely for his asthma. After his successful 400 m, he qualified for the final in 1,500 m where he was the clear favorite to win another gold medal. However, following the positive test, he was removed from the 1,500-m final and lost his gold in the 400 m. Although Rick DeMont had reported the use of ephedrine, this was not accepted on the grounds that he had competed with a prohibited substance in his body. Unfortunately, exemption rules allowing the use of banned substances did not exist at that time to avert this unfortunate situation. In 2001, the US Olympic Committee unsuccessfully appealed to the IOC on behalf of DeMont to reinstate his medal.

The IOC had declared in 1968 that their role would not be to conduct doping controls in the world of sport but to organize for such controls to be conducted at the Olympic Games and alert the National Olympic Committees (NOCs) and international federations (IFs) to take similar action. The IAAF was the first IF to take action by forming an MC at its Congress in Munich in 1972. The IAAF-MC decisively confronted the problem of doping and soon became a leading international sports body in the fight against doping [6].

Further Steps (1973–1999)

The initiation of the fight against the misuse of drugs in sport in the early 1970s revealed decades of widespread drug use in sport and highlighted the need for a concerted response. This allowed the drug takers to establish themselves considerably ahead of those who were trying to combat the use of drugs. Their task was made even more difficult by the inexperience and, at times, unwillingness, both within and outside sport, to decisively tackle the problem of drugs in sport. The generally held view opposing decisive action was: Why could athletes not be allowed to take substances that were not illegal for the public at large? This view exemplified the need for anti-doping education directed not only at the sports world but also at the media and the general public. A number of additional steps were also needed to truly enhance the fight against doping.

List of Prohibited Substances
The first prohibited list presented by the IOC in 1967 did not contain anabolic steroids or anabolic androgenic steroids (AAS) as can be found in the current prohibited list of the World Anti-Doping Agency (WADA). Back then, there was no appetite for and even resistance against banning anabolic steroids given their widespread use by athletes and a general lack of understanding of doping. Instead, there was support for banning a class of strong stimulants like amphetamines, as this class of drug was increasingly being regarded as a narcotic drug and outlawed in numerous countries.

After some campaigning, the IAAF banned steroids in 1974 and used an immunoassay test for their detection at the European Championships in athletics in Rome the same year [7]. There were no positive cases, but the experience paved the way for the IOC to ban steroids before the Montreal Games in 1976 and resulted in 8 positive cases with an improved method. Four decades later, the use of AAS constitutes the vast majority of anti-doping rule violations.

The inclusion of AAS to the list of banned substances was a turning point in anti-doping as the IOC-MC continued to amend the list over time. The inclusion of substances to this list was done without any consultation process, and it is noteworthy that no such process was requested during the IOC management of the prohibited list. This process changed when WADA took over the decision making as from 2004, with the introduction of a consultation process with stakeholders that typically receives several hundreds of submissions during the annual review of the prohibited list.

Standardization of Laboratory Analysis
Since the commencement of the anti-doping process, sampling urine for doping analyses has been the preferred approach as metabolites of most doping substances are excreted via the kidneys. The typical athlete defense to a positive test has

involved contesting the laboratory process. Common claims included the mixing up of samples or following incorrect analytical procedures by laboratories. It soon became apparent that strict laboratory procedures beyond those in existence in standard hospital laboratories with respect to safety and accuracy had to be established for the anti-doping laboratories. In the late 1970s, the IAAF-MC drafted procedural guidelines and identified specific requirements for laboratories used for doping analysis. In 1979, the IAAF Council decided that only laboratories that adhered to these guidelines and requirements would qualify for doping control – the beginning of "accreditation" of doping control laboratories. The IOC adopted the IAAF accreditation system 2 years later, and, for a couple of years, the IAAF and the IOC accredited doping laboratories jointly. In 1986, the IOC took over the full responsibility of accreditation with the aim to encourage all IFs to use accredited laboratories only. Since 2004, WADA has the sole responsibility for accreditation.

Since the introduction of AAS to the prohibited list, it has been argued that this ban would be ineffective since analytical proof of their use would be impossible. While this view was soon proven wrong, a similar argument was made as further substances were added to the prohibited list such as growth hormone and erythropoietin. These hormones are produced by recombinant DNA technology, which make them virtually identical to the naturally occurring form. Yet, differences were identified, which made it possible to detect the administration of the recombinant versions. Similar arguments have also been made about gene doping since the aim is for the body to produce the endogenic versions of the hormones of interest. While gene doping detection methods are early in their development, encouraging results to date have convinced the experts (e.g., WADA Gene Doping Panel) that gene doping will be detectable. In fact, validation procedures of a potential detection method were concluded in 2016 [8].

Introduction of Out-of-Competition Testing
The first list of prohibited substances contained drugs considered performance enhancing when taken before competition. AAS, however, are taken mainly during training periods in order to enhance muscle building and strength. AAS also allow the athlete to train harder and recover quicker. Detecting the use of AAS would, therefore, require testing during training periods, the so-called "out-of-competition testing" (OOCT). The initial concerns raised primarily on ethical grounds (e.g., the appropriateness of visiting an athlete at his/her working place or home to conduct anti-doping tests) were dismissed following investigations in Norway and Sweden that concluded in favor of OOCT as long as the athlete was a member of a sport organization that signed up to these rules.

The Scandinavian countries were the first to start OOCT in the late 1970s to early 1980s, but this idea was met with great resistance when it was being discussed at a more international level. The Ben Johnson scandal at the Seoul Games in 1988 helped sensitize the sporting world to the need for OOCT in the fight against AAS abuse, and this urged the IAAF to introduce the necessary ruling in 1989. Most other federations and countries were quite slow in adopting OOCT. This led the IOC to establish a "Subcommission for Out-Of-Competition Testing" in December 1991 with the objective "to encourage and stimulate IFs and NOCs to carry out their own control programs" [3], but this initiative failed. It is indicative that when WADA was created in 1999, only 12 Olympic IFs had rules that allowed for OOCT, and only a handful of these conducted such testing; 60% of tests were conducted by IAAF, 20% by FINA (Fédération Internationale de Natation), and the remaining 20% by just a few more sports such as rowing, canoeing, and weight lifting. Today, any national anti-doping organization or IF that does not have OOCT included in its program will be declared as not Code compliant by WADA with potentially serious consequences.

An OOCT program can only work if it is known where to find the athletes to be tested at any given time. To that end a "whereabouts rule" was established for all athletes in a registered testing pool whose responsibility was to inform the relevant anti-doping organization where he/she can be found and to keep that information updated. As was the case for OOCT, the introduction of the "whereabouts rule" was controversial. In the end, however, this principle was supported by the Court of Arbitration for Sport (CAS; see further below).

Introduction of Therapeutic Use Exemption
The introduction of exemption for an athlete to use a banned substance for medical reasons was prompted by a Swedish case in the early 1980s [7]. Briefly, a young athlete requested permission from his national anti-doping authority to be allowed to compete despite receiving testosterone replacement therapy after both his testes had been removed (one for testis retention as a baby and the other for testis cancer as a teenager). A juridical analysis concluded that the athlete should be allowed to compete provided that he accepted that his serum levels of testosterone would be monitored in order to make sure that his levels were within the normal range. It was emphasized, however, that in the absence of international rules this decision was valid only in Sweden.

The exemption issue gained considerable international prominence after the inclusion of glucocorticoids, diuretics, and β-blockers to the prohibited list during the years 1985–1988. These substances were commonly used to treat a variety of illnesses, thus aiding individuals suffering from such conditions to compete. In the absence of any rules, 2 athletes were, nevertheless, allowed to take banned substances at the 1988 Olympic Games, one cortisone for chronic inflammatory bowel disease and the other a diuretic for the nephrotic syndrome [9]. These 2 cases polarized opinions within the IOC-MC: some members were in favor of introducing rules, while others strongly opposed this view claiming that an athlete who required treatment with a banned drug should not be allowed to compete, at least not in the Olympic Games.

In 1991, an unofficial group of 3 IOC-MC members was appointed (Medical Advisory Committee – MAC) to develop strict criteria for permitting the use of banned substances, and they proposed the following: (i) evidence that no allowed treatment could be used, (ii) that even temporary withdrawal of the treatment would result in a serious health risk for the athlete, and (iii) that the treatment would not result in further performance enhancement beyond restoration to normal health. The proposal was accepted by the IOC-MC, and MAC started to operate as from the Barcelona Games in 1992. Remarkably, MAC continued to work for 8 years without any official approval by the IOC Executive Board. In 2000, the therapeutic use exemption concept was added in the form of a 1-sentence addendum to the IOC Medical Code that had been published a year earlier. The international standard for therapeutic use exemption is an important part of the current WADA Code, and the criteria that were worked out by MAC remain essentially unchanged.

Introduction of Blood Sampling
After having won the gold medal in team cycling at the Los Angeles Olympic Games in 1984, US cyclists admitted using blood transfusions to enhance oxygen delivery and, thereby, improve endurance performance. During this time, the IOC prohibited list contained only substances and methods for which analytical detection techniques were available. Consequently, blood transfusions were not banned by the IOC, but the confession by the US team sparked a change in the IOC philosophy, and blood doping was banned.

Detection of blood doping would require the analysis of blood samples, but at that time it was generally believed that blood sampling for the purpose of doping control would not be possible on a global basis for religious and cultural reasons. This idea was put to the test in 1992 when the IAAF decided to conduct blood sampling at their great international Galas to conduct blood count analysis [10]. Blood sampling was well tolerated without any protests from the athletes, and no abnormal blood counts were recorded. Analysis of blood samples is an important part of the current full analytical menu, and any anti-doping organization that does not include blood sampling in its testing program will not be in compliance with the WADA Code.

Obstacles on the Way

Lack of Commitment

The general resistance to fight doping during the 1970s and 1980s stems from the fact that East Germany (GDR) had developed a successful state-run doping program in the mid-late 1960s for political gain [11]. The motivation was to demonstrate the superiority of the GDR political system by winning battles on the sports ground, particularly at the Olympic level. The resulting superior sporting performances of this system were widely admired until the full truth behind the success was revealed following the disintegration of the Berlin Wall and the fading of the Cold War. Systematic doping was not confined only to the GDR but was also rife in other countries, both in the East and West, although less sophisticated and extensive than in the GDR. Due to its strength in sport, GDR became powerful also at the international leadership level of sport, and their representatives were well placed to block the fight against doping. For example, Claus Clausnitzer, who was the head of the accredited GDR doping control laboratory in Kreischa, was a member of the IOC-MC, while one of the chief medical engineers of the GDR doping program was Dr. Manfred Höppner, who was a member of the IAAF-MC. Furthermore, when the GDR was invited to join the Nordic Anti-Doping Convention in the mid-1980s, which would have included unannounced OOCT of their athletes, they effectively turned down the offer by suggesting that the GDR would join only if the US and the Soviet Union would also join [12].

Other reasons for the unwillingness to take decisive action at the national and IF levels were the high costs involved in developing and conducting anti-doping programs, the lack of expertise, and the negative publicity that affected those sports and countries that exposed doping in their top athletes.

New Drugs, Designer Drugs, and Food Supplements

Well before WADA was established, the IOC-MC proactively approached the pharmaceutical industry in order to create a process by which the IOC would be alerted to new drugs nearing production that could potentially be misused for doping. The industry was not interested in such a collaboration fearing their drugs would be associated with doping. This reluctance by the industry delayed effective drug testing since analytical methods for the detection of new drugs were usually not available at the time when these drugs reached the market. The situation improved considerably after the creation of WADA, when the pharmaceutical industry became more responsive to the point that today there exists a very good collaboration.

In the 1990s, the IOC-MC was confronted with designer drugs, and, in the early 2000s, the first evidence emerged of the existence of a clandestine industry that produced such doping substances [7]. The BALCO (Bay Area Laboratory Co-Operative) scandal that exploded in 2003 was the most famous example, and the likelihood is high that similar underground activities are in existence today.

Possibly even more problematic were the many claims by athletes from the late 1990s onwards that doping substances found in their urine was the result of the intake of food supplements that had been improperly labeled. A prominent example was the case of Mark Richardson. He was a successful British runner and member of the team that won the silver medal in the 4 × 400 m relay at the Atlanta Games in 1996 and gold at the World Championships in 1997. In 1999, he tested positive for the anabolic steroid nandrolone but blamed the positive test to the intake a particular food supplement. In March 2000, the athlete was suspended by the IAAF and missed the 2000 Olympics in Sydney. In June 2001 and following a heated debate, the athlete was reinstated under the IAAF "exceptional circumstances rule" since contamination of his food supplement could not be excluded. In response, both the IOC and IAAF repeated their earlier warnings against the use of food supplements by athletes and emphasized that the "strict liability" principle would be upheld in the future. Soon thereafter, the Cologne laboratory confirmed that about 15% of food supplements collected from the Internet and food supplement stores contained AAS that were not declared on the label [13]. Unfortunately, the poorly regulated food supplement market today continues to constitute a high risk for inadvertent doping.

Creation of WADA (1999)

The emergence of WADA was to some extent precipitated by cooperation between sport organizations and governments dating back several decades. In the late 1960s, the Council of Europe attempted to address the growing problem of doping in sport by establishing a policy partnership with the IOC. The aim was to harmonize anti-doping activities and rules at domestic and international levels within Europe in the first instance. This partnership soon resulted in the development of a policy document – the European Anti-Doping Charter – that was adopted by the Council in 1984 and committed the European governments to the anti-doping campaign. In 1988, a world conference on anti-doping was convened in Ottawa, Canada, where senior sports leaders and governmental officials from different parts of the world came together and further developed an international anti-doping charter that came to be known as the "International Olympic Charter against Doping in Sport." The IOC adopted this anti-doping charter at the time of the Seoul Games in September 1988 [3].

The Ben Johnson scandal at the Seoul Games in 1988 and the revelations of the GDR system soon thereafter changed attitudes towards doping within sport. As was the case 30 years earlier, it was acknowledged that the reputation of the Olympic movement and sport in general was at stake, and doping became regarded as the greatest threat to the future of competitive sport. Throughout the 1990s, the anti-doping cause received greater attention, respect, and support both inside sport and by the public. As anti-doping activities increased, so did the number of athletes failing doping tests, and this highlighted the urgent need for universally accepted penalties for doping violations. At that stage, the penalties for different anti-doping rule violations varied considerably between the different IFs and between different countries. Thus, athletes from one and the same country could get different penalties depending on the sport, whereas athletes in one and the same sport could get different penalties depending on their nationality.

Inconsistencies in rule violation penalties emerged due to the uncoordinated way in which national and IF rules developed. Generally, these were based on the IOC rules in terms of the list of prohibited substances and procedures for doping control and rule enforcement, but the penalties in the IOC rules were restricted to disqualification from the Olympic Games, and without any consideration given to further penalties. This situation permitted the courts to overturn with ease decisions on penalties taken by the sport authorities; IFs with greatest penalties, such as the IAAF, were most affected. In order to rectify matters, the

IAAF formed an arbitration panel under its own constitution in 1982. The IOC followed this example 1 year later by establishing the CAS, which became operational as from June 30, 1984. However, the Federal Court of Switzerland did not judge CAS sufficiently independent from the IOC until after it had amended its constitution in 1994.

Despite the formation of arbitration procedures in sport, courts continued to become involved in doping cases, sometimes with very serious consequences. For instance, a US district court decided in 1991 to exonerate a doped world champion in athletics and ordered the IAAF to pay the athlete USD 27 million in compensation. Although the verdict was not upheld at the higher level, the 2.5-year-long process was extremely costly for the IAAF. It was clear that a common set of anti-doping rules was needed, particularly with respect to penalties. Creating such rules would require support not only from the world of sport but also by the international legal community and public authorities. This realization and a number of key incidents in 1998 led the IOC to invite the governments to collectively form WADA. One key incident was the intervention by the French police at the Tour de France when doping material was found in the possession of the Festina cycling team, and the other was a scandal with the IOC-accredited laboratory in Rome where doping control samples had been left unanalyzed for anabolic steroids. These incidents and comments made by then IOC President Antonio Samaranch, which were interpreted by the media as signs of leniency towards athletes guilty of doping, led to a world conference with representatives of governments and the world of sport to decide to create WADA in February 1999. WADA was formally established in November the same year.

The creation of WADA is unquestionably an important milestone in anti-doping history as its formation changed the general perspective of the use of doping substances from being a problem for sport alone to being accepted as a problem for the whole of society. A powerful message was sent jointly by the world of sport and the international political establishment that doping is unacceptable.

Early Effects of the Creation of WADA

The WADA Code

The most imminent challenge for WADA was to develop a set of universally accepted rules. After only a few years, a draft code received general support at the WADA World Conference on doping in Copenhagen in March 2003. The IOC compelled the Olympic federations to adopt the Code by stating that those federations that had not adopted the WADA Code by the opening of the 2004 Athens Games would not be allowed to have their sport on the Olympic program. Consequently, all federations adopted the Code in time. The governments also took their own action by producing an anti-doping convention under UNESCO by 2005, which came into operation 2 years later when the necessary 30 states had ratified it. The anti-doping convention assured sport the necessary governmental support to enforce the WADA Code in the fight against doping. The expectation was that the UNESCO convention would be implemented at the national level by the introduction of appropriate domestic legislation in the vast majority of countries where such legislation was not in place, but to date this process has been relatively slow [14].

Stimulation of Anti-Doping Activities

When WADA was created, there were many sports organizations that had no, or ineffective, anti-doping activities, and the same was also true at the domestic level. The Code requires all signatories to have adequate anti-doping programs in place or risk being declared noncompliant with possibly serious consequences. WADA established both a support program for the development of anti-doping activities where needed, in particular in-competition testing and OOCT, and a monitoring system for ascertaining Code compliance. Although more needs to be done, the anti-doping activities in sport today are far more extensive and efficient since WADA was created. New challenges are also emerging, such as the widespread use of AAS outside competitive sport, thereby creating a public health issue [15].

Research

It is surprising that the IOC did not have a fund dedicated to anti-doping research before WADA was created despite doping being regarded as the greatest threat to sport. Only occasionally did the IOC manage to raise money for specific anti-doping projects. One such example is the EU support of the "GH-2000" project, which started in 1996 with the aim to have an analytical method for the detection of human growth hormone in place by the time of the Sydney Olympic Games in 2000. This objective was not met, and the project became too expensive for continued funding. When WADA was formed, however, the IOC made it clear that a substantial part of the annual WADA budget of USD 25 million should go to research, in the beginning about 20–25%. Although that share has dropped in recent years, WADA has distributed close to USD 70 million to about 447 research projects since 2001. In order to support research further, the IOC decided in 2014 to allocate another USD 10 million to research into new detection methods and invited the governments to match that sum. Many governments have responded favorably, and more money will hopefully become available in the future. Research is undoubtedly of utmost importance in ensuring the WADA-accredited laboratories are kept abreast with the very latest testing technologies and the development of new drugs by the pharma industry that can be misused for the purpose of doping.

Conclusions

The history of the anti-doping campaign shows that:
- Sport organizations and governments have to work together in order to combat the use of doping.
- Cooperation with other parties, such as the pharmaceutical industry, is needed.
- The UNESCO convention needs to be implemented by the introduction of appropriate legislation at the domestic level.
- The food supplement market needs to be regulated.
- As new medications come on the market, analytical methods establishing their use will need to be developed.
- A permanent source for the funding of anti-doping research is essential.
- The use of doping substances has spread from sport to society outside sport and become a serious public health issue.

References

1 Groth O: Cykel; in Groth O, Eklöw R (eds): Olympiaboken. Stockholm, Hans Levart Förlag, 1960, p 337.
2 Houlihan B: Dying to Win, ed 2. Strasbourg, Council of Europe Publishing, 2002.
3 Dirix A, Sturbois X: The First Thirty Years of the International Olympic Committee Medical Commission 1967–1997. Lausanne, IOC Olympic Study Center, 1998.
4 Abourashed EA, El-Alfy AT, Khan IA, Walker L: Ephedra in perspective – a current review. Phytother Res 2003;17: 703–712.
5 Mueller RK: History of doping and doping control; in Thieme D, Hemmersbach P (eds): Doping in Sports. Berlin/Heidelberg, Springer, 2004, pp 1–2.

6 Ljungqvist A: The relentless fight against doping; in Watman M (ed): IAAF 100 Years. Monaco, IAAF, 2012, pp 113–119.
7 Catlin DH, Fitch KD, Ljungqvist A: Medicine and science in the fight against doping in sport. J Intern Med 2008;264: 99–114.
8 Baoutina A, Bhat S, Zheng M, Partis L, Dobeson M, Alexander IE, Emslie KR: Synthetic certified DNA reference material for analysis of human erythropoietin transgene and transcript in gene doping and gene therapy. Gene Ther 2016;23: 708–717.
9 Fitch K: Proscribed drugs at the Olympic Games: permitted use and misuse (doping) by athletes. Clin Med (Lond) 2012;12:257–260.
10 Birkeland KI, Donike M, Ljungqvist A, Fagerhol M, Jensen J, Hemmersbach P, Oftebro H, Haug E: Blood sampling in doping control. First experiences from regular testing in athletics. Int J Sports Med 1997;18:8–12.
11 Berendonk B: Doping Dokumente – Von der Forschung zum Betrug. Berlin/Heidelberg, Springer, 1991.
12 Lager G: Doping's Nemesis. Cheltenham, Sports Books, 2011.
13 Geyer H, Parr MK, Mareck U, Reinhart U, Schrader Y, Schänzer W: Analysis of non-hormonal nutritional supplements for anabolic-androgenic steroids – results of an international study. Int J Sports Med 2004;25:124–129.
14 Houlihan B, Garcia B: The use of legislation to controlling the production, movement, importation, distribution and supply of performance-enhancing drugs in sport (PEDS). www.wada-ama.org/en/media/news/2012-11/loughborough-study-supports-doping-specific-legislation (accessed November 15, 2012).
15 Strategy for Stopping Steroids, ed 1. Copenhagen, Anti Doping Denmark, 2012, http://www.antydoping.pl/upload/2012/strategy_for_stopping_steroids_report_web.pdf.

Arne Ljungqvist, MD, PhD
Professor Arne Ljungqvist Anti-Doping Foundation
Birger Jarlsgatan 41A
SE–111 45 Stockholm (Sweden)
E-Mail Arne.Ljungqvist@rf.se

The Development of the World Anti-Doping Code

Richard Young

Colorado Springs, CO, USA

Abstract

This chapter addresses both the development and substance of the World Anti-Doping Code, which came into effect in 2003, as well as the subsequent Code amendments, which came into effect in 2009 and 2015. Through an extensive process of stakeholder input and collaboration, the World Anti-Doping Code has transformed the hodgepodge of inconsistent and competing pre-2003 anti-doping rules into a harmonized and effective approach to anti-doping. The Code, as amended, is now widely recognized worldwide as the gold standard in anti-doping. The World Anti-Doping Code originally went into effect on January 1, 2004. The first amendments to the Code went into effect on January 1, 2009, and the second amendments on January 1, 2015. The Code and the related international standards are the product of a long and collaborative process designed to make the fight against doping more effective through the adoption and implementation of worldwide harmonized rules and best practices.

© 2017 S. Karger AG, Basel

Richard Young is a former member of the World Anti-Doping Agency Foundation Board, a member of the Code drafting team, and lead sport attorney.

The Disharmonized State of Anti-Doping Rules prior to the Code

In the decade before the World Anti-Doping Code (the "Code") went into effect, there was no shortage of anti-doping rules. Most international federations (IFs) and National Olympic Committees (NOCs) had their own anti-doping rules, modeled largely on the International Olympic Committee (IOC)'s Olympic Movement Anti-Doping Code. A number of governments had also adopted their own anti-doping legislation. National anti-doping organizations (NADOs) also had their own rules. The problem was that all of these rules were often inconsistent, ineffective, and uncoordinated, to the point that they undercut the credibility of the anti-doping effort. There was widespread consensus among the stakeholders that harmonization of rules was important for the credibility and effectiveness of anti-doping. The difficulty was that many of the stakeholders with the greatest experience and investment in anti-doping, including governments, NADOs, and IFs, were convinced that harmonization should occur on the basis of their own rules, as opposed to someone else's.

When the World Anti-Doping Agency (WADA) was formed in 1999, it was agreed that one of its most important tasks would be to try to harmonize global anti-doping rules. The lack of harmonization and coordination between the rules of the different anti-doping organizations (ADOs) is illustrated by the following examples.

- Athletes in 2 different sports test positive for the same prohibited substance under the same circumstances. Because the rules of their IFs are different, one gets banned for 6 months; the other gets banned for life.
- Two athletes in different sports inadvertently use a prohibited substance. One is exonerated because the rules of his sport make "intent to enhance performance" an element of an anti-doping rule violation. The other is declared ineligible for 2 years because in their sport the presence of a prohibited substance in an athlete's sample is a strict liability violation regardless of the athlete's intent, fault, or knowing use.
- A young tennis player competing in a foreign national tournament was taking a medication permitted by her NOC, her IF, and the IOC. She was excluded from the tournament and branded a cheat because her medication happened to be prohibited as doping by the laws of the host country and nowhere else.
- An IF and a NADO refuse to recognize each other's anti-doping decisions with respect to a single athlete who is a resident of the NADO's country and a competitor in the IF's sport because of differences in their rules as applied to the athlete's conduct.
- An athlete is tested out of competition twice on the same day, the first by his IF and then several hours later by his NADO. This is not part of a coordinated plan, rather the two ADOs did not coordinate their testing and had no idea what the other was doing.

The 2003 World Anti-Doping Code

WADA was given a clear mandate to harmonize anti-doping rules. The decision was made to accomplish this through the development of a single set of rules entitled the World Anti-Doping Code, which all ADOs would agree to follow.

The 2003 Code Drafting Process
WADA's initial approach to Code drafting was to assemble a large group of representative stakeholders. After several days of extensive deliberation but little progress, this approach was abandoned in favor of a small Code drafting team, which was tasked with soliciting worldwide input and then drafting based on that input. The drafting team included several senior experts from WADA and 2 external team members. One was a process consultant and the other was the author, as primary draftsman. The team started work in September 2001. Before commencing the drafting process, the Code drafting team reviewed the anti-doping rules of virtually all of the Olympic Movement stakeholders (including the IOC, continental federations, other major event organizations, IFs, and NOCs). The team also reviewed the work of the Council of Europe, IADA (International Anti-Doping Arrangement), IICAGDS (International Intergovernmental Consultative Group on Anti-Doping in Sport), and the anti-doping statutes and rules of governments and NADOs.

The key to the development of the Code was the magnitude of the stakeholder consultation process. Before a first draft of the Code was ever circulated, the Code drafting team initiated a comprehensive process to seek feedback from stakeholders and experts on both the framework of the Code (how the Code should interplay with the different facets of anti-doping) and opinions on those key elements of the rules that would form the backbone of the Code. That process included comments from more than 130 different organizations. Thirty experts in anti-doping were involved as content producers on different levels. Numerous meetings were held with athletes, the IOC, IFs, GAISF (General Association of International Sports Federations), governments, NADOs, NOCs, the European Commission, the Council of Europe, the Court of Arbitration for Sport (CAS), IICGADS, and WADA working committees. The consensus of this feedback was that the framework of the Code should include 3 levels of documents, with the Code itself (level 1), international standards that had the effect of rules (level 2), and models of best practice (level 3). Work on the international standards began simultaneously with work on the Code. Stakeholder comments on both the framework and backbone of the Code were incorporated into the first draft of the Code, which was tabled before the WADA Executive Committee, acting as the steering group for the Code drafting project.

During the consultation process following the release of the first draft of the Code, more than 120 additional official comments were received and reviewed. Extensive consultation with stakeholders continued, including, on the sport side, for example, the IOC and European athletes' commissions, the IOC, GAISF, ASOIF (Association of Summer Olympic International Federations), ARISF (Association of IOC Recognized International Sports Federations), AIOWF (Association of International Olympic Winter Sports Federations), the majority of IFs, and some NOCs. On the government side, meetings were held with the Council of Europe, IICGADS chairs, the European Commission, several governments, and many NADOs. Based on this feedback, substantial changes were made, and a second draft of the Code was tabled for review by the WADA Executive Committee and then released for comment in January 2003.

The third and final draft of the Code was circulated in February 2003. During the consultation process, questions had been raised as to whether several different provisions of the Code would survive legal challenges. To address these concerns, WADA obtained a legal opinion from Gabrielle Kaufmann-Kohler and Antonio Rigozzi of the Swiss firm of Levy Kaufmann-Kohler. (Dr. Kaufmann-Kohler chaired the Tribunal Arbitral du Sport/CAS at the Olympic Games from its creation in 1996 through the 2000 Olympic Games.)

The third draft of the Code was presented for consideration at the Second World Conference on Doping in Sport held in Copenhagen in March 2003. By the time of the conference, the document had been downloaded 22,000 times from WADA's website. Representation at the Conference included the IOC, 70 IFs, 60 NOCs, 30 NADOs, 20 athletes, and 80 governments. During the Conference, WADA declared that the Code would be a living document subject to periodic review and amendment, so that if there were aspects of the Code that did not work out in practice as intended, they could be changed. The Code was approved at the World Conference by acclamation without significant modification. Following approval by the Conference, the Code was formally adopted by the WADA Foundation Board. Governments expressed their approval of the Code by executing the Copenhagen Declaration on Anti-Doping in Sport, to be followed by formal legal acceptance through each government's ratification of the UNESCO International Convention against Doping in Sport. The Code and the supporting international standards went into full force on January 1, 2004.

The Substance of the 2003 Code
While there was discussion in the consultation process on every article, indeed every paragraph, of the Code, there were some major provisions within the Code that generated the most discussion and debate, including:
- The strict liability principle was adopted so that a positive test resulted in an anti-doping rule violation regardless of the athlete's intent, fault, negligence, or knowing use.
- Attempts to develop a narrative description of doping that did not require intent to cheat or

to enhance performance and that was also able to incorporate all of the types of conduct that the Code sought to prohibit were abandoned. Instead, doping was defined in terms of the following violations in relation to prohibited substances and methods: (i) a positive test, (ii) use or attempted use, (iii) possession, (iv) trafficking, or (v) administration. Also identified as anti-doping rule violations were refusing to submit to sample collection, violation of out-of-competition testing whereabouts rules, and tampering or attempted tampering with any part of doping control.

- In order for WADA to consider adding a prohibited substance or method on the list, 2 of the 3 following criteria were required to be satisfied: (i) potential to enhance performance, (ii) potential adverse impact on health, or (iii) violation of the spirit of sport. There had been considerable stakeholder feedback in favor of making *potential to enhance performance* a required criterion, but that position was not ultimately accepted. The prohibited list was split into 2 categories – those substances that were prohibited at all times (e.g., steroids) and those substances that were prohibited in competition only (e.g., stimulants and marijuana). The rationale was that because of the way the different substances affect the human physiology, out-of-competition use of the former would affect future competitions, while that would not be the case with the latter.
- The burden of proof by which an ADO was required to prove an anti-doping rule violation was established as "the comfortable satisfaction of the hearing body, bearing in mind the seriousness of the allegation." Presumptions were established in favor of the results obtained by laboratories if they followed the requirements of the international standard for laboratories.
- There was great debate over the subject of sanctions. Athletes generally favored a standard 4-year ban. Many stakeholders, particularly from Europe, feared this would be struck down by the courts. A standard 2-year ban was adopted. A number of stakeholders argued for great flexibility in sanctioning – "individual case management." It was decided that if harmonization of sanctions was to be achieved, flexibility must be limited. Sanctions could be reduced where the athlete could establish "no significant fault" or where the violation involved a "specified substance" (a substance less likely to be abused as a doping agent) where the athlete could establish that the use of the substance was not intended to enhance performance. The sanction for a person charged with an anti-doping rule violation could also be reduced for "substantial assistance" provided to authorities investigating doping.
- The Code established CAS's jurisdiction as the final appellate body in all cases arising from competition in an international event or in cases involving international athletes.
- Stakeholder comments reflected that an important deterrent to cheating by athletes is the realization that the violation will be made public if they are caught. In response to that input, the Code required mandatory public disclosure of an anti-doping rule violation following the opportunity for a hearing.
- To address the concern of athletes who were being tested by and required to provide whereabouts information to multiple ADOs, the Code required coordination of whereabouts and testing information through a central clearinghouse within WADA.
- To resolve what had been ongoing conflicts between IFs and NADOs, the authority to conduct event testing and grant therapeutic use exemptions was clarified. Code signatories were required to mutually recognize each other's decisions.

Beyond these anti-doping rules established in Part 1 of the Code, Parts 2 and 3 of the Code established stakeholders' expectations regarding other parts of effective anti-doping programs, including education, scientific research, and the roles, responsibilities and expectations of each of the different stakeholder groups. To encourage stakeholder acceptance of the Code, the Code also stipulated that failure to accept or comply with the Code by either the government or NOC of a country could have consequences in terms of participation in the Olympic Games, Paralympic Games, World Championships, or other major events.

The 2009 Amendments to the World Anti-Doping Code

The 2009 Amendment Drafting Process
As promised in Copenhagen, WADA initiated a process to review how the Code was working, starting with the formation of another Code drafting team in February 2006. Again, the team included senior experts from within WADA and 2 external experts, a highly regarded CAS arbitrator and law professor, and the author again as primary draftsman. The first task of the drafting team was to review the large body of anti-doping decisions taken during the first 2 years of the Code in order to identify those areas with loopholes, where the Code was unclear or silent in areas where clarity was required, or where hearing panels had reservations applying all or part of the Code provisions. The review process included decisions by CAS, IF, and NADO tribunals, as well as doping cases that came before the Swiss Federal Tribunal and other courts.

The consultation process for the 2009 Code amendments was similar to the process followed in connection with drafting the original Code. Numerous meetings were held with organizations within the Olympic Movement, athletes, governments, NADOs, and intergovernmental organizations. Considerable time was also spent discussing potential changes with lawyers who had experience with cases under the Code before CAS. Three drafts of the Code were disseminated to all stakeholders during a consultation process that lasted more than 1 year. Stakeholders were given an opportunity to comment through both a formal and informal consultation process. Before each draft was published, it was approved by the WADA Executive Committee, which again acted as the steering body for the drafting process. The first consultation phase took place between April and July 2006. WADA received formal submissions from 71 stakeholders during that consultation phase. The second consultation phase took place from January through March 2007. WADA received an additional 81 formal submissions from stakeholders during that phase. The third consultation phase took place from June through July 2007, and WADA received 64 formal submissions from stakeholders during that consultation phase. As was the case with the original Code drafting process, each submission was carefully reviewed by the Code drafting team, resulting in changes to the proposed Code amendment language. Also, as was done with the original Code, an independent legal opinion was obtained to confirm the legal enforceability of the proposed amendments.

The final draft Code amendments were sent to all stakeholders in October 2007 and were tabled without significant change at the Third World Conference on Doping in Sport in Madrid in November 2007. The Code amendments, along with the Madrid Declaration, were accepted at the World Conference by acclamation, and the amendments were subsequently formally approved by the WADA Foundation Board. The amendments were then legally accepted by governments through the UNESCO International Convention against Doping in Sport. The 2009 Code amendments and supporting international standards went into effect on January 1, 2009.

The Substance of the 2009 Code Amendments
The consensus feedback received from stakeholders was that the Code that went into effect on January 1, 2004, was working well and had produced

a substantial degree of harmonization, which was important for the effectiveness of the worldwide anti-doping effort. The proposed Code revisions suggested by stakeholders based on their experience applying the original Code included some substantive changes, particularly in the area of sanctions, and numerous requests for further detail in the Code where it was viewed as being unclear, silent on important issues, or where loopholes had been exposed in the adjudication process. As a result of this stakeholder input, the Code became substantially longer. Significant substantive changes incorporated into the 2009 amendments included:

- Again, sanctions were widely discussed. The sanction article of the original Code was intentionally inflexible to ensure that sanctions would be applied in a harmonized manner. Although there were some ADOs that failed to follow the rules, generally the objective of harmonized sanctions was accomplished. However, the Code Drafting Team received feedback from a considerable number of stakeholders that in some cases the lack of flexibility in sanctions was producing unfair results, which in turn undermined public confidence in the anti-doping process. In response to these concerns, the 2009 Code amendments provided more criteria by which sanctions could be decreased or increased. The definition of "specified substances" was expanded from a finite list to include all prohibited substances except substances in the classes of anabolic agents and hormones and other substances specifically identified on the international standard list of prohibited substances and methods. This change meant that the more flexible sanctioning scheme applicable to specified substances could be considered in more cases. Further, the bottom of the range of sanctions for the use of a specified substance where the athlete was able to establish that the use was not intended to enhance performance was reduced from 3 months to a reprimand.
- Another significant change that had widespread stakeholder support was the addition of the concept of "aggravating circumstances," which allowed the normal 2-year period of ineligibility to be increased up to 4 years where the anti-doping rule violation involved various types of intentional doping.
- Under the original Code, the decision on whether or not athletes or other persons could be provisionally suspended was left to be determined in the rules of each ADO. The 2009 amendments changed this approach by requiring that provisional suspensions be mandatory following an A sample adverse analytical finding for a prohibited substance other than a specified substance.
- Where the original Code left determination of what conduct constituted a whereabouts failure up to the applicable ADOs, the 2009 Code amendments standardized the criteria by defining an anti-doping rule violation as any combination of 3 missed tests and/or filing failures within an 18-month period. Missed tests and filing failures recorded by all organizations with testing jurisdiction over an athlete are combined in applying this criterion. The range of sanctions for a whereabouts failure was increased from a 3-month to 2-year to a 1- to 2-year ineligibility.
- The amount by which an athlete or other person's period of ineligibility could be reduced for substantial assistance was increased from one half to three quarters of the otherwise applicable period.
- A significant number of ADOs complained that they were spending a disproportionate share of their resources dealing with marijuana cases, leaving fewer resources available to combat real doping. The suggestion was again made that "potential to enhance performance" be made a mandatory criterion to put a substance or method on the list. After much stakeholder debate, the list criteria were left unchanged.

- The article addressing consequences of noncompliance with the Code was strengthened to include the provision that the IOC would only accept bids for the Olympic Games from countries where the government has accepted the UNESCO Convention, and the NOC and NADO were in compliance with the Code. After January 1, 2010, IFs and major event organizations would do everything possible to only award events to countries that meet the same requirement. This article also included the provision that noncompliance could result in forfeiture of offices and positions within WADA.

The 2015 Amendments to the World Anti-Doping Code

The 2015 Amendment Drafting Process
In furtherance of its commitment to periodically review the effectiveness of the Code, WADA initiated another Code review process in November 2011. The Code drafting team again included senior experts from WADA and the same 2 external advisors. As was done in connection with the 2009 Code amendments, the drafting team reviewed the anti-doping decisions applied to the Code since 2009. The consultation process for the 2015 amendments took place in 3 phases. The consultation process for the amendments to the international standards coincided with the second and third phases of the consultation process for the Code.

Following a first consultation phase (November 2011 to March 2012), a first draft of the 2015 Code amendments was tabled at the WADA Executive Committee Meeting in May 2012 and then forwarded to all stakeholders for review and comment. A second draft of the 2015 Code amendments was tabled at the WADA Executive Committee Meeting in November 2012; then, it was also forwarded to all stakeholders for review and comment. Based on stakeholder feedback, a third draft of the 2015 Code amendments was tabled at the WADA Executive Committee Meeting in May 2013. After changes were made in response to direction from the Executive Committee, the third draft was circulated to the stakeholders from May through September. During this period, the drafting team engaged in an informal but extensive consultation process with the stakeholders to finalize both concepts and language.

During the final stages of the 2015 Code amendment review process, the drafting team consulted with the Honorable Jean-Paul Costa, who until recently had been the President of the European Court of Human Rights. Judge Costa's opinion was sought on several of the proposed changes to the Code which some stakeholders claimed would be found in court to violate principles of human rights, proportionality, and the right to work. A number of suggestions received from Judge Costa were incorporated into the final draft of the 2015 Code amendments.

The fourth and final draft of the 2015 Code amendments, along with Judge Costa's opinion, was sent to all stakeholders in October 2014. That draft, without significant changes, was presented at the Fourth World Conference on Doping in Sport in Johannesburg in November 2013. It was accepted at the Conference by acclamation, along with the Johannesburg Declaration. The amendments were formally approved by the WADA Foundation Board. Legal acceptance by governments was achieved through the UNESCO International Convention against Doping in Sport. The 2015 Code amendments and corresponding changes to the international standards went into effect on January 1, 2015.

Also like the prior Code consultation processes, the process to consider the 2015 amendments to the Code involved both meetings with stakeholders and opportunities for written comments and suggestions. During the first phase of the process, the drafting team participated in 32 stakeholder meetings and received written submissions from 96 different stakeholders. In the second phase of the process, the drafting team participated in 44 stakeholder meetings and received written submissions from 109 different stakeholders. During the third phase of the consultation process, the drafting team participated in 68 different stakeholder meetings and received 110 written submissions from different stakeholders. Typically, a stakeholder's written submission would make suggestions regarding a number of different Code articles. In total, the stakeholder written submissions offered 3,987 different suggestions regarding various Code articles. The drafting team read and seriously considered all of the written submissions and meeting feedback which were received. It was also quite common for the drafting team to reach out to individual stakeholders and seek clarification on particular points in their submissions or to get their opinion on suggestions made by others. A redline of the 2015 Code amendments to the 2009 Code reflects a total of 22,069 changes.

Substance of the 2015 Code Amendments
The consensus feedback received during the 2015 Code consultation process was that the adoption of the Code had clearly been a good idea, overall it was working well, but there were many constructive suggestions to make it better. While some of the proposed 2015 Code amendments were intended to close loopholes, clarify ambiguities, or address inconsistencies in various anti-doping decisions, in significant part the purpose of this set of amendments was to use the Code as a vehicle to advance the fight against doping to a whole new level.

One of the interesting dichotomies in the Code review process was the sentiment expressed by many stakeholders that the Code should be made shorter and simpler for the benefit of athletes, while the same stakeholders often proposed detailed revisions, which, while appropriate to add clarity in areas where they perceived ambiguity, would make the Code longer and more complex.

Through careful editing, the 2015 amendments managed to incorporate most of the proposed clarifications while shortening the total length of the Code. It was also agreed that the comments to the Code need not be reproduced in each stakeholder's individual rules. In response to the stakeholder suggestions, WADA also produced an athletes' guide to the Code, which was much shorter and focused on those areas of the Code which are of particular importance to athletes.

The following are some of the most significant and widely discussed Code changes made by the 2015 amendments.

- The need to be both tougher and more flexible in imposing sanctions was again a common theme of the stakeholder submissions and meetings. The 2015 Code amendments took very significant steps in both directions. The athletes realized their wish of a 4-year ban for intentional cheaters. (For steroids and hormones, such as erythropoietin, EPO, the burden was on the athlete to establish that the use *was not* intentional. For specified substances, the burden was on ADO to show that the use *was* intentional.) In the absence of intent, the standard sanction remained 2 years, with the possibility that in circumstances where the athlete could establish no significant fault, the sanction could be reduced down to a reprimand for specified substances and 1 year for nonspecified substances such as steroids or EPO. An additional step in the direction of greater flexibility was the addition of an article addressing violations involving contaminated products. Whereas under the 2009 Code, the minimum sanction for an athlete who had inadvertently consumed a contaminated product containing a steroid was a 1-year period of ineligibility, under the new contaminated product article, the sanction could be reduced down to a warning if the athlete could establish no significant fault.
- There was strong stakeholder sentiment that the amendments needed to better target athlete

support personnel under the jurisdiction of the Code. To accomplish this objective, Code amendments direct IFs and NOCs to instruct their national federations to make athlete support personnel involved in their sports subject to their results management jurisdiction. The Code now requires a mandatory investigation of an athlete support person whose minor athlete, or multiple other athletes, commit an anti-doping rule violation. A new article, entitled prohibited association, was also added to the list of conduct that constitutes an anti-doping rule violation. Stakeholders had come forward with examples of athletes still using coaches who had been banned for life or working with other athlete support personnel who had gone to jail for providing illegal prohibited substances to athletes. While the banned coach or drug-pushing support person might be outside the jurisdiction of sport, the prohibited association article of the Code now makes it an anti-doping rule violation by the athlete to continue to associate with such a person after receiving notice not to do so from an ADO.

- In the early days of anti-doping, ADOs only collected samples in competition with notice. Then they improved on the surprise component and started collecting samples in competition without notice, which was more effective. Then, as doping strategies refined, ADOs got smarter still and started collecting samples out of competition without notice. More recently, the most advanced ADOs began target-testing athletes and timing tests to take account of the periods when athletes in a particular sport were most likely to dope. The 2015 changes to Article 5 of the Code are simply an extension of those "smart testing" principles to the "smart analysis of samples." WADA, in collaboration with IFs and NADOs, is charged with developing a technical document which, on a sport-by-sport and discipline-by-discipline basis, identifies those particular prohibited substances and prohibited methods that an athlete intending to dope would be most likely to use. That document then becomes the basis of the analytical methods used by laboratories to analyze each ADO's samples.

- In response to continuing concern on the part of team sports and some individual sports where specialized equipment makes it extremely difficult for an athlete to train on his or her own, the prohibition against ineligible athletes having any involvement with a national federation or club during an athlete's period of ineligibility was softened. Under the 2015 amendments, an athlete is allowed to train with his or her team or to use the facilities of a club during the shorter of: (1) the last 2 months of the athlete's period of ineligibility or (2) the last quarter of the period of ineligibility imposed. During this period, the athlete would remain ineligible to compete.

- Although the principles of proportionality and human rights were implicit in the prior Code and were certainly referenced in CAS and court decisions applying the Code, the 2015 Code amendments included specific references to proportionality and human rights and better account for human right concerns (e.g., special treatment for minors and mandatory public disclosure of anti-doping rule violations delayed until after a final appellate decision).

- There was a strong consensus among the stakeholders that the role of information gathering in the fight against doping should be highlighted in the Code and that cooperation of governments and all stakeholders in anti-doping rule violation investigations is important. Several 2015 Code amendments to accomplish this included greater flexibility in reducing an athlete or other person's period of ineligibility in exchange for providing substantial assistance. The statute of limitations was extended from 8 to 10 years. It was further clarified that the statute of limitations is triggered by notification that an anti-doping rule violation has been asserted. The responsibilities of all stakeholders (including athletes and athlete support personnel) were expanded to require cooperation with ADOs investigating anti-doping rule violations, and the expectation of the signatories with respect to governments were expanded to include governments putting in place legislation, regulation, policies, or practices to cooperate in sharing information with ADOs.

- Interviews with athletes, both clean and those who have acknowledged doping, make clear that long-term storage of samples, in anticipation of further analysis after advances in anti-doping technology, is a significant deterrent to doping. Changes were made to both the Code and the international standard for laboratories to support the additional analysis or reanalysis of stored samples.
- The debate over whether performance enhancement should be made a mandatory criterion in the decision to put a substance or method on the prohibited list intensified from its previously high level during consideration of the 2015 Code amendments. On one hand, many stakeholders believed in principle that sport has no business regulating substances that do not enhance performance. At a practical level, they also argued that their resources were being unnecessarily drained dealing with in-competition adverse analytical findings for marijuana resulting from use out of competition, when marijuana is not prohibited. On the other hand, governments and many sport organizations continued to believe strongly that sport plays a role in society beyond just athletic achievement, and that substances and methods should continue to be added to the list on the basis of a confirmation of their potential detriment to health and violation of the spirit of sport, without requiring the potential to enhance performance. A practical compromise was reached when the WADA Executive Committee increased the laboratory reporting threshold for marijuana to a level likely to eliminate out-of-competition use and, as a result, the list criteria in the Code remained unchanged.
- Monitoring Code compliance by the stakeholders has always proved to be a difficult task for WADA. Primarily, compliance has been assessed through WADA's review of stakeholder rules and self-reporting of anti-doping activities undertaken. While the Code has been able to achieve harmonization of stakeholder rules, the quality of implementation of their anti-doping activities remains far from harmonized. Changes to Article 23 of the Code and the international standards were made to assist WADA in better addressing this problem.

Conclusion

It was often said at the beginning of the initial Code consultation process that getting hundreds of governments and sport organizations to agree on a common set of rules was an unachievable task. At every turn, there were also those who argued that aggressive rules to combat doping were sure to be rejected by courts as violating principles of proportionality, human rights, and the right to work. Indeed, many said the task was simply impossible. As the 1,000 participants at the Fourth World Conference in Johannesburg stood to approve the second amendments to the Code by acclamation, the famous words of Nelson Mandela came to mind: "It always seems impossible until it's done." Now, 14 years later, the Code is viewed, almost universally, as the gold standard in anti-doping. Through each of the 2 sets of amendments, the rules have been made both more fair generally, but tougher for the real cheats. More than 680 sport organizations are signatories to the Code, including the entire Olympic Movement, and 183 governments have accepted the Code through their ratification of the UNESCO Convention. There is still work to be done. The Code will undoubtedly be amended again, and very significant challenges remain in the fight against doping. It would be hard, however, to find a stakeholder today who believes that the World Anti-Doping Code was a bad idea or that it has not been successful in achieving its main goal of harmonizing anti-doping rules.

In the author's view, the success of the Code can be largely attributed to the incredibly collaborative process through which the Code was adopted and amended [1]. Every stakeholder had a chance to express an opinion, and those opinions were listened to. While it is likely that no stakeholder would agree with every provision in the Code, all stakeholders can look at the Code and see their contributions incorporated into the document. The Code has been successful because it is the "world's" anti-doping code, crafted from their input with a collective objective, not a document imposed upon them by WADA or any other organization.

Reference

1 CODE REVIEW PROCESS. http://www.wada-ama.org/en/what-we-do/the-code/code-review-process (accessed May 8, 2017).

Richard Young, Esq.
Suite 1300
90 S. Cascade
Colorado Springs, CO 80903 (USA)
E-Mail richard.young@bryancave.com

Is the Fight against Doping in Sport a Legal Minefield like Any Other?

Ulrich Haas

Rechtswissenschaftliches Institut, University of Zurich, Zurich, Switzerland

Abstract

In the fight against doping, creating a level playing field across all sports is very challenging from a legal perspective. A harmonized approach presupposes first and foremost a supreme regulatory authority on a global level. This task cannot be attributed to the public sector, because there is no supranational authority of public international law capable of dealing with it. Thus, responsibility has to be assumed by a private law entity. This in turn requires complicated contractual agreements by which duties and responsibilities are transferred from the individual to the national level and from there to the top of the pyramid. In practice, this process is not only difficult and cumbersome, it also leads to an accumulation of power at the top of the sports pyramid that must be contained by organizational checks and balances, such as access to justice and the rule of law, accountability, transparency, and possibilities for the respective stakeholders to partake in the decision-making process. The weighting of all these different aspects is demanding and further complicated by the regulatory reach of the various national lawmakers. Since national laws differ considerably and a harmonized legislative approach is nowhere near in sight, a global approach in the fight against doping must push back national laws and legal concepts as much as possible. The purpose of this chapter is to give an overview on all these legal challenges.

© 2017 S. Karger AG, Basel

Introduction

Creating conditions in the field of the fight against doping that are globally uniform and span all sports is a legal minefield. It presents many challenges. These include, as a first step, determining the appropriate regulatory authority. In a second step, the influence of the national law must be downplayed as much as possible, since the different national standards pose the greatest threat to a uniform set of anti-doping rules and regulations, such as the World Anti-Doping Code (WADC). National law can only be effectively suppressed with the help of arbitration. Without arbitration, therefore, a harmonized fight against doping is inconceivable. As a third step, it must be ensured, by organizing the hierarchy of the successive (arbitral) authorities appropriately, that ultimately a single authority has final decision-making power over the interpretation of the WADC. This role of a "supreme world court" in doping cases is assumed by the Court of Arbitration for Sport (CAS). Fourthly, a set of global anti-doping rules and regulations – if accepted by those that will be subjected to it – must have sufficient democratic legitimation. A complicated, time-consuming and costly consultation process is, thus, necessary for this. However, the requisite basis for its legitimation also calls for the WADC to be compatible with core values of the international community, i.e., to take account of fundamental athlete rights in particular. The attempt to steer the WADC back to these fundamental values is not only set out in this code itself, but also in the case law of the CAS. Fifthly, it must ultimately be borne in mind that not even through arbitration can the influence of national law be completely excluded. An Achilles' heel for the values of national law is, in particular, the public policy proviso. In relation to this, threats chiefly arise from European law and competition law in particular. A coherent solution as to how to deal with this latter point has – in spite of the UNESCO International Convention against Doping in Sport – unfortunately not yet emerged in the various countries.

Determining the Appropriate Regulatory Authority

The regulatory challenges in the fight against doping are numerous and complex. This is partly because of the subject matter being governed, where the focus straddles the most diverse disciplines, such as law, medicine, pharmacology, toxicology, social sciences, and sports sciences [1]. Moreover, the rules and regulations have to be structured with sufficient flexibility to enable them to be adjusted to the constantly changing conditions in the field of the fight against doping. The question now is which authority is able to resolve this complex issue. The answer to this seems simple only at first glance.

Organized sport is traditionally hierarchical, i.e. monopolistic and structured in accordance with what German or Swiss doctrine refers to as the *"Ein-Platz-Prinzip"* (the one-place principle) [2–4]. This means that each type of sport is represented at the top level by an international sports association, by which national sports associations and regional sports associations, right down to the individual clubs and sportsmen/women, are governed. Traditionally, decision making in such sports families is a top-down process, i.e., the rules and regulations are established by the international sports association at the top of all the associations and then passed downwards. In the process, the entities at the lower levels of the hierarchy are not really given a choice as to whether they want to adopt the rules and regulations. Rather, the only alternative they are faced with is whether to accept the rules and regulations that have been adopted at the top or refrain from participating in organized sports in the relevant family of associations altogether. This vertical decision-making process, coupled with the wish of all the parties involved to participate in the sports events administered by the top association, ultimately guarantees uniform sports conditions, at least within the respective branch of sport.

In the fight against doping there is a need for the relevant set of rules and regulations to be applied not just within a branch of sport, but uniformly across all branches of sport (in the past, the International Olympic Committee, IOC, had taken the lead role in implementing anti-doping measures within the Olympic family; see Davies [5]). Since, however, leaving aside the IOC for the Olympic sports [5, 6], there is no umbrella organization that is superordinate to the international sports associations, this call for a uniform fight against doping across all professional sports fizzled out long ago. Thus, in the past, the legislative situation in the fight against doping was characterized by a patchwork of anti-doping rules and regulations that varied tremendously from one association to another, and sometimes even from one country to another [7, 8]. This situation did not change until the founding (in 1999) of the World Anti-Doping Agency (WADA), whose purpose was and is, among others, to create uniform sets of rules and regulations for the fight against doping across all sports. The international sports associations undertook, by making relevant declarations to WADA, to accept these anti-doping rules and regulations and to implement them within their branch of sport [9, 10]. Hence, WADA is the top global regulatory authority in the field of the fight against doping. However, the WADC is not directly applicable to the athletes [this is constant CAS jurisprudence, see 11]. Rather, it is a kind of "model law" that applies to the addressees only in so far as it has been incorporated and implemented into the rules and regulations of the respective sports organizations.

For a long time, there was considerable opposition to establishing WADA as the top regulatory authority for doping cases, particularly from the ranks of the international sports associations [12]. It was, to some extent at least, regarded as meddling in the "internal affairs" of the association and thus as undermining the autonomy of the sports associations. Only in the light of the doping scandal of the Tour de France 1998 did the awareness grow that the ability of the international sports organizations to govern themselves in the field of the fight against doping is limited due to conflicts of interest and scarce resources [13–15]. For this reason, and also in view of the imminent danger that otherwise the associations' regulatory autonomy in the fight against doping would be completely revoked by national laws [13] (it is to be noted, however, that even today states are increasingly intervening in sport and, more particularly, in doping matters [16]), the sports associations gave up their opposition to WADA and to a uniform set of rules and regulations across all professional sports.

Democratic Legitimation of Anti-Doping Rules and Regulations

The extremely hierarchical structure in sport, combined with the fact that decision making in sport is generally conducted on a top-down basis, means that the legitimation of the associations' rules and regulations is somewhat lacking. This is because rules are ultimately established at the level of the most powerful association by individuals who themselves are not affected, or hardly affected, by such rules and regulations. The parties that are directly affected by them (generally the athletes) have, however, no influence whatsoever, or at least hardly any influence, on their content [17]. The international sports associations endeavor to make up for this lack of democracy and legitimation. Hence, for instance, many international sports associations have set up athletes' commissions and involved them in key decision-making processes in order to ensure that the interests of the lower levels of the hierarchy are also adequately represented in the administration of the sport at the highest level. After all, the more levels of hierarchy there are between the addressees of the rules, the more problematic the lack of legitimation becomes. Even more so, since those subjected to the rules have no scope whatsoever for circumventing them if they want to participate in organized sports events.

To prevent the WADC from becoming a set of rules and regulations of a small elite, WADA has established a – truly unique – procedure for making rules and regulations. Namely, the WADC is the product of a global consultation process, which is coordinated by WADA [18]. Every stakeholder can take part in this, essentially web-based, consultation process by submitting relevant input [19]. In principle, 3 time frames are available for participating in this roughly 20-month-long legislative process. Participation is open to everyone, regardless of whether they belong to a level of the sport's hierarchy or what such level might be. This consultative opportunity has always had a high take-up rate. In the process for establishing the new WADC 2015 alone, the various participants contributed over 3,900 proposed amendments. Ultimately, therefore, the WADC is a set of international rules and regulations that is widely supported and legitimated within (and outside) the entire world of sport.

Curtailing National Law

The establishment of a set of rules and regulations such as the WADC does not – in legal terms – take place in a vacuum. Instead, the autonomy to establish such rules and regulations is set within a legal framework, which stipulates the limits of the autonomy. A universally applicable international legal framework covering the limits of sports organizations' regulatory autonomy and making them transparent does not exist in principle. Rather, the limits of international sports organizations' regulatory competence only transpires from the respective national legal systems. The limits set by national law vary considerably from country to country. Essentially – leaving aside hybrid forms – 2 national regulatory models can be identified, namely a sports model that tends to be more "state led" and one that tends to be more "liberal" [20, 21]. The state-led sports model is based on the notion that sport is a public good, the provision and administration of which is in principle one of the state's tasks. According to this conception, regulatory autonomy should be based on the relevant legal standards for state action. Thus, in this scenario, the sports organizations that establish the sets of rules and regulations are ultimately regarded as an extended arm of the state.

In contrast, the "liberal" sports model is based on the notion that the establishment and administration of sport is in principle the private matter of the sports associations. In this scenario, the source of the regulatory autonomy is, initially, freedom of contract, which is familiar in the private law of most countries, i.e., the freedom to govern one's own affairs autonomously and free from state influence. Admittedly, countries that follow the "liberal" sports model also set limits to sports associations' regulatory authority. This is because these countries are aware that, due to their monopolistic structure, sports organizations acquire an immense power, which requires limitation and control for the protection of the structurally weaker party. The organization of such control varies considerably in the individual countries, both in terms of the legal point of reference and in terms of the intensity of the control. The points of departure for controlling regulatory autonomy are – usually in addition to the general limits under private law – personality rights [22], association law, labor law, competition law, consumer law, or even national constitutional law.

The varying influence of the national legal systems on the regulatory sovereignty claimed by the sports organizations presents great challenges for the latter [23]. For example, when establishing globally uniform conditions for practicing sport, these organizations are not faced with a single international legal standard. Instead, the sports organizations are confronted with numerous very disparate national legal standards. A consequence of this regulatory patchwork may be, for instance, that taking a blood sample for anti-doping testing purposes is deemed admissible before the courts in one country but inadmissible in another country. Also, a doping ban (based on identical facts) may be legally valid before the courts in one country but not in another country. This regulatory fragmentation calls the essence of the transnational practice of sport into question, since this presupposes that the same conditions apply to all the participants practicing the sport. Indeed, in the final analysis, an athlete only subjects himself to the doping rules because he believes that his competitors from another country are similarly bound. Therefore, the fact that there is no uniform international legal standard constitutes the greatest challenge for establishing a set of anti-doping rules that claims globally uniform validity.

If there is no desire to make the (useless) lowest common denominator of the various national legal systems the basis for the fight against doping, then the influence of the state must be curtailed as much as possible. The options for achieving this are limited. Under no circumstances do the various legal systems accept the exclusion of any kind of judicial control. Clauses in the rules and regulations whereby measures adopted by a sports association on the basis of the rules and regulations are immune from any kind of judicial review are invalid. Nor can sports organizations escape the application of the various national control standards by, for instance, transferring their head office to a particularly liberal legal system. This stems from the fact that due to "forum shopping" it is often possible for the various stakeholders to sue a sports organization outside their country of incorporation – with the result that in such a case a national control standard that diverges from the one in the country of incorporation is then generally applied. The most effective way to suppress the application of national law is to strip the national courts of their jurisdiction to resolve doping-related disputes by way of arbitration. Not only is arbitration familiar to most legal systems as an alternative to state jurisdiction that is autonomously agreed upon by the parties, but also the New York Convention on the Recognition and Enforcement of Foreign Arbitral Awards of 1958 (NYC) provides a universally recognized international legal framework, with over 150 countries having ratified it to date. Whilst the NYC does not harmonize all the aspects of international arbitration, it does set out a uniform international legal framework for 2 particularly important cross-border issues, namely the recognition of arbitration agreements, and the recognition and enforcement of foreign arbitral awards. Establishing a uniform set of rules and regulations in the fight against doping is, consequently, absolutely inconceivable without a dispute resolution mechanism favoring arbitration.

Centralization of Jurisdiction

Uniform rules and regulations are not the only prerequisite for a harmonized global fight against doping. Rather, it is also necessary for these rules and regulations to be applied uniformly [24]. If a uniform application is not ensured, this will lead, sooner or later, to legal practitioners attributing different content to the body of rules and regulations, and, consequently, the uniform standard being lost through legal practice. These dangers can hardly be avoided, since the uniform application of the law is already jeopardized by the fact that the various legal practitioners have become socially integrated into different legal worlds and, therefore, approach the interpretation of the body of rules and regulations with a differently formed preconception. The latter may result in key concepts in the WADC, such as "fault" or "strict liability," being construed and applied differently by the various legal practitioners.

The options for preventing regulatory fragmentation from occurring through legal practice are limited. The WADC tries to counteract this by, for instance, defining some key concepts itself [25] and also by sometimes commenting on provisions. In addition, the WADC specifies that the interpretation of the provisions must be undertaken autonomously, i.e. without recourse to the respective national law [26–28]. The most important contributing factor for uniform legal practice, however, is based on the assumption that the WADC designates the CAS (for the history of the CAS, see Mavromati and Reeb [29]) [30, 31] as the highest authority for questions of interpretation relating to doping (Article 13 WADC) [32–34] (for the significance of the CAS as an instrument of harmonization in relation to the application of the law, see McLaren [34]). This applies irrespective of where in the world the dispute originated. Thus, the CAS takes on the role of a "World Supreme Court" in the field of the fight against doping. Its task is to ensure uniformity in the application of the rules and regulations, and to ensure the legal development of the WADC [35, 36].

Such uniform application by the CAS, however, is bound by (practical) limits. The CAS's closed list of arbitrators makes only a limited contribution to uniform case law, since in practice the composition of the CAS formations varies from case to case. The CAS's list of arbitrators contains several hundred arbitrators from widely varying legal and cultural backgrounds [37]. In the light of such a group of arbitrators, which is relatively inhomogeneous from the outset, the call for uniform case law is consequently relatively ambitious. The basic instrument for achieving this objective is, nevertheless, the publication of all CAS decisions [38]. In this regard, Article 59(6) of the Code of Sports-Related Arbitration and Mediation Rules ("CAS Code") states as follows:

> The award, a summary and/or a press release setting forth the results of the proceedings shall be made public by the CAS, unless both parties agree that they should remain confidential.

The arbitral awards are thus accessible to everyone, including the parties to the arbitration [39]. The latter make heavy use of the art of drawing an analogy or "distinguishing" in their statements of case, thereby compelling the CAS formations to grapple intensively with the uniformity of the application of the law. Indeed, for proceedings before the CAS, there is no such thing as a rigid "case doctrine" [40]. A CAS panel is neither obliged to follow a (previous) CAS arbitral award in relation to a particular legal issue, nor are any of the many national or sports-specific anti-doping arbitral tribunals [41–45] compelled to stop at the legal interpretation of a CAS panel. Nevertheless, the respective CAS formations go to great lengths to achieve a uniform and consistent application of the law [46]. The following extract from a decision by a CAS formation is cited as a representative example of this [47]:

> In CAS jurisprudence there is no principle of binding precedent … However, a CAS panel will try, if the evidence permits, to come to the same conclusion on matters of law as a previous CAS panel. Whether that is considered a matter of comity, or an attempt to build a coherent corpus of law, matters not.

The principle of party disposition inherent to arbitration, according to which the parties dispose of the beginning, the contents, and the end of any dispute, constitutes an additional challenge for a uniform application of the law. Whether or not a case is brought before the CAS is determined solely by the parties, as is the question of the subject matter of the case. Sometimes, however, it is in the interest of neither the sports organization that issued the (doping-related) decision nor the sportsman/sportswoman "affected" thereby to have the decision comprehensively reviewed by an independent arbitral tribunal (in this context the CAS). Thus, at first glance, it primarily depends on the individual directly affected by the measure/decision as to whether the WADC standards are to be implemented or not. However, the principle of the uniform practice of sport would be critically undermined thereby. For this reason, the WADC provides for the entitlement of WADA (among others) to file an "appeal" with the CAS against all doping-related decisions by (national and international) anti-doping organizations, even where WADA is not adversely affected by the decision or was not even involved in the initial proceedings as a party, respectively (of course it should not be overlooked that WADA's right of appeal may not only be exercised to the detriment of athletes but also in their favor [48]). WADA's special "right to appeal" is an essential driver for the harmonization and uniformity of the application of the law [49], and, in addition, it should also help to take account of the particular conflicts of interest facing many sports organizations in connection with handling doping offences involving "their" athletes.

It stands to reason, however, that – despite all the effectiveness of the instruments described above – not all the inconsistencies between the individual CAS decisions can be eliminated (for an analysis of what constitutes "intent to enhance performance" as per the meaning of Article 10.4 WADC 2009, see de La Rochefoucauld [50]) [51–56]. Indeed, the WADC throws up questions of law and interpretation that have given rise to differences in opinion and different "schools of thought" among the CAS arbitrators. On the whole, however, so far, the CAS has lived up to the responsibility assigned to it by the WADC to ensure the uniform application of the law [40].

The centralization of jurisdiction for doping-related disputes by the CAS, however, does not only serve to further the uniform application of law, but also to further the legal development of the WADC. Many of the principles underpinning the WADC can be traced back to the case law of the CAS. This applies, for instance, to the so-called principle of "strict liability" in relation to the disqualification of doped sportsmen/sportswomen in competitions.

> The Panel is of the opinion that the system of strict liability of the athlete must prevail when sporting fairness is at stake. This means that, once a banned substance is discovered in the urine or blood of an athlete, he must be automatically disqualified from the competition in question, without any possibility for him to rebut this presumption of guilt. [57]

The principle (of guilt) for imposing periods of ineligibility that is enshrined in the WADC as well as the differentiated distribution of the burden of presentation and proof in respect of the prerequisites for the existence of a doping offence can be traced back to the CAS case law.

> Having established the principle that the suspension of an athlete for a doping offence requires fault on his/her part, this does not, in the Panel's view, mean that it is for the federation to provide full proof of every element of the offence, as is necessary in respect of a criminal act for which a presumption of innocence operates in favor of the accused. [58]

Control Standard before the Court of Arbitration for Sport

As a general rule, doping-related disputes are dealt with before the CAS in the so-called appeal arbitration procedure. This is governed by Article R47ff of the CAS Code. These provisions stipulate, in Article R58 of the CAS Code, that the

> Panel shall decide the dispute according to the applicable regulations and, subsidiarily, to the rules of law chosen by the parties or, in the absence of such a choice, according to the law of the country in which the federation, association, or sports-related body which has issued the challenged decision is domiciled or according to the rules of law the Panel deems appropriate. [59, 60]

Therefore, in accordance with this provision, doping-related disputes are primarily decided on the basis of the WADC or the relevant sets of anti-doping rules and regulations adopted by the sports organizations, respectively. The question is, however, whether there are also overarching legal standards to which the doping-related case law must be aligned. Consequently, this requires verifying the legality of the WADC itself [61]. The WADC 2015 itself unequivocally points in this direction and specifies in its introduction that the provisions of the WADC "are intended to be applied in a manner which respects the principles of proportionality and human rights." This finding, however, has not only existed since the WADC 2015, since WADA has always strived to ensure that the WADC respects the "fundamental rights of athletes" [19]. In particular, this is reflected by the fact that WADA has had the compatibility of the various versions of the WADC with "fundamental rights" reviewed by independent experts [62, 63].

The dogmatic principle for taking account of these "fundamental rights" in the case law of the CAS is not easy to identify. This is the case, firstly, for the sources of the athletes' fundamental rights [64]. There is a large number of international legal texts dealing with human rights [64]. These include at their core, where the CAS is concerned, the Council of Europe's Convention for the Protection of Human Rights and Fundamental Freedoms (ECHR), since the headquarters of the CAS are in Switzerland, which in turn is a member state of this convention. However, the ECHR does not allude specifically to either arbitration or sport. Moreover, the ECHR is directed at governments (see Article 1 ECHR); therefore, it intends to limit the extent of their power for the purpose of protecting individuals. In horizontal legal relationships between private individuals on the other hand – which is what arbitration proceedings before the CAS concern – the prevailing opinion is that the ECHR does not directly apply [65, 66].

Ultimately, however, the question can be left open, since the correct opinion is that in doping-related disputes the CAS is, at least indirectly, bound by the ECHR [67]. The CAS shares this view [68–71]. Thus, in one of its opinions it states [68]:

The Panel is of the view that even though it is not directly bound by the provisions of the ECHR (cf. Article 1 ECHR), it should nevertheless account for their content within the framework of procedural public policy.

Equally, in CAS 2011/A/2433 (§58) the panel held:

However, the Panel is conscious of the fact that certain procedural guarantees enshrined in Article 6(1) of the ECHR, in disputes relating to civil rights and obligations, are indirectly applicable even before an arbitral tribunal – even more so in disciplinary matters. This follows from the fact that Switzerland, being a member state of the ECHR, the judges must ensure that when implementing arbitral awards (in the stage of enforcement of the arbitral award or in the context of an appeal against the latter), that the parties to the arbitral proceeding had the benefit of an equitable procedure, that was conducted within reasonable time by an independent and impartial tribunal.

Besides these legal sources, Swiss law also plays an important role as an overarching legal standard in doping-related disputes. This is because the headquarters of most international sports associations are in Switzerland and Article R58 of the CAS Code provides that, absent any agreement of the parties to the contrary, the law of the country in which the federation that has issued the challenged decision is domiciled applies on the merits on a subsidiary basis [72]. It must be added that arbitral awards by the CAS are subject to a public policy control before the Swiss Federal Supreme Court as part of an action for annulment, which public order control is based on Swiss law. At the same time, the protection of personality pursuant to Articles 27(2) and 28 of the Swiss Civil Code lies at the core of Swiss standards, which CAS panels additionally invoke [22, 73, 74].

From these overarching legal standards, the CAS has derived a number of general legal principles that are applied to the WADC, sometimes by way of a supplement, sometimes by way of clarification, and sometimes also by way of correction. These include for example:

- The principle of interpretation contra proferentem: according thereto, the lack of clarity of a rule cannot go to the detriment of an athlete; as a general rule, any provision with an unclear wording is to be interpreted against the author of the wording; this principle has been upheld by numerous CAS panels [75–81].
- The principle of legal certainty according to which disciplinary measures must find a clear and unambiguous basis in rules of the federation in order to be admissible [82–84].
- The principle of hierarchy of norms, whereby subordinate sets of rules and regulations must be consistent with superordinate sets of rules and regulations, particularly the statutes of the association [85–87].
- The principle of proportionality: according thereto, the severity of a penalty must be in proportion with the seriousness of the infringe-

ment; the CAS has evidenced the existence and the importance of the principle of proportionality on numerous occasions [88–96].
- The principle of equal treatment of the athletes [97].
- The principle of fairness or the right to be heard [68, 98–100].

Remaining Influence of National Law

The influence of national law cannot be completely excluded by arbitration [101]. Instead, intersections remain between national law and arbitration, which serve as an entry point for national law. This applies in particular to the phase after arbitration, namely to challenging the arbitral award as well as its recognition and enforcement [102]. In particular, the recognition and enforcement of CAS arbitral awards outside Switzerland sometimes cause problems [103]. This is especially true where recognition and enforcement in EU countries is sought. Namely, in this case, EU law is increasingly threatening to become an obstacle to recognition and enforcement.

For example, in the Meca-Medina case, the European Court of Justice (ECJ) decided that sports associations' anti-doping rules must be measured against the yardstick of European competition law [104–108]. Admittedly, in the "Eco Swiss" decision the ECJ held that not every provision under European law is automatically part of the (national) public policy [109, 110]. When the latter state of affairs is the case, however, is not easy to answer [111]. To this extent, the ECJ requires that the matter must concern a "fundamental provision" which "is essential for the accomplishment of the tasks entrusted to the Community and, in particular, for the functioning of the internal market" [112–114]. What is "essential" in this sense, according to the ECJ, is European competition law (Article 101ff; Treaty on the Functioning of the European Union) [112, 115] and consumer protection [113, 116]. The fundamental freedoms and the general prohibition of discrimination will also have to be regarded as "fundamental provisions" in the sense of the public policy (§1061) [117].

The aforementioned provisions of European law are complex provisions. This is particularly so in the case of the European fundamental freedoms (in relation to their application to sport, see the overview of the case law of the ECJ by Halgreen [118]) and the European competition law. For example, whether an anti-doping rule for sportsmen/sportswomen established by a sports association infringes specific discrimination prohibitions, the freedom of establishment or the freedom of movement of workers is – as a glance at the "Meca-Medina" decision of the ECJ shows – a complex legal issue both in fact and in law. Attributing these provisions to public policy carries the risk that reviewing the arbitral award in terms of compliance with these principles of European law will degenerate into a "révision au fond" (review of the merits) [119] of the arbitral award, which is undesirable and incompatible with the meaning and purpose of arbitration [120–122]. Consequently, there is no lack of proposals and attempts to limit the depth of reviews by the national courts in the phase after arbitration [123–125]. A coherent approach as to how this threat to the uniformity of the practice of sport, which arises from European law, is to be dealt with at the stage of recognition and enforcement has unfortunately yet to evolve. Furthermore, it has been seen that the UNESCO International Convention against Doping in Sport [28] has so far seemingly failed to induce the courts to exercise greater restraint in relation to public policy control [103].

Conclusion

The fight against doping is particularly legally challenging. This is partly due to the dynamics in the field of (anti-)doping, which are evidenced, inter alia, by the fact that since their first enactment in 2003 the anti-doping rules (WADC) had to be revised twice already in order to adapt to developments in the complex and ever-changing environment. The main problem, however, arises from the application of basically national legal instruments to a globalized world, in an environment that is based on and demands the equal and uniform application of rules with respect to athletes' rights and the need of an efficient fight against doping.

References

1 McLaren RH: CAS doping jurisprudence: what can we learn? Int Sports Law Rev 2006, pp 4, 7ff.
2 Halgreen L: European Sports Law: A Comparative Analysis of European and American Models of Sports, ed 2. Stockholm, Karnov, 2013, p 64ff.
3 Nafziger JAR: A comparison of the European and North American models of sports organisation. Int Sports Law J 2008, p 10ff.
4 Mitten MJ: The Court of Arbitration for Sport and its global jurisprudence: international legal pluralism in a world without national boundaries. CAS Bull 2014; 2:48, 51ff.
5 Davies P: A Guide to the World Anti-Doping Code, ed 2. Port Melbourne, Cambridge University Press, 2013, p 2ff.
6 Lewis A, Taylor J (eds): Sport: Law and Practice, ed 3. London, Bloomsbury Professional, 2014, B1.21ff.
7 Lewis A, Taylor J (eds): Sport: Law and Practice, ed 3. London, Bloomsbury Professional, 2014, B.122.
8 Davies P: A Guide to the World Anti-Doping Code, ed 2. Port Melbourne, Cambridge University Press, 2013, p 15ff.
9 Niggli O: Code mondial antidopage: processus de révision et principales modifications. Jurisport 2013;137:20.
10 Davies P: A Guide to the World Anti-Doping Code, ed 2. Port Melbourne, Cambridge University Press, 2013, p 3.
11 Court of Arbitration for Sport 2011/A/2601, §8.4.5ff.
12 Report of the Cycling Independent Reform Commission, http://www.uci.ch/mm/Document/News/CleanSport/16/87/99/CIRCReport2015_Neutral.pdf, p. 107.
13 Pound R: The World Anti-Doping Agency: an experiment in international law. Int Sports Law Rev 2002, p 53.
14 Davies P: A Guide to the World Anti-Doping Code, ed 2. Port Melbourne, Cambridge University Press, 2013, p 1.
15 Lewis A, Taylor J (eds): Sport: Law and Practice, ed 3. London, Bloomsbury Professional, 2014, B1.23.
16 Kaufmann-Kohler G, Malinverni G, Rigozzi A: Doping and fundamental rights of athletes – comments in the wake of the adoption of the World Anti-Doping Code. Int Sports Law Rev 2003, pp 39, 43.
17 Mitten MJ: The Court of Arbitration for Sport and its global jurisprudence: international legal pluralism in a world without national boundaries. CAS Bull 2014; 2:48, 49ff.
18 Rigozzi A, Viret M, Wisnosky E: Does the World Anti-Doping Code revision live up to its promises. Jusletter November 11, 2013 (annex).
19 Niggli O: Code mondial antidopage: processus de révision et principales modifications. Jurisport 2013;137:20ff.
20 Halgreen L: European Sports Law: A Comparative Analysis of European and American Models of Sports, ed 2. Stockholm, Karnov, 2013, p 63.
21 Haas U: Die Streitbeilegung durch Schiedsgerichte im internationalen Sport; in Gilles P, Pfeiffer T (eds): Neue Tendenzen im Prozessrecht. Baden-Baden, Nomos, 2008, pp 9, 17ff.
22 Baddeley M: Droits de la personnalité et arbitrage: le dilemma des sanctions sportives; in Gauch P: Mélanges en l'honneur de Pierre Tercier. Geneva, Schulthess, 2008, p 707ff.
23 Haas U: Die Streitbeilegung durch Schiedsgerichte im internationalen Sport; in Gilles P, Pfeiffer T (eds): Neue Tendenzen im Prozessrecht. Baden-Baden, Nomos, 2008, pp 9, 18ff.
24 Blackshaw I, Siekmann RCR, Soek J (eds): The Court of Arbitration for Sport 1984–2004. The Hague, Asser, 2006, p 42.
25 World Anti-Doping Code. Appendix 1. Montreal, WADA, 2015, https://www.wada-ama.org/sites/default/files/resources/files/wada-2015-world-anti-doping-code.pdf, pp 129–142.
26 World Anti-Doping Code. Article 24 Interpretation of the Code. 24.3. Montreal, WADA, 2015, https://www.wada-ama.org/sites/default/files/resources/files/wada-2015-world-anti-doping-code.pdf, p 128.
27 Davies P: A Guide to the World Anti-Doping Code, ed 2. Port Melbourne, Cambridge University Press, 2013, p 6.
28 Rigozzi A, Haas U, Wisnosky E, Viret M: Breaking down the process of determining a basic sanction under the 2015 World Anti-Doping Code. Int Sports Law J 2015;15:3, 5ff.
29 Mavromati D, Reeb M: The Code of the Court of Arbitration for Sport. Alphen aan den Rijn, Kluwer Law International, 2015, p 1ff.
30 Rigozzi A: L'arbitrage international en matière de sport. Basel, Helbing & Lichtenhahn, 2005, p 216ff.
31 Lewis A, Taylor J (eds): Sport: Law and Practice, ed 3. London, Bloomsbury Professional, 2014, E3.1ff.
32 Lewis A, Taylor J (eds): Sport: Law and Practice, ed 3. London, Bloomsbury Professional, 2014, B1.2, B1.26.
33 Davies P: A Guide to the World Anti-Doping Code, ed 2. Port Melbourne, Cambridge University Press, 2013, p. 11.
34 McLaren RH: CAS doping jurisprudence: what can we learn? Int Sports Law Rev 2006, p 4ff.
35 Davies P: A Guide to the World Anti-Doping Code, ed 2. Port Melbourne, Cambridge University Press, 2013, pp 5, 8ff.
36 Mitten MJ: The Court of Arbitration for Sport and its global jurisprudence: international legal pluralism in a world without national boundaries. CAS Bull 2014; 2:48, 54ff.
37 http://www.tas-cas.org/en/arbitration/list-of-arbitrators-general-list.html.
38 http://www.tas-cas.org/jurisprudence-archives.

39. Davies P: A Guide to the World Anti-Doping Code, ed 2. Port Melbourne, Cambridge University Press, 2013, p 8.
40. Davies P: A Guide to the World Anti-Doping Code, ed 2. Port Melbourne, Cambridge University Press, 2013, p 19.
41. http://www.dis-sportschiedsgericht.de/.
42. www.irb.com.
43. www.usantidoping.org.
44. www.cces.ca.
45. www.uksport.gov.uk.
46. Mitten MJ: The Court of Arbitration for Sport and its global jurisprudence: international legal pluralism in a world without national boundaries. CAS Bull 2014; 2:48, 69ff.
47. Court of Arbitration for Sport 2004/A/628, §19.
48. Article 13.2.3 World Anti-Doping Code.
49. Lewis A, Taylor J (eds): Sport: Law and Practice, ed 3. London, Bloomsbury Professional, 2014, B1.2.
50. de La Rochefoucauld E: CAS jurisprudence related to the elimination or reduction of the period of ineligibility for specified substances. CAS Bull 2013;2: 18ff.
51. Court of Arbitration for Sport 2012/A/2747, §7.5ff.
52. Court of Arbitration for Sport 2011/A/2645, §§79–81.
53. Court of Arbitration for Sport 2011/A/2495, §8.31.
54. Court of Arbitration for Sport 2012/A/2822, §§8.9–8.12.
55. Court of Arbitration for Sport 2A/2011, §47.
56. Court of Arbitration for Sport 2012/A/2804, §9.15ff.
57. Court of Arbitration for Sport 95/141, §15.
58. Court of Arbitration for Sport 2001/A/317 (v.2.3).
59. Rigozzi A: L'importance du droit Suisse de l'arbitrage dans la résolution des litiges sportifs internationaux. ZSR 2013, pp 301, 317ff.
60. McLaren RH: CAS doping jurisprudence: what can we learn? Int Sports Law Rev 2006, pp 4, 6ff.
61. Rigozzi A: L'importance du droit Suisse de l'arbitrage dans la résolution des litiges sportifs internationaux. ZSR 2013, pp 301, 318.
62. Costa JP: Legal opinion regarding the draft 3.0 revision of the World Anti-doping Code. https://www.wada-ama.org/sites/default/files/resources/files/WADC-Legal-Opinion-on-Draft-2015-Code-3.0-EN.pdf.
63. Kaufmann-Kohler G, Malinverni G, Rigozzi A: Legal opinion on the conformity of certain provisions of the draft World Ant-Doping Code with commonly accepted principles of international law. 2003, https://www.wada-ama.org/sites/default/files/resources/files/kaufmann-kohler-full.pdf.
64. Kaufmann-Kohler G, Malinverni G, Rigozzi A: Doping and fundamental rights of athletes – comments in the wake of the adoption of the World Anti-Doping Code. Int Sports Law Rev 2003, pp 39, 40ff.
65. Court of Arbitration for Sport 2012/A/2862, §106.
66. Kaufmann-Kohler G, Malinverni G, Rigozzi A: Doping and fundamental rights of athletes – comments in the wake of the adoption of the World Anti-Doping Code. Int Sports Law Rev 2003, pp 39, 46ff.
67. Haas U: Role and application of the European Convention on Human Rights in CAS procedures. Int Sports Law Rev 2012, pp 43, 45ff.
68. Court of Arbitration for Sport 2011/A/2384, 2386, §172ff.
69. Court of Arbitration for Sport 2006/A/1063, §42ff, §55ff.
70. Court of Arbitration for Sport 2012/A/3031, §68.
71. Court of Arbitration for Sport 2013/A/3274, §65.
72. Morgan M: The relevance of Swiss law in doping disputes, in particular from the perspective of personality rights – a view from abroad. ZSR 2013, pp 341, 342ff.
73. Morgan M: The relevance of Swiss law in doping disputes, in particular from the perspective of personality rights – a view from abroad. ZSR 2013, pp 341, 344ff.
74. Court of Arbitration for Sport 2011/A/2325, §195.
75. Court of Arbitration for Sport 98/222, §31.
76. Court of Arbitration for Sport 99/A/223, §§25, 48.
77. Court of Arbitration for Sport 2006/A/1025, §10.7ff.
78. Court of Arbitration for Sport 2010/A/2268, §140ff.
79. Court of Arbitration for Sport 2012/A/2997, §32.
80. Court of Arbitration for Sport 2011/A/2612, §107.
81. Court of Arbitration for Sport 2013/A/3274, §81.
82. Court of Arbitration for Sport 2011/A/2612, §103ff.
83. Court of Arbitration for Sport 1995 94/129, §§30, 34.
84. Court of Arbitration for Sport 2009/A/1752, 1753, §4.8ff.
85. Court of Arbitration for Sport 2011/O/2422, §8.33ff.
86. Court of Arbitration for Sport 2011/A/2612, §101ff.
87. Court of Arbitration for Sport 2011/A/2562, §7.6.
88. Court of Arbitration for Sport 1996/56.
89. Court of Arbitration for Sport 1999/A/246.
90. Court of Arbitration for Sport 2000/A/270.
91. Court of Arbitration for Sport 2002/A/396.
92. Court of Arbitration for Sport 2004/A/690, §86.
93. Court of Arbitration for Sport 2005/C/976, 986, §138ff.
94. Court of Arbitration for Sport 2005/A/830, §10.24.
95. Court of Arbitration for Sport 2010/A/2268, §133ff.
96. Morgan M: The relevance of Swiss law in doping disputes, in particular from the perspective of personality rights – a view from abroad. ZSR 2013, pp 341, 347ff.
97. Morgan M: The relevance of Swiss law in doping disputes, in particular from the perspective of personality rights – a view from abroad. ZSR 2013, pp 341, 349ff.
98. Haas U: Role and application of the European convention on human rights in CAS procedures. Int Sports Law Rev 2012;12:43, 48ff.
99. Mitten MJ: The Court of Arbitration for Sport and its global jurisprudence: international legal pluralism in a world without national boundaries. CAS Bull 2014;2:48, 61ff.
100. Nafziger JAR: The principle of fairness in the Lex Sportiva of CAS awards and beyond; in Siekmann RCR, Soek J (ed): Lex Sportiva: What Is Sports Law? The Hague, Asser, 2012, p 588ff.
101. Haas U: Loslösung des organisierten Sports aus der Umklammerung des nationalen Rechts. SJZ 2010;106:585, 590ff.
102. Rigozzi A: L'importance du droit Suisse de l'arbitrage dans la résolution des litiges sportifs internationaux. ZSR 2013, pp 301, 311ff.

103 Decision of the Higher Regional Court of Munich SpuRt 2015, p 78ff.
104 European Court of Justice (March 23, 2006) C-519/04, David Meca-Medina and Igor Majcen v/ Commission of the European Communities.
105 Coccia M: Applicable law in CAS proceedings: what to do with EU law; in Bernasconi M, Rigozzi A (ed): Sport Governance, Football Disputes, Doping and CAS Arbitration. Bern, Weblaw, 2009, pp 69, 75ff.
106 Adolphsen J: Challenges for CAS decisions following the adoption of the new WADA Code; in Bernasconi M, Rigozzi A (eds): Sport Governance, Football Disputes, Doping and CAS Arbitration. Bern, Weblaw, 2009, pp 175, 182ff.
107 Subiotto R: The adoption and enforcement of anti-doping rules should not be subject to European competition law. Int Sports Law Rev 2010, p 32ff.
108 Subiotto R: Antitrust and antidoping do not mix. Jusletter July 16, 2012.
109 Haas U: The influence of EU law on international arbitration, in particular in Switzerland; in Müller C, Rigozzi A (eds): New Developments in International Commercial Arbitration 2012. Zurich, Schulthess, 2012, pp 47, 58.
110 Oberhammer P: Europäisches Beihilferecht und schiedsrechtlicher ordre public. Festheft für Karl Hempel zum 75. Geburtstag. GesRZ 2012, pp 29, 30.
111 Coccia M: Applicable law in CAS proceedings: what to do with EU law; in Bernasconi M, Rigozzi A (eds): Sport Governance, Football Disputes, Doping and CAS Arbitration. Bern, Weblaw, 2009, p 69.
112 European Court of Justice (June 1, 1999) C-126/97, Eco Swiss China Time Ltd v/ Benetton International NV, §36.
113 European Court of Justice (October 6, 2009) C-40/08, Asturcom Telecomunicaciones SL v/ Cristina Rodríguez Nogueira, §51.
114 European Court of Justice (October 26, 2006) C-168/05, Elisa Maria Mostaza Claro v/ Centro Movil Milenium SL, §37.
115 European Court of Justice (July 13, 2006) C-295/04 to C-298/04, Vincenzo Manfredi and Others v/ Lloyd Adriatico Assicurazioni SpA and Others, §31.
116 European Court of Justice (October 26, 2006) C-168/05, Elisa Maria Mostaza Claro v/ Centro Movil Milenium SL, §36.
117 Böckstiegel K-H, Kröll SM, Nacimiento P (eds): Arbitration in Germany: The Model Law in Practice, ed 2. Alphen aan den Rijn, Kluwer Law International, 2015.
118 Halgreen L: European Sports Law: A Comparative Analysis of European and American Models of Sports, ed 2. Stockholm, Karnov, 2013, pp 43ff, 79ff.
119 German Supreme Court. SchiedsVZ 2014, p 98.
120 Haas U: The influence of EU law on international arbitration, in particular in Switzerland; in Müller C, Rigozzi A (eds): New Developments in International Commercial Arbitration 2012. Zurich, Schulthess, pp 47, 61ff.
121 Higher Regional Court of Thüringen. SchiedsVZ 2008, pp 44, 45.
122 Cour d'Appel de Paris (18.11.2004), SA Thalès Air Defence v/ Le GIE Euromissile and SA EADS France. Rev Arb 2005, pp 751, 758.
123 Landolt P: Limits on court review of international arbitration awards assessed in light of states' interests and in particular in light of EU law requirements. Arbitration Int 2007;23:63, 81ff.
124 Oberhammer P: Europäisches Beihilferecht und schiedsrechtlicher ordre public. Festheft für Karl Hempel zum 75. Geburtstag. GesRZ 2012, pp 29, 32.
125 Haas U: The influence of EU law on international arbitration, in particular in Switzerland; in Müller C, Rigozzi A (eds): New Developments in International Commercial Arbitration 2012. Zurich, Schulthess, 2012, pp 47, 62ff.

Prof. Dr. Ulrich Haas
Rechtswissenschaftliches Institut
Universität Zürich
Freiensteinstrasse 5
CH-8032 Zurich (Switzerland)
E-Mail ulrich.haas@rwi.uzh.ch

How Will the Legal and Sport Environment Influence a Future Code?

Olivier Niggli

World Anti-Doping Agency (WADA), Montreal, QC, Canada

Introduction

When the World Anti-Doping Agency (WADA) was created in 1999, the most urgent and important matter was to harmonize rules and regulations linked with anti-doping. The hope was that all athletes, whatever their sport or country, would be treated equally. Following 2 years of consultations, national governments and the international sports movement adopted the first World Anti-Doping Code (the Code) in 2003 in Copenhagen. Since then, it has been amended twice, in 2009 and most recently in 2015.

From the outset, it was always clear that the Code would be a "living" document requiring amendments from time to time to adapt to the evolution of the fight against doping in sport. Cheaters are becoming more sophisticated, and it is quite obvious that the anti-doping community and the Code need to adapt in order to become more effective. Furthermore, the application of the Code in practice, and its interpretation by arbitral institutions, such as the Court of Arbitration for Sport (CAS) or other tribunals, highlight possible loopholes in the rules that need to be addressed and fixed from time to time.

Although the Code was designed to evolve over the years, in order to avoid too many changes, the system was also designed to allow mandatory documents under the Code. These are called the international standards, and they can be amended on a more regular basis. This is the case for the international standard of the list of prohibited substances and methods, which is reviewed and amended yearly.

Both the legal and sports environments have influenced the latest revision of the Code. The legal environment had a major influence with more emphasis put on the question of the athletes' fundamental rights and, more precisely, the respect of the principles outlined in the European Convention on Human Rights.

The sport environment also had an influence on the revisions to the 2015 Code. First and foremost, there was a strong call from the athletes for harsher penalties. Standard sanctions for an intentional infraction were increased from 2 years in the previous versions of the Code to 4 years in the 2015 Code. Furthermore, there was also an expectation from sport that the new Code would provide the tools and the mechanisms to deal not only with the athletes, but also with their entourage. The new provision on prohibited association resolved this concern. In addition, the new Code embodied a general philosophy to support the collection and management of information and gave WADA new investigative powers, too.

Going forward, revisions of the World Anti-Doping Code will continue to be influenced both by the legal and sport environments. This chapter aims to summarize the main factors that could influence the Code and the fight against doping in the coming years.

How Will the Sport Environment Influence the Fight against Doping?

Current Environment
It is important to realize that we have entered an era where doping is no longer the only threat to the integrity of sports. In the past 5 years, the risk of match fixing, illegal betting, and, more generally, bad governance of sport have been top-of-mind concerns in the sporting community. As the fight against doping continues to grow, others have taken on match fixing and corruption.

In 2014, a number of countries ratified a Council of Europe convention against match fixing. This is both an opportunity and a risk for the fight against doping. With sports integrity on the agenda of international federations (IFs) and sports organizations, the time is ripe for anti-doping advocates to advance the cause. However, there is a concern. Match fixing may become more complicated to understand and complex to resolve. With limited resources available to address issues of sports integrity, the focus on anti-doping may be reduced. Those of us in the anti-doping community do not believe that match-fixing provisions will find their way into the World Anti-Doping Code. We see the issues and challenges of doping and match fixing to be quite distinct. Some have suggested that a new organization be created – an agency for the integrity of sport. This body could combine both anti-doping and match fixing. At the moment, there are no plans to move forward with such an integrity agency.

Where match fixing may influence the World Anti-Doping Code and the fight against doping, however, is in the establishment of closer relationships with law enforcement and other state agencies in the fight against organized crime. Doping, like match fixing, is often organized by clandestine, and often criminal, organizations and can only be apprehended by state organizations whose powers have been defined by law. The creation within police forces and customs of sport integrity units which could deal with both anti-doping and match fixing may enhance the already robust cooperation between sports and law enforcement in the fight against doping. This cooperation should be reflected either in the Code or the related international standards.

It is well known that "bad guys" tend to do "bad things." In other words, an investigation into a doping ring might also highlight issues of match fixing and other illegal activities and vice versa. For example, in the recent investigation into doping in Russia, it became clear from the start that some individuals were engaged in other criminal activities such as extortion and bribery. By sharing information with the relevant law enforcement authorities, WADA was able to provide sufficient evidence for a criminal investigation in France. The exchange and sharing of information is undoubtedly going to be one of the key priorities in an effective fight against doping. Of course, this also requires appropriate follow-up and the allocation of resources to perform these investigation tasks both at the sport and government levels.

The Athletes
Those who should have the most influence on a future Code and on the evolution of the fight against doping are the athletes – the clean athletes, of course. The entire fight against doping is

built around the idea that the clean athlete deserves to be protected so that they can perform on a level playing field free of doping. It is their voice that has the most impact on sports and government leaders. Clean athletes should continue to speak out and demand more action and more resources for the fight against doping.

The players' unions will also have a role to play. So far, these unions have generally hampered the fight against doping. Their position is that they mainly represent team sports in which the problem of doping is, according to them, relatively minor. It is to be hoped that in the future such an attitude will evolve and that a constructive collaboration will arise between the anti-doping organizations and the athlete unions. The future of the Code and how strict the rules can be will heavily be influenced by the attitude of the athletes and by their readiness and willingness to accept a number of constraints (and sometimes restrictions to their freedom) in order to protect the sport for which they have invested so much of their time, energy, and hope.

The Governance of Sport
Along with the athletes, it is important that the leadership of the sports community ensures that the highest ethical standards are applied across their sports and their organizations. Recent FIFA (Fédération Internationale de Football Association) and IAAF (International Association of Athletics Federations) scandals have illustrated the magnitude of the issue. Furthermore, as was revealed by the report from the CIRC (Commission for Cycling), ethics within sports organizations is not always at the highest level [1]. One would hope that these unfortunate events remain the exception, and that the governance of sport globally will keep supporting and pushing for strong rules to be written and enforced. In the revision of the 2015 Code, there was a strong commitment from sports towards harsher sanctions. It was reflected in the submissions received from the IOC (International Olympic Committee) and ASOIF (Association of Summer Olympic International Federations), the organization that represents all International Olympic Summer Federations, during the Code review process. It is to be hoped that the influence of sports on a future Code will continue along the path of reinforcing and ensuring an efficient fight against doping. Sports leadership also has the responsibility to allocate enough resources to this fight, which should not be seen by them as a burden on their budget, but rather as an investment in clean athletes and in the future of their sports. Consequently, the evolution of the Code will be influenced by the global politics of sports in the coming years. The IFs must show a clear commitment to the fight against doping. The hope remains that a future Code will be allowed to go even further in the fight against doping without being impeded by political battles and personal ambitions.

At the moment, the IOC is pushing for WADA to take over all testing for all IFs. If the IOC is able to convince the IFs to delegate their testing to WADA and is ready to find a mechanism to fund such a program, this will be another push for a more independent, more transparent, and more efficient system. This may require some Code changes to ensure that the roles and responsibilities of all parties are well defined.

The Court of Arbitration for Sport
At present, there are a number of question marks surrounding the CAS and, in particular, the recognition of its decisions by state courts. This situation comes as a result of a recent German decision in the Claudia Pechstein case, which questioned the way CAS is structured and established. Without debating the validity of the decision, which is currently under appeal, it is certain that this case may have a tremendous influence on the future evolution of the Code. The nonrecognition of CAS decisions would mean that the entire sport system could become unmanageable very quickly. Not only for doping disputes but for all

the other matters that fall under CAS's purview such as football transfers and commercial deals. If all the disputes currently adjudicated by CAS were to end up in front of civil courts in various jurisdictions of the world, not only would the cost of such litigation rapidly become unsustainable for the world of sports, but it would also mean very inconsistent decisions across the world and a very slow resolution of matters in total incompatibility with the requirements of sports calendars. Therefore, it is absolutely key that CAS not only be maintained but also recognized by all as the "Supreme Court of Sport." If, however, CAS were to be challenged further, this would require the World Anti-Doping Code to address this issue and to see if other alternatives are possible for resolving disputes related to anti-doping. The creation of a permanent court for anti-doping, with the help of governments, could be an avenue to be explored and was a possibility mentioned recently during one of the WADA Foundation Board meetings. The international anti-doping community is not yet at that stage; however, if such a perspective were to be considered further, this may have an important impact on any future Code revisions.

The Legal Environment

Human Rights
One of the key features of the revised 2015 Code was the introduction of more principles linked to human rights in general and the rights of athletes in particular. An opinion from Judge Jean-Paul Costa, the former President of the European Court of Human Rights, had significant influence on the final draft of the 2015 Code. It is likely that the legal evolution of the case law from the Court of Human Rights will continue to influence the fight against doping. Any future revisions to the Code will have to balance provisions that truly protect the clean athlete and that maximize the chances of detecting cheaters while ensuring that the fight is conducted within the boundaries that are set by fundamental principles of law and human rights. Experience will show how the application of the current Code unfolds and whether there are any areas which will require improvement in order to be compatible with the above-mentioned principles.

Data Protection
Anti-doping activities, by their very nature, require the collection of vast amounts of data. Athletes provide information on their whereabouts, laboratory results, biological passport data, and therapeutic use exemptions. The protection of these data is of paramount importance. Future Code revisions will be impacted by new national legislation on data protection. For example, current European Union directives were taken into account for the 2015 Code; however, it did create some challenges. The main difficulties arising from these directives stem from the collection and the sharing of information and the publication of anti-doping sanctions. Currently, the trend is towards reinforcing legislation for data protection through regulations that would apply in all member states. This regulation is very restrictive and may further complicate the exchange of information to support the fight against doping. The anti-doping movement is hoping that some exceptions may be granted that take into account the specificity of anti-doping.

The Evolution of National Legislation
As previously mentioned, investigations are key to the fight against doping. While sport and WADA can initiate some investigations under the new 2015 Code, their power and jurisdiction is limited. Only state agencies, namely police and custom forces, can have a true legal basis to conduct proper investigations. For this to happen, it is necessary that each country has a law allowing for such investigations, therefore granting law enforcement agencies the power to act. A few coun-

tries, including Italy and Germany, have, therefore, criminalized doping at various degrees. Some have limited criminalization to trafficking and manufacturing of doping substances, while others have gone further and made the use of a prohibited substance a criminal offense. The Code deals with athletes who cheat by banning them from sport for 4 years (and more in case of a second offense); however, WADA does not see a need for them to be sent to jail. What is necessary is that a strong criminal legislation deals with all those surrounding the athletes who help them dope, whether they are coaches, doctors, agents, or other athletes. WADA must encourage governments to put proper legislation in place, and, when this happens, this may also influence the next version of the Code.

Conclusion

Sport is at the crossroads. Either good governance, ethics, and values will prevail or the entire landscape will change rapidly. The Code provides a solid framework for the fight against doping, but its rules must be implemented in practice. WADA's role in enforcing compliance with the rules of the Code will be a key factor in the success of the fight against doping. One thing is certain, in 5 years' time sport will be very different than it is today. Those of us in the anti-doping community certainly hope it is for the better.

Reference

1 CIRC Report: http://www.uci.ch/mm/Document/News/CleanSport/16/87/99/CIRCReport2015_Neutral.pdf.

Olivier Niggli
Director General of the World Anti-Doping Agency
Stock Exchange Tower
800 Place Victoria, Suite 1700
Montreal, QC H4Z 1B7 (Canada)
E-Mail olivier.niggli@wada-ama.org

Structure and Development of the List of Prohibited Substances and Methods

Audrey Kinahan[a, d, e] · Richard Budgett[a, b, g] · Irene Mazzoni[c, d, f]

[a]Prohibited List Expert Group, [b]Working Group on World Anti-Doping Agency (WADA) Governance Matters, and [c]Science Department, [d]WADA, Montreal, QC, Canada; [e]Eipharm, Ennis, and [f]Sport Ireland, Dublin, Ireland; [g]Institute of Sport Exercise and Health, University College London Hospital, London, UK

Abstract

The list of prohibited substances and methods (the List) is the international standard that determines what is prohibited in sport both in- and out-of-competition. Since 2004, the official text of the List is produced by the World Anti-Doping Agency (WADA), the international independent organization responsible for promoting, coordinating, and monitoring the fight against doping in sport. Originally based on the prohibited lists established by the International Olympic Committee, the List has evolved to incorporate new doping trends, distinguish permitted from prohibited routes of administration, and adjust to new analytical and pharmacological breakthroughs. In this chapter, the elements that compose the List as well as the updates over the years are presented.

© 2017 S. Karger AG, Basel

Introduction

"Is this drug prohibited?" Every day athletes all over the world ask this question to their doctors, trainers, sports federation, or anti-doping organization. The answer can be found in the list of prohibited substances and methods (the List), yearly published and updated by the World Anti-Doping Agency (WADA). The List is a legal document that defines what drugs or procedures are prohibited for athletes, in which instances they are prohibited and, in some cases, in which sport. Although it is full of scientific and pharmacological terminology and chemical names that may be a good subject for a spelling bee competition, it is, at the same time, the clean athlete's best friend. This chapter will address how the List has evolved, the processes that make this possible, and look at what new drugs and methods may find their way into future Lists.

Legal Context – The Code

The structure and contents of the List are defined in the 2003, 2009, and 2015 World Anti-Doping Codes (the Code). The Code is the overarching document on which the anti-doping program is based and harmonizes rules and regulations throughout sports. Only those sport organizations and public authorities that are signatories of the Code are bound to it. To date, the vast majority of governments (183 countries out of 195 possible) and sports authorities (e.g., the International Olympic Committee, IOC, International Paralympic Committee, and IOC-recognized and -nonrecognized organizations) have accepted the Code and enforce its rules and policies accordingly.

The Code outlines the principles that constitute the framework of the List, briefly:
- *Publication and Revision of the List:* the Code establishes the timing and process involved in the preparation of the List.
- *Prohibited Substances and Methods Included:* the Code outlines what is prohibited in sports and when.
- *Criteria for Including Substances and Methods:* the 3 criteria used to consider whether a substance or method should be included in the List are defined in the Code.
- *Therapeutic Use Exemptions:* the Code explains the procedures to follow if an athlete needs to use a prohibited substance for a medical reason.
- *Monitoring Program:* the Code states the procedures to follow the patterns of use of non-prohibited substances that are suspected to be used in doping.

Publication and Revision of the List

The first List published by WADA came into effect in January 2004. Immediately following the 2nd World Conference on Doping in Sport that took place in Copenhagen in March 2003, the newly formed List Expert Group (LiEG) met and drafted the 2004 List. This List was based on the 2003 IOC prohibited List and was modified and adapted to the requirements of the Code. One of those requirements was the need for consultation with WADA's stakeholders (governments and sports authorities – signatories of the Code). As stated in the Code, the draft List should be circulated among the stakeholders for comments, making this, for the first time in the history of lists of prohibited drugs in sport, a highly interactive and participative process. Every year, the LiEG meets to discuss the contents of the List and modifies it according to new doping trends and new drugs with doping potential. This draft is sent to WADA's stakeholders, who have a period of about 3 months to send their comments on the changes made as well as other changes they may consider pertinent. In a subsequent meeting, the LiEG discusses the stakeholders' comments, modifies the draft List if needed, and makes their recommendations to WADA's Health, Medical, and Research Committee (HMRC). The HMRC can amend the recommendations made by the LiEG on the List. Finally, the draft List is submitted to WADA's Executive Committee, who can approve the draft List as presented by the HMRC or make further modifications before its approval. As a matter of principle, modifications introduced after the consultation period with stakeholders are avoided as much as possible, to preserve the spirit of the consultation process.

The Code also has a provision to modify the List at any time of the year if a substance or method in question requires immediate action. This "fast track" mechanism was used for the first time in 2014, when reports during the Winter Olympic Games in Sochi of the abuse of hypoxia-inducible factor (HIF) activators like xenon prompted the LiEG to revise the 2014 List in June. The modified List came into effect on September 1, 2014.

Prohibited Substances and Methods Included

The Code establishes in general terms that there exist substances and methods which are considered as doping both in- and out-of-competition, i.e., at all times, others that are only prohibited in competition, and finally a smaller number that are prohibited in certain sports. The distinction is based on the fact that some substances or methods can have long-term effects and, even if taken during the training period, can impact future competitions so they should be always prohibited, while the effects of others are more restricted in time. It is up to the LiEG to determine the categories of drugs or methods to be included in the List and to determine the periods of time in which they should be prohibited. Examples of substances prohibited at all times include those that can affect the quality and quantity of muscles, like anabolic steroids, growth hormone, and $β_2$-agonists, as well as substances and methods that affect the number of red blood cells, erythropoietin (EPO), or blood transfusion. Masking agents, as they can conceal the use of doping substances, are also included in this category. On the other hand, drugs that increase arousal, like stimulants, or curtail pain, like narcotics, are examples of substances prohibited in-competition only. To date, only 2 groups of substances are prohibited in particular sports: alcohol and β-blockers. The use of these substances would be detrimental for or incompatible with the practice of most sports but, for example, the use of β-blockers could be an advantage in the practice of sports requiring precision, such as shooting, archery, or darts. In the first List published by WADA in 2004, there were 9 categories of prohibited substances and 3 categories of prohibited methods until 2011, where the category S0 (non-approved substances) was introduced. The other categories have evolved in time and new subcategories added, as will be described later.

Another classification defined by the Code is that of specified substances. Except for all the anabolic agents and hormones, as well as some stimulants and hormone antagonists and modulators, which one can think of as substances more likely to be used for doping, all other substances included in the List are considered "specified." But what is exactly a "specified substance?" In the original 2003 Code, "specified substances" were those that could be easily accessible as medicinal products, for example, over-the-counter medications, or those that were potentially less likely to be used for doping. When the World Anti-Doping Code was revised in 2009, this distinction was strictly linked to sanctions. However, the definition of "specified substances" in the revised 2015 Code resembles more that of 2003, as they are defined as substances more likely to be consumed for purposes other than performance enhancement [1–3]. In any case, there is a misconception that an athlete doping with a "specified substance" will automatically get a reduced sanction. This is not necessarily the case and if it can be proven that the athlete had the intention to dope with a "specified substance," a full-term sanction can be applied. Alternatively, an athlete can get a reduced sanction if he/she can prove that there was no intention to dope with a non-specified substance. In brief, "specified substances" are not less important or less dangerous doping substances.

The categories included in the List can be closed or open. In the closed categories, only the drugs or methods listed are prohibited; an example of this is the Narcotics section. In the open categories, only some typical examples are shown on the List, so there are many other substances or methods that are not shown that are part of these categories. One of the reasons to do this is space, as it would take many pages to name all the drugs and methods prohibited. The other reason is that there are new pharmacological and illegal drugs entering the market that are included in these open categories, so if all the prohibited substances must be listed, this would require a constant updating of the List. Therefore, these open categories can be identified in the List by phrases like "including but not limited" or "similar chemical structure and/or biological effect." Nevertheless, each year, the LiEG adds examples to help the athlete and entourage identify what is prohibited or allowed. In any case, it is always better for an athlete to ask an anti-doping organization or sports federation rather than risk a sanction.

Criteria for Including Substances and Methods

The Code also defines 3 criteria, 2 of which need to be fulfilled before a substance or method can be considered for the inclusion in the List. These criteria are: proven or potential performance-enhancing abilities of the candidate drug or method, actual or proven health risk, and violation of the spirit of sport. The 3 criteria and their equal importance have remained unaltered since the first Code in 2003. During the consultation process of the latest Code revision, some stakeholders suggested that performance enhancement should be made a mandatory criterion. However, since experiments to prove performance enhancement may be difficult to perform in humans, especially for designer and unapproved drugs, in the end it was decided not to introduce any modifications.

Monitoring Program

There are some substances that are not prohibited but which WADA closely monitors to detect patterns of use or abuse in sport that would suggest a perceived competitive advantage. Substances may be monitored because they have a mechanism of action that is not well defined but could attract the attention of cheating athletes. Other substances, like the stimulant caffeine, are in the program because they are consumed by the majority of the population, and it is difficult to distinguish normal use from doping abuse. Medications with mild doping potential, but which are broadly used, can also be placed in the Monitoring Program. Such is the case for bupropion used for smoking cessation. This means that despite being a recognized stimulant, such substances are not prohibited, but instead the risk of abuse for doping is monitored.

Substances placed in the Monitoring Program are included in the routine doping analysis, and results of their presence in urine are reported to WADA. The results are compiled by region and/or by sport, and the LiEG monitors any change in use by athletes year by year. One of the substances included in the first Monitoring Program published in 2004, pseudoephedrine (PSE), has made its way back onto the List in 2010. Originally included in the IOC Lists, it was removed from the first List published by WADA in 2004 and placed in the Monitoring Program. It was reasoned that it was a medication widely used for the treatment of symptoms of cold and sold over the counter in most countries, so it could easily result in inadvertent doping. In addition, there were studies showing that at therapeutic doses, the ergogenic effects of PSE were limited [4–9]. The monitoring of PSE over subsequent years showed that there was an upward trend of usage after its withdrawal from the List. The PSE concentrations in urine were in many instances significantly higher than those expected with therapeutic use of the substance. In addition, 3 scientific articles that appeared between 2000 and 2010 indicated that PSE could be ergogenic when used at supratherapeutic doses [10–12]. In view of this, the LiEG decided to reintroduce PSE following a clinical study ordered by WADA, in which the urinary concentration to distinguish therapeutic from supratherapeutic use of PSE up to 24 h before competition (150 μg/mL) was established [13]. Continued monitoring of PSE at lower concentrations since 2010 has not shown any increase in use; so, this was stopped from 2015 onwards.

Meldonium was included in the 2015 Monitoring Program. The information gathered over 2015 demonstrated clear evidence of abuse and led to the inclusion of meldonium in the 2016 List. Other substances have been added to the Monitoring Program over the years, and data continue to be gathered, and trends analyzed.

Each section in the List and how these have evolved since the first WADA List of 2004 is described below based on IOC Lists 1968–2003 and WADA Lists and Explanatory Notes 2004–2017 [14–23]. The sections are presented in the same order as the current 2017 List.

The Prohibited List

General Considerations

To ensure consistency, substances are included in the List in accordance with their international non-proprietary name (INN) or when the INN is not known, the common name with the corresponding International Union of Pure and Applied Chemistry (IUPAC) nomenclature. There have been many nomenclature changes over the years in line with this practice, e.g., in the absence of an INN, the substance methylhexaneamine is also declared by its IUPAC name, 4-methylhexan-2-amine in the 2017 List.

Substances and Methods Prohibited in- and out-of-Competition

S0 Non-Approved Substances

This section was not in the 2004 WADA List and was only introduced in the 2011 List. To address the possibility of abuse in sport of substances not currently included in any section of the List, including those which would be embraced by virtue of being of "similar chemical structure and/or biologic effect," a prologue section named S0 was introduced. It is intended that this section now addresses substances currently or previously in development, those substances not intended for human use, and the potential synthesis of "designer drugs" to circumvent the List itself.

S1 Anabolic Agents

S1.1 Anabolic Androgenic Steroids. The WADA 2004 List subdivided "S1.1 Anabolic Androgenic Steroids (AAS)" into "S1.1a Exogenous AAS" and "S1.1b Endogenous AAS." Over the years the number of examples have grown, and now S1.1a Exogenous AAS includes some of the older examples of methandienone, stanozolol, and oxymetholone, the newer designer steroids, such as tetrahydrogestrinone and desoxymethyltestosterone (added as examples in 2005 and 2006, respectively), and substances found in the flourishing supplement industry such as 5α-androst-2-ene-17-one, commonly known as "delta-2" or 2-androstenone, which was added for the 2017 List. S1.1b Endogenous AAS substances include androstenediol, androstenedione, dihydrotestosterone, prasterone (dehydroepiandrosterone, DHEA), and testosterone, with many of their metabolites and isomers included as examples. The 1996 IOC List introduced the concept of the testosterone/epitestosterone (T/E) ratio. T/E ratios of greater than 6:1 were subject to further scrutiny, including a review of previous/subsequent tests, and any results of endocrine investigations. This concept was included in the WADA 2004 List as a T/E ratio of 6:1, with a tightening of the T/E ratio in the 2005 List to 4:1. The 2006 WADA List indicated that isotope ratio mass spectrometry was regarded as a "reliable method" in the detection of testosterone of exogenous origin, and that this complex analysis should be performed in all cases of high T/E ratios. There were several rewordings and clarifications over the years with the ever lengthening of the text associated with the T/E ratio. From the 2010 List, the T/E ratio was removed from the List and instead addressed in technical documents, and from 2014 onwards the T/E ratio is evaluated in accordance with the steroidal module of the athlete biological passport technical document, to better target the use of this sophisticated test [24]. For the 2017 List, as some anabolic steroids listed in the exogenous section (S1.1a) can be produced endogenously at very low doses, boldenone, boldione, 19-norandrostenedione, and nandrolone were transferred from S1.1a to S1.1b and 19-norandrostenediol added to S1.1b. Such a change did not alter the prohibited status of these substances but instead ensured that WADA laboratory documents were synchronized with the List.

S1.2 Other Anabolic Agents. Prior to the WADA 2004 List, this section was called "β$_2$-Agonists" and included clenbuterol, salbutamol, terbutaline, salmeterol, fenoterol, and related substances as examples. The heading "Other Anabolic Agents" was used for the 2003 IOC List whereby only clenbuterol and salbutamol at a urinary concentration in excess of 1,000 ng/mL of non-sulfated salbutamol was listed, and it was this heading that was used in the WADA 2004 List. The 2004 List removed salbutamol to its own category as a β_2-agonist, and the only substances listed in 2004 were clenbuterol and the growth promoter zeranol. Since then the list of examples has expanded with the addition of zilpaterol (2005), the synthetic steroid tibolone (2006), and selective androgen receptor modulators (2008).

S2 Peptide Hormones, Growth Factors, Related Substances, and Mimetics

No other pharmacological area has evolved more since the inception of the idea of a list of prohibited substances and methods. The 1996 IOC List first included the heading of "Peptide and Glycoprotein Hormones and Analogues." Substances included human chorionic gonadotrophin (hCG), corticotrophin, growth hormone (GH), and "all respective releasing factors for such substances" and EPO. In 2000, this section expanded to include insulin-like growth factor (IGF) and insulin, which was "permitted only to treat athletes with certified insulin-dependent diabetes." Pituitary and synthetic gonadotrophins were also added, of which luteinizing hormone (LH) was only prohibited in males. Likewise, men were also prohibited from using hCG in the 2000 List. Releasing factors and analogues were also included for all substances except insulins and EPO.

When WADA introduced its List in 2004, the heading was simplified to "S5 Peptide Hormones"; it included the same substances as the 2000 IOC List and declared that "substances with similar chemical structure or similar pharmacological effect(s), and their releasing factors were also prohibited." For the 2005 WADA List, the prohibition of hCG and LH were combined in one subgroup as gonadotrophins (LH/hCG), and the prohibition was for both men and women. This decision was reversed for the 2006 List, with the LiEG explaining that

Despite the scientific rationale to prohibit these substances in women, the experience during 2005 has led, in some cases, to detect elevated hCG levels due to physiological (pregnancy) or pathological conditions with potentially significant psychological or social consequences for the athlete, in addition to the difficulty, to date, to discriminate at the laboratory level these cases from doping abuse.

The 2005 List also saw the addition of mechano-growth factors (MGFs) and the heading of this section now changed to "S2 Hormones and Related Substances." The heading expanded for the 2010 List, to "Peptide, Hormones, Growth Factors and Related Substances" to reflect the subsection on GH, IGF-1, and MGFs, in addition to the inclusion of platelet-derived growth factors, fibroblast growth factors, vascular endothelial growth factor, and hepatocyte growth factor as well as "any other growth factor affecting muscle, tendon or ligament protein synthesis/degradation, vascularisation, energy utilization, regenerative capacity or fibre type switching." To reflect the requests from stakeholders to include examples of releasing factors, S2.5 of the 2015 List included examples of GH-releasing hormone and its analogues and GH secretagogues in addition to stating the types of growth factors that were prohibited.

The List is updated to reflect developments both in science and doping practices, and this development has led to the evolution of the subsection now referred to as EPO receptor agonists. It was for the 2009 List that EPO was renamed as EPO-stimulating agent (ESA), and that darbepoetin and hematide were included as examples of this class, while CERA (methoxy polyethylene glycol-epoetin β) was added as a specific example to this subgroup in 2010. HIF stabilizers were included in the 2011 List with the addition of HIF activators xenon and argon in September 2014, as already discussed.

In the 2015 List, EPO receptor agonists were subdivided into "S2.1.1 Erythropoiesis-Stimulating Agents (ESAs)," which, in addition to EPOs, also included examples of EPO-mimetic peptides, and into "S2.1.2 Non-Erythropoietic EPO-Receptor Agonists." HIF stabilizers and activators were listed as their own subclassification of S2. The title of S2 was updated to include mimetics to highlight the fact that synthetic analogues were also prohibited. For the 2017 List, to extend the scope of EPO-stimulating agents, GATA inhibitors (e.g., K-11706) and transforming growth factor-β inhibitors (e.g., sotatercept and luspatercept) were added as further examples.

The intramuscular administration of platelet-derived preparations, known as platelet-rich plasma, or "blood spinning," was prohibited under S2 for the 2010 List only. From the 2011 List onwards, these products were removed as there was a "lack of any current evidence concerning the use of these methods for purposes of performance enhancement notwithstanding that these preparations contain growth factors." The LiEG explained that "Despite the presence of some growth factors, current studies on platelet-rich plasma do not demonstrate any potential for performance enhancement beyond a potential therapeutic effect" and clarified that individual growth factors are still prohibited when given separately as purified substances. Insulins were removed from S2 in the 2013 List and reclassified as metabolic modulators under "S4 Hormone and Metabolic Modulators," which was deemed more appropriate given their mechanism of action. This also clarified that only insulin and not any respective releasing factor was prohibited.

For the 2016 and 2017 Lists, there were some noteworthy stakeholder comments to include thyroid hormone as a prohibited substance. However, the LiEG felt that there was no clear evidence of its performance enhancement since consumption of thyroid hormone decreases the level of TSH to appropriately lowering the endogenous production of T_3/T_4, therefore staying within the normal range. Thus, exogenous thyroid hormone should in the end have no impact on performance.

As newer pharmacological classes evolve, it is anticipated that there may be restructuring of S2 for future Lists including a reevaluation of the nomenclature used with respect to HIF regulators to keep it more focused upon activity in the EPO pathways.

S3 Beta-2 Agonists

Prior to the WADA 2004 List, $β_2$-agonists were initially included in the 1996 IOC List for their anabolic and stimulant properties, being included under both anabolic agents and stimulant headings. A specific exemption was included for salbutamol, salmeterol, and terbutaline, which were "Permitted by inhaler only to prevent and/or treat asthma and exercise-induced asthma." The List referenced the fact that "Written notification of asthma and/or exercise-induced asthma by a respiratory or team physician is necessary to the relevant medical authority." The IOC 2000 List provided a summary of urinary concentrations above which the laboratory must report a positive finding. For salbutamol, it was above 100 ng/mL as a stimulant and above 1,000 ng/mL as an anabolic agent. The WADA List in 2004 categorized these substances into their own pharmacological class. The 2004 List declared that

> All beta-2 agonists including their D- and L-isomers are prohibited except that formoterol, salbutamol, salmeterol and terbutaline are permitted by inhalation only to prevent and/or treat asthma and exercise-induced asthma/bronchoconstriction.
>
> A medical notification in accordance with section 8 of the International Standard for Therapeutic Use Exemptions is required.

A medical notification was referred to as an abbreviated therapeutic use exemption (TUE), which enabled these 4 $β_2$-agonists to be used by inhalation only.

The urinary threshold limit of 1,000 ng/mL of salbutamol (free plus glucuronide) was continued from previous Lists, whereby the athlete with levels in excess of 1,000 ng/mL was considered a positive finding unless the athlete proved that the abnormal result was the consequence of the therapeutic use of inhaled salbutamol. The 2010 List also clarified that the maximum dose for a controlled pharmacokinetic study should be 1,600 μg.

In compliance with the 2009 Code, references to abbreviated TUEs were removed for the 2009 List and instead required those wishing to use inhaled $β_2$-agonists to apply for a full TUE. This resulted in a very significant increase in the number of TUE applications. In order to address this increasing burden to TUE committees and also because research pointed to the fact the inhaled $β_2$-agonists at therapeutic doses were not performance enhancing, inhaled salbutamol (to a maximum 1,600 μg over 24 h) and inhaled salmeterol were permitted once a declaration of use (DOU) was provided from the 2010 List onwards. In 2011, in response to concerns expressed by stakeholders, the DOU requirement was removed for these two $β_2$-agonists, and a maximum inhalation limit for salmeterol was set as in accordance with the manufacturer's recommended therapeutic regime.

For the 2017 List, to ensure that a full-day dose of salbutamol was not administered all at one time, the maximum inhaled dose was clarified as a maximum of 1,600 μg over 24 h with no more than 800 μg every 12 h; the maximum salmeterol dose was set according to the manufacturer's recommendations as 200 μg over 24 h.

In the 2012 List, the LiEG allowed inhaled formoterol be permitted at maximum-delivered dose of 36 μg/24 h, which corresponded to maximum urinary levels of 30 ng/mL formoterol. In 2013, this exemption was expanded further and higher doses of formoterol were allowed, covering temporary asthma exacerbations, where the inhaled maximum-delivered dose was increased to 54 μg/24 h with a corresponding increase in the urinary threshold to a maximum of 40 ng/mL.

While studies have been conducted to develop thresholds to distinguish between oral and inhaled terbutaline, this has proven difficult, so this substance currently remains prohibited at all doses and routes.

For the 2017 List, the examples of prohibited $β_2$-agonists were expanded to include higenamine (a non-selective $β_2$-agonist found in dietary supplements), indacaterol, olodaterol, and vilanterol (these are ultra-long-acting $β_2$-agonists which are increasingly used in medicine) in addition to fenoterol, formoterol, procaterol, reproterol, salbutamol, and terbutaline.

S4 Hormone and Metabolic Modulators

The first reference to substances now classified as "S4 Hormone and Metabolic Modulators" was in the IOC 2000 List, which included clomiphene, cyclofenil, and tamoxifen as examples of substances prohibited in men only under the category of "Peptide Hormones, Mimetics and Analogues." While the 2001 List added aromatase inhibitors to this section as an example, it was not until the 2003 List that agents with anti-estrogenic activity were assigned their own category, and this same nomenclature was used for the 2004 WADA List. The 2005 WADA List subdivided this pharmacological class into 3 categories: (1) aromatase inhibitors, (2) selective estrogen receptor modulators, and (3) other anti-estrogenic substances. The prohibition of use by men only was also removed in 2005. The title was changed in 2008 to "Hormone Antagonists and Modulators" in conjunction with the addition of a 4th category of agents modifying myostatin function(s).

Metabolic Modulators. Peroxisome proliferator-activated receptor δ (PPARδ) agonists (e.g., GW1516) and PPARδ-AMP-activated protein kinase axis agonists (e.g., AICAR) were added as a 5th category in the 2012 List. This pharmacological class was reclassified from gene doping, which is a prohibited method, to substances that modify cellular metabolism. To reflect the addition of this category, the title of this section was modified to "Hormone and Metabolic Modulators." The subsection metabolic modulators expanded in the 2013 List with inclusion of insulins, which has been reclassified from "Peptide Hormones, Growth Factors and Related Substances." Insulin mimetics were added to subsection S5.2 to include all insulin receptor agonists for the 2016 List. The angina treatment trimetazidine was the third addition to metabolic modulators. This substance had initially been categorized as a stimulant based on its chemical structure but was reclassified in the 2015 List under "Metabolic Modulators" to reflect its activity as a modulator of cardiac metabolism and was included in subsection S5.4.

Meldonium. Meldonium, also known by the brand name Mildronate, was included as its own subsection (S5.3) in the 2016 List because of evidence of clear abuse of the substance while it was on the List's 2015 Monitoring Program, as already outlined.

S5 Diuretics and Masking Agents

Diuretics were first prohibited in the 1996 IOC List with examples including spironolactone, mannitol, bumetanide, acetazolamide, furosemide, hydrochlorothiazide, and related substances, while epitestosterone and probenecid were included in the list of examples of masking agents. For the 2003 List, "Diuretics and Masking Agents" were listed as 2 separate categories. In this List, masking agents "are products that have the potential to impair the excretion of prohibited substances or to conceal their presence in urine or other samples used in doping control." The WADA 2004 List combined diuretics and masking agents into one section entitled "Masking Agents" including an extensive list of diuretics in addition to epitestosterone, probenecid, and plasma expanders. The title changed for the 2005 List to "Diuretics and Other Masking Agents," which remained for 10 years, when it was modified slightly to "Diuretics and Masking Agents" reflecting that diuretics are not just included for their masking effects, but they can be abused for other purposes, such as achieving rapid weight loss, too.

While the use of plasma expanders has been included as a prohibited method since the 2000 IOC List, plasma expanders were first listed by name as masking agents with hydroxyethyl starch included in the 2003 IOC List. By the 2009 WADA List, plasma expanders included albumin, dextran, hydroxyethyl starch, and mannitol when administered by intravenous routes only. Glycerol was prohibited as a plasma expander by all routes in the 2010 List, and assurances were included in the explanatory notes to the 2011 and 2012 Lists that normal exposure to this substance from foodstuffs and toiletries would not cause a positive test.

A urinary threshold limit of 200 ng/mL of epitestosterone was set for the 2003 List, where it was noted that levels in excess would be regarded as an "anti-doping violation unless there is evidence that it is due to a physiological condition" and investigation would be carried out using isotope ratio mass spectrometry. From the 2009 List onwards, epitestosterone was reclassified as an endogenous anabolic androgenic agent (S1.1a) as an isomer of testosterone, and also because under this class it would be regarded as a non-specified substance, with those substances potentially achieving a higher sanction. α-Reductase inhibitors (e.g., finasteride and dutasteride) were included as masking agents on the WADA Lists from 2006 onwards until the 2009 List, when they were removed having "been rendered ineffective as masking agents by closer consideration of steroid profiles" according to the accompanying explanatory note. Additions of note to the diuretic subclass are desmopressin, an antidiuretic hormone analogue (2011), with the topical application of felypressin in dental anesthesia as exception (2012), and the inclusion of vasopressin V2 antagonists (vaptans) (2014). Exceptions from the diuretics class due to their milder diuretic properties have been indicated for the topical application of the carbonic anhydrase inhibitors dorzolamide and brinzolamide (2009), and weak diuretic pamabrom (2010) and for drospirenone (2005), a progestogen, commonly used in contraceptive medication.

Since 2004, the List has always included a warning note in this Diuretics and Masking Agents section requiring that even if an athlete has a TUE to use a diuretic, if that athlete wishes to use a threshold substance, i.e., a substance with a urinary limit associated with its use, such as formoterol, then another TUE approval is required for the second substance. The wording was updated in 2009, 2011, and 2013 for the purposes of clarity.

Prohibited Methods

The format of this section of the 2004 WADA List has significantly evolved from the IOC Lists. For the IOC 1996 List, prohibited methods were indicated as blood doping and pharmaceutical, chemical, and physical manipulation, but it was the 2002 IOC List that most closely resembles the current format and includes the following:
- Enhancement of oxygen transfer with (a) blood doping and (b) "The administration of products that enhance the uptake, transport or delivery of oxygen, e.g., modified haemoglobin products including but not limited to bovine and cross-linked haemoglobins, microencapsulated haemoglobin products, perfluorochemicals, and RSR13."
- Pharmacological, chemical and physical manipulation.
- Gene doping, which was defined as "the non-therapeutic use of genes, genetic elements and/or cells that have the capacity to enhance athletic performance."

This format was adopted by the first WADA List in 2004 and was reclassified as M1, M2, and M3.

"M1 Enhancement of Oxygen Transfer," the first subsection "Blood Doping" was defined as "including the use of autologous, homologous or heterologous blood or red blood cell products of any origin, other than for legitimate medical treatment" with this definition changing only in 2013 to "The administration or reintroduction of any quantity of autologous, homologous or heterologous blood or red blood cell products of any origin into the circulatory system." The second subsection refers to artificially enhancing oxygen uptake, transport, or delivery, and since 2004, the only modification of note is that supplemental oxygen is no longer prohibited (2010) by inhalation (2017).

The 2011 List included "Sequential withdrawal, manipulation and reinfusion of whole blood into the circulatory system" as a third subcategory of "M2 Chemical and Physical Manipulation." The explanatory note commented that it is not intended to prevent plasmapheresis, rather it specifically addresses the process in which an *athlete's* blood is removed, treated, or manipulated, and then reinjected. Those undergoing hemodialysis as part of the treatment of chronic kidney disease will require a TUE for such procedures. This subsection was reclassified as the third subsection under "M1 Manipulation of Blood and Blood Components" in 2013, the new heading reflecting the change and prohibited "any form of intravascular manipulation of the blood or blood components by physical or chemical means." The 2005 List reexamined "Chemical and Physical Manipulation" removing reference to the already prohibited substances and reworded it as follows: "*Tampering,* or attempting to tamper, in order to alter the integrity and validity of *Samples* collected in *Doping Controls.* These include but are not limited to intravenous infusions, catheterisation, and urine substitution." Catherization was removed as an example from the 2012 List, the explanatory note confirming that while it could be necessary for medical purposes it still remained prohibited if used to tamper with the integrity of samples. A specific exemption for intravenous infusions when used as a "legitimate acute medical treatment" was included in the 2005 List, and this section was divided into "Tampering" and "Intravenous Infusions" for the 2006 List, whereby "intravenous infusions are prohibited, except as a legitimate acute medical treatment." While the word "acute" was removed in 2007, in 2008, it was explained that in "an acute medical situation where this method (i.e. infusions) is deemed necessary a retroactive therapeutic use exemption will be required."

The 2009 List stated that "Intravenous infusions are prohibited except in the management of surgical procedures, medical emergencies or clinical investigations." The accompanying explanatory note clarified that "the intent of this section is to prohibit hemodilution, overhydration and the administration of prohibited substances by means of intravenous infusion. An intravenous infusion is defined as the delivery of fluids through a vein using a needle or similar device" and that "injections with a simple syringe are not prohibited as a method if the injected substance is not prohibited and if the volume does not exceed 50 mL." The 2012 explanatory notes referred readers to the medical information to support the decisions of the TUE Committee, and the 2012 List clarified that it was 50 mL per 6-hour period.

"M3 Gene Doping," the third section, had been first included in a 2003 IOC List. While this definition was expanded in the 2005 List to include the modulation of gene expression, it was the 2009 List which redefined gene doping as the "transfer of cells or genetic elements or the use of cells, genetic elements or pharmacological agents to modulating expression of endogenous genes having the capacity to enhance athletic performance." The definition was reworded in 2010 and remains unchanged as of 2015, stating:

The following, with the potential to enhance sport performance, are prohibited:

1 The transfer of polymers of nucleic acids or nucleic acid analogues
2 The use of normal or genetically modified cells

The final amendment to Gene Doping was the inclusion of PPARδ and AMP-activated protein kinase axis agonists as part of M3 in the 2009 List. However, these were subsequently reclassified in 2012 as metabolic modulators in "S4 Hormone and Metabolic Modulators."

Substances and Methods Prohibited in-Competition

Prohibited Substances
S6 Stimulants
Stimulants were prohibited from an early stage in the development of anti-doping, and the first IOC List in 1968 included "sympathomimetic amines (e.g., amphetamine), ephedrine and similar substances" and "stimulants of the central nervous system (strychnine) and analeptics." The IOC List of 1996 included $β_2$-agonists and prohibited caffeine at a urinary concentration of greater than 12 μg/mL and PSE at all concentrations.

The 2004 WADA List prohibited stimulants in-competition only and provided an extensive list of examples, while $β_2$-agonists were reclassified in their own section. Exceptions to the 2004 List were cathine, ephedrine, and methylephedrine, which were only prohibited at urinary concentrations greater than 5, 10, and 10 μg/mL, respectively, which was unchanged from the 2000 IOC List. Notably, there were significant changes from the IOC approach for phenylpropanolamine and PSE, both of which previously had been only prohibited at urinary concentrations greater than 25 μg/mL and for caffeine which was previously prohibited on IOC Lists at urinary concentrations in excess of 12 μg/mL. These 3 stimulants were now not prohibited at all and only listed in the Monitoring Program. Although clarified in the 2005 update, co-administration of epinephrine (adrenaline) with local anesthetics or by local administration (e.g., nasal or ophthalmologic), which had been included in IOC Lists since 1996, were not included in the 2004 WADA List. Similarly, the exemption for topical imidazoles was not included in the 2004 List but clarified from 2007 onwards. The 2006 List added new examples to include octopamine, fenbutrazate, and sibutramine.

From 2009 onwards, stimulants were subdivided into "S6a Non-Specified Stimulants" (a closed list) and "S6b Specified Stimulants" (examples) in accordance with article 4.2.2 of 2009 WADA Code as previously discussed. The LiEG classified each stimulant example as specified or non-specified using some of the following criteria:

- The ability to enhance performance in sports
- The risk to health
- General use in medicinal products
- Legitimate market availability
- Their illicit use
- Legal/controlled status
- History and potential of abuse in sports
- Their breakdown pattern, such as metabolism into amphetamine and/or methamphetamine
- The likelihood of approval of a TUE

The LiEG changed the status of PSE in 2010, prohibiting urinary PSE concentrations in excess of 150 µg/mL, as discussed under the Monitoring Program.

The 2010 List indicated methylhexaneamine was a non-specified stimulant, but reclassified it the following year in recognition of its deliberate inclusion in some nutritional supplements and confusion associated with the name of the substance.

As part of its review of the division for the 2014 List, substances such as benzphetamine that metabolize to amphetamine or metamphetamine were reclassified due to improved analytical techniques that allow differentiation between parent and metabolites, while MDMA and MDA were also reclassified specified stimulants (S6b) as they were regarded as less likely to be used as doping agents. In a similar manner, the 2015 List reclassified phenmetrazine to S6b to reflect its metabolism to fenbutrazate which is classified under S6b and lisdexamfetamine, an inactive prodrug of amphetamine, was added to S6a for the 2017 List.

To reflect increased availability of illegal stimulants mainly as street drugs, cathinone and its analogues (e.g., mephedrone, methedrone, and α-pyrrolidinovalerophenone) were added as examples of stimulants to the 2014 List and phenethylamine and its derivatives were included as examples in the 2015 List.

S7 Narcotics

Narcotics have always been regarded as doping substances and were included on the very first list of prohibited products published by the IOC in 1968 as "Narcotics and Analgesics (e.g., Morphine), Similar Substances." The examples expanded for the 1971 IOC Medical Commission List to include "heroin, methadone, dextromoramide, dipipanone, pethidine, and related compounds."

The narcotics included in the first WADA List in 2004 were similar to the 2016 List except for the inclusion of "fentanyl and its derivatives," which was added the following year. While there has been much debate on the inclusion of the class of narcotics on this List, this section of the List has remained unchanged from 2005 until an update to the 2017 List, whereby the morphine prodrug nicomorphine was added.

S8 Cannabinoids

The WADA List (2004) clearly stated that cannabinoids (e.g., hashish and marijuana) are prohibited in-competition and in all sports. This was a change in approach from the IOC, which from 1996 onwards categorized these substances as a class of drugs subject to certain restrictions. "In agreement with the International Sports Federations and the responsible authorities, tests may be conducted for cannabinoids (marijuana, hashish...). The results may lead to sanction [18]." The 2000 IOC List defined doping as a concentration greater than 15 ng/mL of 11-nor-Δ^9-tetrahydrocannabinol-9-carboxylic acid (carboxy-THC).

The WADA 2004 text remained unchanged until 2010, when it was clarified that synthetic cannabinoids were included. From 2011 onwards cannabimimetics were also included in this List with the 2017 List referring to the prohibition of

- Natural, e.g., cannabis, hashish and marijuana, or synthetic Δ^9-tetrahydrocannabinol (THC).
- Cannabimimetics, e.g., "spice", JWH-018 and -073, and HU-210.

The concentration for cannabinoids which is regarded as a positive test now is not stated in the WADA List itself, but instead is found in the WADA technical documents, where the threshold concentration of carboxy-THC is 150 ng/mL since May 2011.

S9 Glucocorticoids

Glucocorticoids, as per the scientific name of this class in the 2015 List, were first included as "Corticosteroids" in the 1996 IOC List as a class of drugs subject to certain restrictions. These were prohibited except for topical use (aural, dermatological, and ophthalmological) and administration by local or intra-articular injection or by inhalation which required written notification. For the 2000 IOC List, it was simply stated that the systemic use of glucocorticosteroids is prohibited when administered orally, rectally, or by intravenous or intramuscular injection, with the addition in 2001 that "When medically necessary, local and intra-articular injections of glucocorticosteroids are permitted. Where the rules of a responsible medical authority so provide, notification of administration may be necessary." The introduction of the WADA 2004 List maintained the prohibition of these 4 systemic routes of administration and stated that all other (i.e., non-systemic) routes required an abbreviated TUE. The 2005 List did clarify that dermatological preparations were not prohibited at all. This exemption was extended in 2006 to topical preparations, to treat aural, otic, nasal, buccal cavity, and ophthalmic ailments, due to the "absence of doping potential for these routes of administration" according to the accompanying explanatory note. The 2007 List further extended the topical use exemption to include buccal, gingival, and perianal administration, and iontophoretic and phonophoretic administration as a dermatological route. All of the other non-systemic routes of intra-articular, periarticular, peritendinous, epidural, or intradermal injections and/or by inhalation required an abbreviated TUE. With the removal of abbreviated TUEs from the 2009 Code, these non-systemic routes instead required a DOU, while topical administration of glucocorticosteroids required neither TUE or DOU. This remained the situation until 2011, when the DOU requirements were removed, and thus glucocorticosteroids were prohibited when administered by the 4 systemic routes, while administration by all other routes was permitted. While there was much debate in the anti-doping community regarding a proposal in the draft 2017 List which would have resulted in the prohibition of intra-articular glucocorticoid injections 72 h before the competition period due to the elevated systemic concentrations attained by this and similar routes of administration, the LiEG decided not to recommend such a change in its final draft and to further evaluate the situation. In summary, the prohibition on glucocorticoids as per the 2017 List is in reality unchanged from the 2000 position.

Substances Prohibited in Particular Sports

In the first version of the Code, it was the pertinent sports federation alone that decided and requested to prohibit alcohol or β-blockers in their sport. In the subsequent versions of the Code, WADA took a more proactive role and now works with the corresponding federation to decide the prohibition of alcohol or β-blockers in a particular sport. Furthermore, WADA alone can decide which sports are included. This new procedure allows for a better harmonization between different sports.

P1 Alcohol
The first WADA List in 2004 provided a list of international federations that prohibited alcohol in-competition only as detected in blood or by breath analysis. Previously, alcohol was only subject to certain restrictions, and the prohibition was dependent on the specific international sports federation and the responsible authorities. The 2004 List designated thresholds in the range of 0.0–0.40 g/L as indicated for each specific sport. Where there was no threshold, the presence of any quantity of alcohol was regarded as a doping violation. The sports involved were aeronautics, archery, automobile, billiards, boules, gymnastics, karate, modern pentathlon (for the modern pentathlon disciplines), motorcycling, roller sports, skiing, triathlon, and wrestling. Gymnastics, roller sports, triathlon, and wrestling were removed from the 2005 List, skiing in 2006, billiards in 2007, boules in 2008 (added 2006), 9- and 10-pin bowling in 2012 (added in 2009), karate in 2015, and motorcycling in 2016. Due to changes in the format of the modern pentathlon, alcohol was no longer prohibited for disciplines involving shooting from 2011. In 2006, powerboating (Union Internationale Motonautique) and archery were added. The 2007 List clarified that the doping violation thresholds corresponded to hematological values. The threshold for automobile and motorcycling (Federation Internationale Motocycliste) increased from 0.00 to 0.10 g/L for 2005 and 2006 Lists, respectively, and this level was harmonized for all international federations from the 2009 List onwards.

For the 2016 and 2017 List discussions, the LiEG regarded that alcohol use is primarily a safety issue, and it ultimately will be individual sporting organizations that will assume responsibility for addressing alcohol use within their own rules, and who will decide how best to manage testing and infractions. It was felt that this will permit more effective application of safety regulations than is possible when alcohol use is addressed via anti-doping regulations. As of 2017, 4 sports prohibited alcohol on the List: air sports (formerly known as aeronautics), archery, automobile, and powerboating.

P2 Beta-Blockers
β-Blockers were prohibited in the WADA 2004 List in-competition in a list of specific sports. Prior to this, the 1996 IOC List had included examples of commonly used β-blockers of atenolol, metoprolol, propranolol, and the likes, and testing was at the discretion of the responsible authorities. The 18 sports in which the in-competition use of β-blockers was prohibited in 2004 were aeronautics, archery, automobile, billiards, bobsled, boules, bridge, chess, curling, gymnastics, motorcycling, pentathlon (for the modern pentathlon disciplines), 9-pin bowling, sailing (for match race helms only), shooting, skiing (for ski jumping and freestyle snowboard), swimming (diving and synchronized swimming), and wrestling. Archery and shooting also prohibited their use out-of-competition, and this has remained unchanged ever since. Changes over the years involved the removal of this prohibition in swimming (2006), chess (2007), and gymnastics (2011). The LiEG reevaluated the prohibition of β-blockers in certain sports for the 2012 and 2013 Lists, removing bobsled and skeleton, curling, modern pentathlon, motorcycling, sailing, and wrestling in 2012, and aeronautic, boules, bridge, 9- and 10-pin bowling, and powerboating the following year. Additions to the List included expansion of the skiing/snowboarding disciplines (2006), powerboating (added 2008 but removed 2012), 9- and 10-pin bowling (added 2009 but removed

2012), golf (2009), darts (2011), skeleton added to bobsled (added 2011, whole sport removed 2012), and certain disciplines governed by the World Underwater Federation (added 2015). β-Blockers are prohibited in the 2017 List in 8 sports, and the list of examples of β-blockers has remained unchanged from the 2004 List to the 2017 List.

Conclusions

The List has evolved significantly since its inception in 1968 as an IOC document. For 35 years, the sporting movement followed the IOC List of prohibited substances and methods, until the creation of WADA (a partnership of sport and governments) and the first WADA List in 2004. Over the next 13 years, the List further evolved to reflect advancements in science and medicine, and improved insight into changes in doping practices. The determination of stakeholders to protect clean athletes with an effective prohibited list has enabled the LiEG to maintain a list harmonized across all sports while evolving and improving its effectiveness. The evolution of this document over the years is due to the contributions of the sporting movement, medical and scientific stakeholders, and, since 2004, governments (through national anti-doping organizations). It is the responsibility of all stakeholders through WADA, and in particular the work of the WADA LiEG, to ensure that the List remains an effective tool in the fight against doping.

References

1. World Anti-Doping Code (2003). Montreal, World Anti-Doping Agency, 2003.
2. World Anti-Doping Code (2009). Montreal, World Anti-Doping Agency, 2009.
3. World Anti-Doping Code (2015). Montreal, World Anti-Doping Agency, 2015.
4. Chester N, Reilly T, Mottram DR: Physiological, subjective and performance effects of pseudoephedrine and phenylpropanolamine during endurance running exercise. Int J Sports Med 2003;24: 3–8.
5. Chu KS, Doherty TJ, Parise G, Milheiro JS, Tarnopolsky MA: A moderate dose of pseudoephedrine does not alter muscle contraction strength or anaerobic power. Clin J Sport Med 2002;12:387–390.
6. Clemons JM, Crosby SL: Cardiopulmonary and subjective effects of a 60 mg dose of pseudoephedrine on graded treadmill exercise J Sports Med Phys Fitness 1993;33:405–412.
7. Gillies H, Derman WE, Noakes TD, Smith P, Evans A, Gabriels G: Pseudoephedrine is without ergogenic effects during prolonged exercise J Appl Physiol 1996;81:2611–2617.
8. Hodges AN, Lynn BM, Bula JE, Donaldson MG, Dagenais MO, McKenzie DC: Effects of pseudoephedrine on maximal cycling power and submaximal cycling efficiency. Med Sci Sports Exerc 2003; 35:1316–1319.
9. Swain RA, Harsha DM, Baenziger J, Saywell RM Jr: Do pseudoephedrine or phenylpropanolamine improve maximum oxygen uptake and time to exhaustion? Clin J Sport Med 1997;7:168–173.
10. Gill ND, Shield A, Blazevich AJ, Zhou S, Weatherby RP: Muscular and cardiorespiratory effects of pseudoephedrine in human athletes. Br J Clin Pharmacol 2000;50:205–213.
11. Hodges K, Hancock S, Currell K, Hamilton B, Jeukendrup AE: Pseudoephedrine enhances performance in 1500-m runners. Med Sci Sports Exerc 2006;38:329–333.
12. Pritchard-Peschek KR, Jenkins DG, Osborne MA, Slater GJ: Pseudoephedrine ingestion and cycling time-trial performance. Int J Sport Nutr Exerc Metab 2010;20:132–138.
13. Barroso O, Goudreault D, Carbó Banús ML, Ayotte C, Mazzoni I, Boghosian T, Rabin O: Determination of urinary concentrations of pseudoephedrine and cathine after therapeutic administration of pseudoephedrine-containing medications to healthy subjects: implications for doping control analysis of these stimulants banned in sport. Drug Test Anal 2012;4:320–329.
14. Annex VIII, Doping, Report of the Medical Commission, Minutes of the 66th Session of the International Olympic Committee, New Town Hall, Grenoble, February 1–5, 1968.
15. List of Doping Substances, Meeting of the International Olympic Committee Medical Commission, Munich, May 19, 1971.
16. List of Doping Substances, International Olympic Committee Medical Controls, Games of the XXI Olympiad, Montreal, 1976.
17. List of Doping Substances, International Olympic Committee Medical Controls, Games of the XXII Olympiad, Moscow, 1980.

18 Prohibited Classes of Substances and Prohibited Methods, Lausanne. International Olympic Committee Medical Commission, 1996.
19 Prohibited Classes of Substances and Prohibited Methods, 2000, Olympic Movement Anti-Doping Code, Appendix A. Lausanne, International Olympic Committee Medical Commission, 2000.
20 Prohibited Classes of Substances and Prohibited Methods, 2001–2002, Olympic Movement Anti-Doping Code, Appendix A. Lausanne, International Olympic Committee Medical Commission, 2001.
21 Prohibited Classes of Substances and Prohibited Methods, 2003 Olympic Movement Anti-doping Code, Appendix A. Lausanne, International Olympic Committee Medical Commission, 2003.
22 The Prohibited List International Standard, 2004, 2005, 2006, 2007, 2008, 2009, 2010, 2011, 2012, 2013, 2014, 2015, 2016, 2017. Montreal, World Anti-Doping Agency, 2003–2016.
23 The Prohibited List Summary of Major Modifications and Explanatory Notes 2004, 2005, 2006, 2007, 2008, 2009, 2010, 2011, 2012, 2013, 2014, 2015, 2016, 2017. Montreal, World Anti-Doping Agency, 2003–2016.
24 WADA Technical Document – TD-2017DL, WADA Laboratory Expert Group (LabEG). Montreal, World Anti-Doping Agency, 2016.

Audrey Kinahan
Eirpharm
21 Parnell Street
Ennis, Co. Clare V95 RK3C (Ireland)
E-Mail pharmacy@eirpharm.com

Therapeutic Use Exemptions

David Gerrard[a] · Andrew Pipe[b]

[a]Dunedin, New Zealand, and World Anti-Doping Agency (WADA) Therapeutic Use Exemption (TUE) Expert Group, Montreal, QC, Canada; [b]Division of Prevention and Rehabilitation, University of Ottawa Heart Institute, and Faculty of Medicine, University of Ottawa, Ottawa, ON, Canada

Abstract

The introduction, in 2004, of the World Anti-Doping Code and a standardized "prohibited list" of substances and methods proscribed in sport represented a consistent, international response to the escalating challenge of drug misuse in contemporary sport. Simultaneously, it was recognized that athletes experiencing illness or injury might legitimately require the use of "prohibited" medications or procedures, and the concept of the "therapeutic use exemption" (TUE) was introduced. The mechanisms of the TUE process are carefully defined and described in a specific WADA "international standard" (IS). As a consequence, anti-doping organizations (ADOs) were empowered to establish "Therapeutic Use Exemption Committees" (TUECs) whose membership and responsibilities were clearly delineated in the IS, and to whom an athlete and treating physician(s) could make appropriate application for a TUE. A careful review of such an application by a TUEC panel of physicians might allow permission for an otherwise prohibited course of treatment, provided that appropriate criteria had been met. Sport physicians have a clear responsibility to ensure accurate and complete documentation of the clinical circumstances requiring a TUE when completing such applications. Typically, applications for consideration by TUECs are forwarded to a national ADO, but depending on an applicant's level of competition, it may become necessary to involve an international federation or major event organization (e.g., International Olympic Committee, or Commonwealth Games Federation). Such organizations may receive, review, and grant TUEs specific to the competitions over which they preside. Increasingly, there is recognition of TUEs granted by other ADOs. However, this is not always the case; in certain circumstances, the decisions of other TUECs to grant or deny an application may be appealed. The advent of the TUE process ensures that an athlete with a genuine medical condition that necessitates the use of a prohibited substance or procedure can apply for permission to use such treatments and is not denied access to competition or training.

© 2017 S. Karger AG, Basel

David Gerrard is professor emeritus of the Faculty of Medicine, University of Otago, Dunedin, New Zealand; he holds the vice-chair of the FINA (Fédération Internationale de Natation) Sport Medicine Committee and the chairs of the World Rugby TUEC and FINA TUEC.

Andrew Pipe holds currently the chair of the FIBA (International Basketball Federation) TUEC and was previously chairman of the WADA Prohibited List Expert Group; he is also Medical and Scientific Advisor at the Canadian Centre for Ethics in Sport.

Introduction

Since the late 19th century, some athletes have, sadly, sought to derive competitive advantage by the administration of various chemicals, compounds, medications, or other forms of physiological manipulation [1, 2]. The hazards of such approaches to both the health of the athlete and the integrity of sport have become increasingly obvious through a number of highly publicized incidents [3]. Sport authorities have, since the late 1960s, attempted to address these behaviors through a combination of regulation and the imposition of drug testing programs. Drug-related deaths in international cycling (Rome 1960 and Tour de France 1967), evidence of drug-based cheating, and the reports of state-sponsored experimentation with potent ergogenic substances to enhance sports performance (German Democratic Republic 1960–1980, Russia 2014–2016) continue to focus the minds of many physicians, sport organizations, and, in particular, the International Olympic Committee (IOC) on this disturbing, seemingly escalating trend in elite sport [4, 5]. Notwithstanding the initial leadership of the IOC Medical Commission in addressing these issues in the late 1960s, early policies and programs were inconsistently developed and varied greatly in their application across various sport disciplines.

The doping-tainted results of the Canadian track sprinter, Ben Johnson, in the 100-m final at the 1988 Seoul Olympic Games not only resulted in his disqualification but also catalyzed intense discussions regarding the need for more robust anti-doping efforts. Sport organizations at every level recognized that doping practices had become increasingly common, with the frequent involvement of collaborating physicians and scientists [6]. It became increasingly clear that to combat doping practices in sport required a comprehensive, coordinated international effort. By the late 1990s, when existing inadequacies and limitations were more completely understood, governments and sport organizations decided to pool their existing knowledge and resources – a collaboration that saw the emergence of the World Anti-Doping Agency (WADA). The WADA Code (the Code) "is the core document that harmonizes anti-doping policies, rules and regulations within sport organizations and among public authorities around the world." [7] It includes 5 "international standards" (ISs) "which aim to foster consistency among anti-doping organizations in various areas."

Fundamental to this coordinated, pan-sport strategy for anti-doping was the creation of the "international standard for the list of prohibited substances and methods" (the List) [8] that identified the "substances and methods" to be prohibited in all sporting disciplines subjected to the scrutiny of the IOC [see chapter by Kinahan et al., this vol., pp. 39–54]. Subsequent to that original decision, the List has since been accepted by several non-Olympic sport organizations. At the same time that WADA was determining the "substances and methods" to be included in the List, it recognized that the use of prohibited substances or methods might also be required for the legitimate treatment of illness, injury, or long-standing medical conditions experienced by athletes. A process was subsequently established to permit athletes to apply for an exemption to use a prohibited substance – a therapeutic use exemption (TUE) – carefully described in the "International Standard for Therapeutic Use Exemptions." [9] The TUE process provides a specific mechanism by which permission is granted to use a prohibited substance or method where that use could be demonstrated to be necessary for the appropriate treatment of a documented clinical condition. Since the introduction of the TUE process, condition-specific diagnostic criteria reflecting best-practice guidelines have been developed to facilitate the review of TUE applications.

In the late 1980s, a process of granting athletes permission to use banned substances for justified clinical purposes had been initiated by Prof. Ken Fitch, a leading anti-doping expert and past member of the IOC Medical Commission. Prof. Fitch championed this concept – the forerunner of the modern TUE. He initiated the early TUE process by linking prohibited substances with common clinical conditions requiring their use. Though not clearly codified or publicized (due to a concern that athletes and physicians might abuse this knowledge), the early provisions for "medical dispensation" subsequently introduced by the IOC required the treating physician to provide written, clinical justification for the use of a banned drug by an athlete [10]. In the event of a subsequent "positive" urinalysis, evidence of legitimate medical use of a prohibited substance would be sought. In some cases, this information was accepted retroactively, and there was frequently no demand placed upon the attending doctor to make advanced notice to a sport governing body. The limitations of the approaches of that time are self-evident; they have resulted in today's more formalized, consistent rules and procedures.

Therapeutic Use Exemptions: The International Standard

The World Anti-Doping Code provides, as noted above, for the publication of an IS for TUE (ISTUE) – which defines, describes, and delineates the processes that must be undertaken to ensure that an athlete's right to receive appropriate medical treatment is considered within the context of sport and the associated anti-doping rules [8]. The ISTUE outlines: the conditions that must be satisfied in order for a TUE to be granted; the responsibilities imposed upon anti-doping organizations (ADOs) to ensure that the TUE process is appropriately communicated, supported, and administered, and the approach that must be taken by an athlete when applying for a TUE. It also specifies the organization to which that application should be made, depending on the level of competition of the athlete (i.e., international competition or other levels of sport). The ISTUE also defines the membership and responsibilities of a TUE Exemption Committee (TUEC); outlines the processes for appealing TUE decisions; and, provides for the ability of WADA to review such decisions.

Sport administrators should be familiar with the ISTUE and its provisions; sport physicians should be aware of their particular responsibilities regarding TUEs and, in particular, the need to ensure that the athletes for whom they care are assisted with the TUE application process when necessary.

TUEC members must be particularly cognizant of the criteria for granting a TUE and aware of the critical role they play in ensuring access to appropriate treatment for an athlete; a 'level playing field' for sporting competition; and, doping-free sport.

Therapeutic Use Exemption Committees

National ADOs (NADOs), international federations (IFs), and major event organizations (MEOs) must establish a TUEC comprised of at least 3 clinicians with experience in the care and treatment of athletes and a broad knowledge of sports medicine. Typically, members of TUECs are senior physicians drawn from a spectrum of clinical disciplines with extensive experience in the care of elite athletes. In cases involving athletes with impairment, the ISTUE provides that at least 1 member of a TUEC should have specific experience in what has become widely referred to as "disability sport."

The standard also mandates that a majority of the members of any TUEC should have clinical independence with no potential for any conflict of interest when considering any application for a TUE. The ISTUE mandates that clinical judgement be the most important resource brought to

Table 1. Medical information to support the decisions of the Therapeutic Use Exemption Committees (TUECs)/therapeutic use exemption (TUE) physician guidelines

The WADA TUE Expert Group has published the following documents which greatly assist TUECs in the review of applications submitted regarding the use of medications for the treatment of these conditions:

ADHD	Infertility/polycystic ovarian syndrome
Adrenal insufficiency	Inflammatory bowel disease
Anaphylaxis	Intravenous infusion
Androgen deficiency – male hypogonadism	Intrinsic sleep disorders
Arterial hypertension	Musculoskeletal conditions
Asthma	Neuropathic pain
Diabetes mellitus	Postinfectious cough
Female-to-male transsexual athletes	Renal transplantation
Growth hormone deficiency	Sinusitis/rhinosinusitis
Adults	
Children and adolescents	

This information can be accessed electronically at: www.wada-ama.org/en/resources/science-medicine/medical-information-to-support-the-decisions-of-tuecs-list-of.

---

the deliberations of a TUEC. All TUECs are empowered to seek additional expertise, at their discretion, to enhance the assessment of any application; they may also request additional relevant information from the athlete and treating physician(s). The ISTUE emphasizes that clinical judgement is a fundamental element in the activities of a TUEC. Finally, all TUEC deliberations must respect complete confidentiality consistent with the highest standards of professional and institutional practice to reflect the obvious sensitivity that surrounds matters of personal health. Confidentiality agreements must be signed annually by members of a TUEC and by those in a sport organization entrusted with the administration of TUE processes.

The decisions of a TUEC are clinical, and the responsibility for such decisions must always reside with clinicians, not sport administrators. The activities of TUECs are greatly assisted by the WADA TUE Expert Group who publishes documents which provide specific "medical information to support the decisions of TUECs" addressing a range of clinical conditions commonly linked to applications for a TUE [11].

Therapeutic Use Exemption Applications

An athlete competing at the international level (as defined by their IF) should apply to that federation for a TUE; an athlete competing at any other level of sport should ordinarily apply to their NADO. The ISTUE provides for "recognition"; increasingly, IFs are recognizing, while retaining the right of review, TUEs granted by NADOs. It should be noted that TUEs granted by NADOs are valid only for domestic competition – they must be reviewed and recognized, as noted above, by an IF or MEO to have validity for purposes of international competition. An IF and MEO must publish a notice indicating which athletes under their jurisdictions are required to apply for a TUE and the organizations whose TUE approvals it will automatically recognize. The reader is directed to the ISTUE for greater detail and clarity regarding these important jurisdictional matters.

TUE applications are submitted by the athlete but must be signed by a treating physician who is expected to provide a succinct summary of the relevant clinical details including, when appro-

> Monkland Family Medicine Centre,
> Kapuskasis, Ontario
>
> Date
>
> To Whom It May Concern:
>
> **RE: TUE Application – Mr. Arnold Armstrong. DOB February 27, 1995**
>
> Mr. Armstrong, a member of our national fencing team, has been a patient of mine since 2007. He was initially diagnosed with ADD/ADHD in 2006 at the age of 11 by Dr. I. M. Echspert, a child psychiatrist at the University Medical Centre in Sydney. Psychological testing had supported the diagnosis.
>
> School performance and behavioural issues were noted to improve immediately following the initiation of treatment -- 5 mg methylphenidate given twice daily.
>
> The dose was increased to 10 mg twice daily at the age of 14 and has remained stable. Mr. Armstrong is seen by me every three months. His condition has remained stable.
>
> Arrangements have been made for him to be re-assessed by Dr. Jack Hopkin, a specialist in the management of ADD/ADHD in the adult, in 2 months time. Copies of Mr. Armstrong's relevant clinical records have been attached to this application.
>
> Please contact me if I can be of any further assistance.
>
> Yours sincerely,
>
> David Redbank, MD, CCFP
> Monkland Family Medicine Centre

Fig. 1. A sample clinical note to accompany a TUE application.

priate, specialist endorsement. Unfortunately, it is not uncommon for such applications to be incompletely prepared, resulting in delays, while additional, often basic, clinical information is obtained in order to facilitate an appropriate review. All sport physicians should be familiar with the "Medical Information to Support the Decisions of TUEC Physician Guidelines" which delineates, for many common conditions, the criteria for granting a TUE [11] (Table 1). The provision of a short note, emphasizing key elements in the diagnosis, treatment, and plan of management of the particular clinical condition, greatly facilitates a timely review of a TUE application and is a basic expectation of clinicians preparing such applications (Fig. 1).

Reviewing a Therapeutic Use Exemption Application

The criteria defining the basis for TUE approval are clearly identified in the ISTUE. The specified treatment must be necessary to manage the condition in question; not result in an enhancement of performance other than that expected by a return to the athlete's "normal" state of health; be necessary in the absence of a reasonable permitted therapeutic alternative; and not required as a consequence of prior use of a prohibited substance (Table 2). Careful consideration of the application and the accompanying documentation is then undertaken by the physicians constituting the TUEC guided by the criteria noted above and

Table 2. Criteria for granting a therapeutic use exemption (TUE) [9]

The athlete would experience a significant impairment in health if the prohibited substance or prohibited method were to be withheld in the course of treating an acute or chronic medical condition
The therapeutic use of the prohibited substance or prohibited method would produce no additional enhancement of performance other than that which might be anticipated by a return to a state of normal health following the treatment of a legitimate medical condition The use of any prohibited substance or prohibited method to increase "low-normal" levels of any endogenous hormone is not considered an acceptable therapeutic intervention
There is no reasonable therapeutic alternative to the use of the otherwise prohibited substance or prohibited method
The necessity for the use of the otherwise prohibited substance or prohibited method cannot be a consequence, wholly or in part, of the prior use, without a TUE of a substance or method which was prohibited at the time of use

found on the WADA website showing medical information to support the decisions of TUECs [11]. The guidelines permit an efficient review of a TUE submission and, more importantly, serve to enhance the quality of care provided to the athlete.

Decisions regarding an application for TUE must be rendered promptly and forwarded to the athlete in writing. An approval for a TUE will specify details of "dose" and "duration" and may require the provision of monitoring details or other clinical updates required by the TUEC.

When an application has been approved, it must be entered within the anti-doping administration and management system (ADAMS) operated by WADA or otherwise approved by WADA. Such registration facilitates recognition of the existence of a TUE and facilitates any review by WADA (or a MEO) to ensure it has been granted in accordance with the ISTUE criteria. The use of ADAMS also ensures that an athlete has a centralized record of therapeutic exemption that might facilitate any subsequent reapplication. At the present time, unfortunately, not all ADOs are utilizing ADAMS.

Retroactive Therapeutic Use Exemption Applications

It is recognized that medical emergencies may require urgent treatment with the use of prohibited substances or methods. The ISTUE provides for such circumstances by permitting a "retroactive" TUE application at the time of, or immediately following, such incidents. Such applications are only permitted following emergency treatment or when, as a consequence of other exceptional circumstances, there was "insufficient time or opportunity for the athlete to submit or the TUEC to consider an application" prior to a sample collection. Further details are contained within the ISTUE and on the WADA website.

Appeals of Therapeutic Use Exemption Committee Decisions

The ISTUE specifies that both athletes and sport organizations may appeal decisions rendered by a TUEC. WADA must review denials of TUE applications rendered by an IF following the granting of a TUE by a NADO; in addition, WADA must review an IF decision to approve a TUE following submission by a NADO; and, finally, WADA has the right to review at any time any other TUE decision on its own initiative. In considering appeals, WADA will mandate a special WADA TUEC to review the case in question.

The Therapeutic Use Exemption Expert Group of the World Anti-Doping Agency

Responsibility for the ongoing development, oversight, and review of the TUE process is vested in the WADA TUE Expert Group. This panel, with its international membership of experienced sport medicine clinicians, initiates the publication of the "TUE physician guidelines" noted above, monitors the patterns of TUE applications and approvals, and remains sensitive to emerging clinical practices and changing patterns of care. The composition of the WADA Expert Group is detailed on the website; its members have particular expertise in the area of therapeutic exemptions. It remains the only WADA "subcommittee" comprised solely of physicians and is administered by the Office of the WADA Medical Director. The Chair of the TUE Expert Group is, ex officio, a member of the WADA Health, Medicine, and Research Committee.

A Historical Perspective

As the TUE process evolved following the creation of WADA, it became clear that a substantial administrative burden can be imposed on sport organizations and their TUECs by the requirement to review applications for TUEs for commonly prescribed medications. This was particularly evident in the choice of medications used in the management of asthma, a common clinical condition, with an incidence in some parts of the world of between 12 and 15% and elevated rates in athletes in certain sport settings [12]. To address this challenge, the concept of an abbreviated TUE was introduced requiring only the submission of documentation of the diagnosis of asthma and the use of an anti-asthmatic medication. This too proved an onerous process requiring the time-consuming review of large numbers of applications received worldwide to comply with this new "category" of therapeutic use. Some ADOs were processing, filing, and reviewing hundreds of such applications each year. This required a disproportionate use of limited resources, and a sensible resolution of this challenge was achieved with the establishment of analytical thresholds for the most commonly prescribed asthmatic medications – the detection of evidence of use of such medications above the analytical threshold requiring further investigation by testing authorities. Athletes using certain inhaled asthma medication appropriately were no longer identified as using a prohibited substance. Today, through this vastly improved process, there is no longer a requirement for athletes to submit TUE applications when selected anti-asthma medication is prescribed. Those prescribed less commonly used alternatives must submit an application for a TUE demonstrating clear evidence of the diagnosis of asthma in accordance with the criteria expressed in the *medical information* document distributed by the WADA TUE Expert Group [11]. As a result, the burden previously imposed on asthmatic athletes, physicians, sport organizations, and their TUECs has been appropriately reduced. No evidence has emerged demonstrating the inappropriate use of asthma medication by athletes seeking to misuse these drugs for performance enhancement.

Emerging Challenges

Emerging challenges regarding the submission and review of applications for TUE reflect changing demographics – particularly the emergence of *masters*' or veterans' sport. The greater use of medication to treat established medical conditions in this group and their participation in events at which random drug testing takes place have the potential to overburden TUECs. At present, there is no universal application of the ISTUE across masters' sport. There has been, however, an increasing call from some athletes in these age-related categories for a robust application of TUE processes in such settings. Their concerns reflect increasing levels of competitiveness, the kudos attached to records or titles and the significant financial rewards afforded masters' athletes in some disciplines. The application of the ISTUE to senior age categories in sport will likely result in an unpredictable demand on human and financial resources, an increase in costly clinical justification processes and a very significant increase in reviews and appeals. The authors suggest a very cautious approach when considering the introduction of TUE processes to masters' level sport.

Patterns of medical practice in some locales have led to an increase in the controversial use of testosterone and androgenic precursors to treat males with "low levels" of testosterone. While applications for TUE to address this phenomenon have increased, they attract considerable and careful scrutiny from TUECs. A guiding principle for the diagnosis of true hypogonadism in an athlete is that the etiology must have a clear organic genesis [13]. Similarly, among female athletes, the use of hormones and related agents (e.g., dehydroepiandrosterone/DHEA) has become a more frequent challenge to TUE processes, particularly where there is the potential for ergogenesis through the use of a potent androgenic precursor. Evidence of adrenal suppression secondary to the use of systemic glucocorticoids also remains a contentious issue that may challenge a TUEC when application is made for the use of a combination of glucocorticoids and DHEA [14].

The use of androgens and other hormones to manage the transgendered athlete, though an uncommon clinical consideration in elite sport, also demands very careful consideration by TUECs [15].

The use of "medical marijuana" has become more common in certain jurisdictions and poses special challenges for TUECs. Typically used to assist in the management of pain and spasticity, clinical guidelines are now emerging for the use of cannabinoids in clinical practice with little standardization of products or dosage [16–19]. This issue is of particular relevance for elite athletes competing with disability under the auspices of the International Paralympic Committee.

The diagnosis and treatment of attention deficit disorder (ADD)/attention deficit hyperactivity disorder (ADHD) has increased in many communities and remains challenging for physicians in many parts of the world [20]. The standard treatment of this condition involves the prescription of amphetamines or other stimulants. From the perspective of WADA, the number of applications for the use of such medications continues to increase, perhaps in response to the increasing recognition and diagnosis of this disorder. The review of applications for permission to use stimulant medication in the treatment of this disorder can be complicated by the incomplete nature of many of the applications submitted by athletes and their physicians. Not infrequently, basic information concerning the diagnosis and management of ADD/ADHD is incomplete or missing, underscoring the important responsibility of physicians to ensure an appropriately completed application for TUE. In its *TUE physician guidelines,* the WADA Expert Group makes specific reference to the DSM-V criteria for the diagnosis of ADD/ADHD emphasizing that these international guidelines are the minimum requirements for a successful TUE application [21].

The Scope and Scale of Therapeutic Use Exemption Processes

In recent years, the number of TUECs has increased, and the number of successful applications for TUEs has augmented proportionally. In this light, the statistics of FINA (Fédération Internationale de Natation), an IF, and NADOs (Canadian Centre for Ethics in Sport [CCES] and

Table 3. Applications for therapeutic use exemptions (TUEs): the FINA (Fédération Internationale de Natation) experience from 2009 to 2014

Substances (S) and methods (M)		n	%[1]
S1	Anabolic agents	0	0
S2	Peptide hormones, growth factors, related substances, and mimetics	4	0.6
S3	β_2-Agonists[2]	454[2]	72
S4	Hormone and metabolic modulators	6	0.9
S5	Diuretics and masking agents	5	0.7
S6	Stimulants	47	7.4
S7	Narcotics	9	1.4
S8	Cannabinoids	0	0
S9	Glucocorticoids	99	16
M1	Manipulation of blood and blood components	1	0.15
M2	Chemical and physical manipulation	3	0.4
Total		628	

FINA is the world governing body for the 6 aquatic disciplines and is responsible for the receipt and review of TUE applications from international caliber athletes in swimming, open water swimming, synchronized swimming, water polo, diving, and high diving.
[1] Approximate percentages are shown.
[2] Note the changing incidence of TUE applications for β_2-agonists following changes to the prohibited list introduced in 2010: S3 β_2-Agonists: 2009: *346*; 2010: *62*; 2011: *31*; 2012: *6*; 2013: *5*; 2014: *4*.

Table 4. Applications for therapeutic use exemptions (TUEs): the CCES (Canadian Centre for Ethics in Sport) experience from 2009 to 2014

Substances (S) and methods (M)		n	%[1]
S1	Anabolic agents	26	6
S2	Peptide hormones, growth factors, related substances, and mimetics	9	2
S3	β_2-Agonists[2]	155[2]	35
S4	Hormone and metabolic modulators	34	8
S5	Diuretics and masking agents	10	2
S6	Stimulants	131	30
S7	Narcotics	22	5
S8	Cannabinoids	12	3
S9	Glucocorticoids	39	9
M1	Manipulation of blood and blood components	0	
M2	Chemical and physical manipulation	1	0.2
Total		439	

CCES is the Canadian National Anti-Doping Organization with responsibility for the receipt and review of TUE applications from athletes in the Canadian sport system.
[1] Approximate percentages are shown.
[2] Note the changing incidence of TUE applications for β_2-agonists following changes to the prohibited list introduced in 2010: S3 β_2-Agonists: 2009: *102*; 2010: *26*; 2011: *17*; 2012: *5*; 2013: *1*; 2014: *4*.

Table 5. Applications for therapeutic use exemptions (TUEs): the Drug-Free Sport NZ experience from 2009 to 2013

Substances (S/P) and methods (M)		n	%[1]
S1	Anabolic agents	1	0.6
S2	Peptide hormones, growth factors, related substances, and mimetics	3	0.2
S3	β_2-Agonists[2]	5[2]	0.3
S4	Hormone and metabolic modulators	18	10
S5	Diuretics and masking agents	23	13
S6	Stimulants	14	8
S7	Narcotics	25	14
S8	Cannabinoids	0	
S9	Glucocorticoids	82	47
M1	Manipulation of blood and blood components	0	
M2	Chemical and physical manipulation	1	0.6
P1	Substance prohibited in a particular sport (β-blocker)	1	0.6
Total		173	

The Drug-Free Sport NZ is the New Zealand National Anti-Doping Organization with responsibility for the receipt and review of TUE applications from athletes in the New Zealand sport system.
[1] Approximate percentages are shown.
[2] NZ Data relating to TUE applications for β_2-Agonists following changes to the prohibited list introduced in 2010 are not available.

Table 6. Therapeutic use exemption (TUE) approvals: the World Anti-Doping Agency (WADA) experience 2014

Substances (S/P) and methods (M)		n	%[1]
S1	Anabolic agents	20	2
S2	Peptide hormones, growth factors, related substances, and mimetics	18	2
S3	β_2-Agonists	56	6
S4	Hormone and metabolic modulators	117	12
S5	Diuretics and masking agents	76	8
S6	Stimulants	237	25
S7	Narcotics	55	6
S8	Cannabinoids	5	0.5
S9	Glucocorticoids	317	34
M1	Manipulation of blood and blood components	2	0.2
M2	Chemical and physical manipulation	22	2
M3	Gene doping	1	0.1
P2	Substance prohibited in a particular sport (β-blockers)	19	2

WADA oversees the coordinated international approach to doping control in sport and maintains a registry of TUEs granted by many sport organizations. These figures represent a partial compilation of such TUE approvals assembled by WADA in 2014.
[1] Approximate percentages are shown.

> Dear Colleagues,
>
> **RE TUE 15-001**
>
> Attached please find documents in support of a retroactive application for permission to use the otherwise prohibited substance *prednisone*, administered orally in declining doses to treat an exacerbation of asthma.
>
> To initiate discussion, it is my recommendation that:
>
> **"The application be approved. Dose and duration as per the application."**
>
> Your kindness in responding to this message in the next 5 days indicating: your approval of the recommendation; your disapproval of the recommendation; or, suggesting another recommendation is greatly appreciated.
>
> Thank you for your assistance with this matter.
>
> Yours sincerely,
>
> Charles Adamson, MD, Dip Sport Med
> Chair, National TUE Committee

Fig. 2. Sample electronic correspondence to facilitate the review of TUE applications.

Drug-Free Sports NZ) reveal an increase in applications for TUE as well as current patterns of prescribing. Dominant classes of medication and a description of the nature and number of applications are shown in Tables 3–5. Recent data from WADA provide a more global perspective, but data are limited as many NADOs and several major IFs do not register their TUE experiences using ADAMS (Table 6). It will be noted that, subsequent to the changes in the prohibited list in 2010, glucocorticoids and stimulants are the classes of medication for which TUEs are most commonly sought – the former being ubiquitous in the treatment of many common medical conditions, and the latter typically used in the treatment of ADD/ADHD, the diagnosis of which is increasingly common [20].

Management of a Therapeutic Use Exemption Committee – Practical Considerations

The effective and efficient administration of a TUE process – at any level – begins with the selection of a TUEC. This is usually accomplished by identifying and recruiting broadly experienced sport medicine physicians; national and international sport organizations typically have knowledge of clinicians appropriate for this important role. In some settings, NADOs fulfil the role for the national sport community. They are typically assisted in recruiting appropriately experienced practitioners by national sport medicine organizations. Appropriate, professional administrative support is usually provided by the ADO – whose staff must, like members of the TUEC itself, sign confidentiality agreements on an annual basis.

One approach to the efficient administration of the TUE process is to conduct all reviews electronically. Copies of the application and supporting documents are first reviewed for legibility and completeness, names and other identifying elements are redacted, and they are then forwarded to the TUEC chair. The chair will then electronically forward a letter with a recommendation to initiate discussion to all members of the TUEC (Fig. 2). TUEC members are asked to reply, indicating their response to the recommendation or suggesting an alternate recommendation within a specified time period. Typically, such responses are received quickly. If consensus exists regarding the recommendation, the sport organization is notified of the panel's decision, and the TUE documents and accompanying correspondence are prepared and distributed to the athlete and the relevant physician(s) by the administrative staff. Where consensus does not exist initially, relevant revisions can be made to the original recommendation, and the process repeated until there is consensus as to the decision that should be rendered.

In other settings, the distribution of the application serves as the stimulus to broader discussion regarding merits of the application, and a decision is developed more collectively electronically via teleconference or by in-person meetings. The decision is then conveyed to the sport organization, and administrative staff prepare and distribute the appropriate documentation and correspondence.

At all times, it must be realized that, consistent with the ISTUE, conditions or expectations can be placed upon the athlete regarding the TUE. A requirement to provide laboratory results on a regular basis or to deliver annual updates by treating physicians regarding the progress and ongoing management of the underlying clinical condition are typical of the conditions that might be imposed by a TUEC.

The Future

As clinical practices evolve, and as new medications are introduced, the need to ensure that athletes continue to receive optimal health care in the context of a commitment to doping-free sport will pose interesting challenges for clinicians involved in TUECs [22]. It will remain the responsibility of WADA, IFs, NADOs, and their TUECs to ensure that no unfair pharmacologically mediated performance enhancement follows as a consequence of athlete care. The commitment of sport medicine practitioners is central to ensuring the scientific integrity and clinical credibility of TUE processes. In so doing, they will protect the rights of all athletes to doping-free sport while contributing to a universally high standard of care for athletes.

References

1. Reardon CL, Creado S: Drug abuse in athletes. Subst Abuse Rehabil 2014;5: 95–105.
2. Momaya A, Fawal M, Estes R: Performance-enhancing substances in sports: a review of the literature. Sports Med 2015;45:517–531.
3. McGrath JC, Cowan DA: Drugs in sport. Br J Pharmacol 2008;154:493–495.
4. Franke WW, Berendonk B: Hormonal doping and androgenization of athletes: a secret program of the German Democratic Republic government. Clin Chem 1997;43:1262–1279.
5. Hoberman JM: Mortal Engines. The Science of Performance and the Dehumanization of Sport. New York, Free Press, 1992.
6. Hoberman J: Physicians and the sports doping epidemic. Virtual Mentor 2014; 16:570–574.
7. World Anti-Doping Agency: The Code. Montreal, WADA, 2015, https://www.wada-ama.org/en/resources/the-code/world-anti-doping-code.
8. World Anti-Doping Agency: The 2015 Prohibited List – International Standard. Montreal, WADA, 2015, https://www.wada-ama.org/en/resources/science-medicine/prohibited-list-documents.
9. World Anti-Doping Agency: International Standard for Therapeutic Use Exemptions. Montreal, WADA, 2015, https://www.wada-ama.org/en/resources/therapeutic-use-exemption-tue/international-standard-for-therapeutic-use-exemptions-istue.
10. Fitch KD: Therapeutic use exemptions (TUE's) at the Olympic Games 1992–2012. Br J Sports Med 2013;47:815–818.
11. World Anti-Doping Agency: Medical Information to Support the Decisions of TUECs – List of Contributors. Montreal, WADA, 2017, www.wada-ama.org/en/resources/science-medicine/medical-information-to-support-the-decisions-of-tuecs-list-of.
12. Boulet LP, O'Byrne PM: Asthma and exercise-induced bronchoconstriction in athletes. N Engl J Med 2015;372:641–648.
13. Bhasin S, Cunningham GR, Hayes FJ, et al; Task Force, Endocrine Society: Testosterone therapy in men with androgen deficiency syndromes: an Endocrine Society clinical practice guideline. J Clin Endocrinol Metab 2010;95:2536–2559.
14. Gerrard DF, Handelsman DJ: Adrenal insufficiency in female athletes: the place of DHEA supplementation. NZ J Sport Med 2014;41:79.

15 Fabris B, Bernardi S, Trombetta C: Cross-sex hormone therapy for gender dysphoria. J Endocrinol Invest 2015;38: 269–282.
16 Moulin D, Boulanger A, Clark AJ, et al: Pharmacological management of chronic neuropathic pain: revised consensus statement from the Canadian Pain Society. Pain Res Manag 2014;19:328–335.
17 Wright S, Yadav V, Bever C Jr, et al: Summary of evidence-based guideline: complementary and alternative medicine in multiple sclerosis: report of the Guideline Development Subcommittee of the American Academy of Neurology. Neurology 2014;83:1484–1486.
18 Koppel BS, Brust JC, Fife T, et al: Systematic review: efficacy and safety of medical marijuana in selected neurologic disorders: report of the Guideline Development Committee of the American Academy of Neurology. Neurology 2014; 82:1556–1563.
19 Lynch ME, Campbell F: Cannabinoids for treatment of chronic non-cancer pain; a systematic review of randomized trials. Br J Clin Pharmacol 2011;72:735–744.
20 Thomas R, Sanders S, Doust J, Beller E, Glasziou P: Prevalence of attention-deficit/ hyperactivity disorder: a systematic review and meta-analysis. Pediatrics 2015;135:e994–e1001.
21 American Psychiatric Association: Diagnostic and Statistical Manual of Mental Disorders, ed 5. Arlington, American Psychiatric Association, 2013.
22 Towns CR, Gerrard DF: A fools game: blood doping in sport. Perform Enhancement Health 2014;3:54–58.

Prof. Andrew Pipe
Division of Prevention and Rehabilitation
University of Ottawa Heart Institute
40 Ruskin Street
Ottawa, ON K1Y 4W7 (Canada)
E-Mail apipe@ottawaheart.ca

Challenges in Modern Anti-Doping Analytical Science

Christiane Ayotte[a] · John Miller[b] · Mario Thevis[c]

[a]Laboratoire de contrôle du dopage, INRS-Institut Armand-Frappier, Laval, QC, Canada; [b]Institute of Pharmacy & Biomedical Science, Strathclyde University, Glasgow, UK; [c]Institute of Biochemistry/Center for Preventive Doping Research, Cologne, Germany

Abstract

The challenges facing modern anti-doping analytical science are increasingly complex given the expansion of target drug substances, as the pharmaceutical industry introduces more novel therapeutic compounds and the internet offers designer drugs to improve performance. The technical challenges are manifold, including, for example, the need for advanced instrumentation for greater speed of analyses and increased sensitivity, specific techniques capable of distinguishing between endogenous and exogenous metabolites, or biological assays for the detection of peptide hormones or their markers, all of which require an important investment from the laboratories and recruitment of highly specialized scientific personnel. The consequences of introducing sophisticated and complex analytical procedures may result in the future in a change in the strategy applied by the Word Anti-Doping Agency in relation to the introduction and performance of new techniques by the network of accredited anti-doping laboratories.

© 2017 S. Karger AG, Basel

Historical Background

In the 1960s, testing for the presence of banned substances from a list prepared by a few international sports federations, e.g., IAAF (International Association of Athletics Federations) and UCI (International Cycling Union), was restricted to narcotics and some stimulants. By the end of the decade, the newly formed Medical Commission of the International Olympic Committee (IOC) took over the responsibility of drafting a common list to be adopted by member sports federations and, most importantly, of establishing a network of laboratories capable of testing athletes' samples collected during major competitions. In the following years, with reports of drug abuse and the development of high-resolution gas chromatography (GC) or high-performance liquid chromatography (HPLC)/mass spectrometry (MS) techniques, the list of banned drugs and methods was gradually expanded to include androgenic anabolic steroids (1974), blood doping by transfusions (1982), diuretics, β-blockers, corticosteroids, peptide hormones, and masking agents (1988 and 1992) [1].

In the 1970s, stimulants and a few narcotics were detected in urine samples with GC and nitrogen phosphorus detectors and confirmed by GC-MS after pretreatment of urine samples: conjugated metabolites were hydrolyzed, and amino and hydroxyl groups were often converted to trifluoroacetyl (TFA) or mixed trimethylsilyl-TFA derivatives to improve chromatography and generate more characteristic mass spectra. In the next decade, diuretics were first screened with HPLC with ultraviolet detection followed by the complex confirmation of the permethylated derivative by GC-MS. The limits of detection of such techniques were relatively high, often around 100–250 ng/mL. From the beginning of the 1970s to mid-1980s, a few anabolic androgenic steroids could be tested but with very limited efficiency, utilizing antibodies developed against their C-19-nor position (nortestosterone) and C-17α-methyl groups. The commercialization of benchtop mass spectrometers coupled to high-resolution gas chromatographs with highly efficient software revolutionized the anti-doping tests allowing the automated analysis of batches of samples with greatly improved sensitivity after suitable pretreatment (extraction from the matrix, hydrolysis, and derivatization). The contemporary testing approaches employed to detect and identify synthetically produced chemical substances in urine involve a combination of LC-MS/MS and GC-MS/MS techniques on enzymatically hydrolyzed or intact conjugates with limits of detection reaching a few picograms per milliliter. This testing approach has allowed the detection of long-lasting metabolites at very low concentration, hence increasing the detection window for some prohibited substances. Thus, evidence of doping in some cases can be obtained long after the administration of the prohibited substance. Many adverse analytical findings (AAF), resulting in sanctions and withdrawal of Olympic medals, have been widely reported in the media as a result of retrospective testing of stored athlete samples for these previously unknown long-lasting metabolites.

Since 2004, the World Anti-Doping Agency (WADA) has had the responsibility of the review and annual publication of the list of prohibited substances and methods, which includes therapeutic agents and methods which have been used, or have the potential to be used, by athletes to improve their performance. In the past 20 years, new classes of substances, including β_2-agonists, veterinary growth promoters, selective androgen receptor modulators, inhibitors of aromatase, selective estrogen receptor modulators, anti-estrogenic substances, insulins, and peroxisome proliferator activated receptor δ, all of which have specific performance-enhancing properties, have been developed by pharmaceutical companies and have been included in the list of prohibited substances and methods [2, 3]. Additionally, many of these substances and their related compounds as well as stimulants, anabolic steroids, and hormones can either be purchased from suppliers on the Internet, sometimes labelled for "research only" or as active ingredient(s) or contaminant(s) of dietary supplements.

Over the years, the laboratories have introduced an increasing number of sophisticated and complex procedures and techniques to identify these doping agents. In the same period, both the number of laboratories has increased from less than a dozen recognized anti-doping laboratories to 34 in 2017, and the number of samples analyzed has increased substantially from 30,000 urine samples from certain major competitions to more than 325,000 blood and urine samples collected in and out of competition, during training, or at rest.

Accreditation by the International Organization for Standardization and the World Anti-Doping Agency

Laboratories accredited by WADA must, as a prerequisite, be audited and found compliant with the *ISO/IEC17025:2005 General Requirements for the*

Competence of Testing and Calibration Laboratories published by the International Organization for Standardization (ISO) and in addition comply with the requirements of the WADA international standard for laboratories (ISL) and its associated technical documents (TDs) and guidelines that are specific to anti-doping laboratories. The various TDs comprise mandatory scientific, technical, and forensic requirements covering all aspects of the work of the anti-doping laboratories to ensure good practice and harmonization. The requirements included in the ISL and the associated TDs indicate the minimum acceptable standards to be applied by the laboratories. Guidelines are precursors of TDs which are published, on the approval of a novel methodology by WADA, to aid their introduction by all anti-doping laboratories. Technical notes, giving more detailed advice and examples of good practice in the application of particularly complex methodologies, e.g., GC carbon isotope ratio MS (GC/C/IRMS), are also distributed by WADA to the laboratories.

Laboratories do not necessarily employ identical and normalized methods, but they must demonstrate that the methods employed are fit for purpose, validated, and approved for inclusion in the scope of the ISO accreditation.

The laboratories must hire suitably qualified and competent scientific personnel and be equipped with state-of-the-art analytical instrumentation to perform the full array of analyses required, not only for the physicochemical techniques commonly applied in forensic sciences but also for the molecular biological assays comprising isoelectric focusing, sodium dodecyl sulfate (SDS) and SAR (sodium N-lauroylsarcosinate) polyacrylamide gel electrophoresis (PAGE), and immunoassays with specific antibodies. The procedures applied must unequivocally identify any of the prohibited substances or methods, their metabolites, or markers of use in a given matrix, usually urine but also plasma or serum for particular analyses. Laboratories are required to report an adverse AAF when a prohibited substance and/or its metabolite(s) is detected at any concentration. However, minimum required performance levels have been set for the various classes of prohibited substances, which is the minimum concentration to be detected and identified by the laboratories. In addition, there are a few substances for which a threshold concentration has been adopted so that a quantitative determination is necessary to ascertain whether the threshold has been exceeded to be able to report an AAF.

Under the pressure of legal challenges, it is essential that the stringent requirements, contained in the ISL and chain of custody guidelines, are applied to ensure the adequate control and accountability of the samples from receipt, through testing, reporting, and final disposal. All anti-doping laboratory staff must agree to the code of ethics, as described in the ISL, which includes clauses to exclude the risk of conflict of interest and external influence as well as assuring confidentiality. Access to anti-doping laboratories is strictly controlled and monitored, and a list is established of persons allowed to enter. Visitors can be given restricted access, but they mainly only enter when accompanied by a member of staff and are chaperoned throughout their stay in the facility. Doping control officers or couriers, delivering samples, are not permitted access. The laboratory must assiduously document the movements of the sample bottles and aliquots throughout the process from receipt to disposal of the sample. Records must show the analytical steps followed during the initial and confirmation tests, clearly identifying the staff involved at each stage.

The analytical procedures employed must include appropriate negative and positive quality control samples (reference materials) to ensure the unambiguous detection, identification, and, when required, quantification of prohibited substances. For threshold substances, the laboratory must estimate the uncertainty of the method.

WADA monitors the performances of its accredited and probationary laboratories with an external quality assessment scheme; each trimester,

5–6 blind samples are received for analysis containing zero or up to 3 prohibited substances. The laboratories also receive double-blind samples together with routine athletes' samples. The results are evaluated, and points are lost in function of the gravity of the mistake made; it is understood that reporting a false-positive result may lead to immediate suspension and disciplinary process.

The external quality assessment scheme also distributes samples for educational purposes to the anti-doping laboratories when new analytical methods/technologies have been approved by WADA and are to be implemented. The laboratories are aware of the composition of the samples and may be provided with a protocol. The purpose of the exercise is twofold – to give the laboratories experience in the application of the analytical methodology/technique and eventually demonstrate their competence to permit inclusion in their scope of accreditation – to demonstrate the fitness for purpose of the analytical procedure.

Scope of Modern Testing Assays

The tests must be efficient – errors are not permitted; reports are requested within 10 working days and within 48–72 h during major international events.

The laboratories are continually striving to incorporate a variety of substances which have been added to the WADA list of prohibited substances and methods, including new therapeutic agents, designer steroids, stimulants, "research" peptides, or so-called supplements, and prohormones, into existing initial testing procedures or developing new analytical procedures for their detection. A well-characterized chemical substance can often be incorporated into an existing initial testing procedure provided that the metabolism and pharmacokinetics are known, and reference standards of the substance and/or its major metabolites are available. It is then sufficient to demonstrate there is adequate selectivity and sensitivity (i.e., meets the minimum required performance levels). In the presence of sufficiently high levels, the GC-MS analysis in the full scan mode provides sufficient evidence for the identification. However, in many instances, particularly when recently minimum required performance levels for the different classes of prohibited substances were lowered, the initial testing procedures and confirmation analysis requires more sensitive LC- or GC-MS/MS techniques in the selected or multiple reaction monitoring modes. Negative control and appropriate reference material (pure compound or well-characterized collection of specimens from an administration study) form part of each confirmatory assay.

Detecting doping is nowadays a refined cat-and-mouse game that requires not only an important initial investment but constant technological improvements; laboratories must be staffed with highly specialized and trained scientists in molecular biology and analytical chemistry, and maintain the best and up-to-date analytical instruments to keep abreast of the demand to increase the effectiveness of the testing.

Detection of Potentially Endogenous Hormones

Anabolic Androgenic Steroids
One of the most complex analytical challenges sports drug testing has been facing for decades is the identification of xenobiotics for which endogenously produced and naturally occurring analogues exist. The first indicator, which was first proposed in the early 1980s, of pharmaceutical medications of synthetically derived testosterone (T) is the increased level of urinary testosterone in comparison to epitestosterone (E) resulting in abnormally high values of the T/E ratio [4 and references cited herein]. This measured ratio in the athlete's sample is compared to reference ranges established in populations of athletes. A confounding factor, however, is that a small per-

centage of males and females normally and systematically excrete urine samples with higher testosterone concentrations so that the established threshold for the T/E ratio may be exceeded leading to a risk of a false-positive result. A more efficient approach, referred to as steroid profiling, is presently applied whereby the individual athlete's T/E values, metabolites of testosterone, and their relative ratios are monitored and recorded regularly over time. These longitudinal studies are part of the athlete biological passport. Nonetheless, in a small number of cases, there are some limitations which preclude this approach from being definitive in establishing an AAF. Consequently, in the late 1990s, a direct method to establish doping with certainty was developed, which is based on the different isotope ratios ($^{13}C/^{12}C$) obtained from endogenously produced testosterone, including its metabolites, and synthetically produced testosterone present in pharmaceutical preparations. Ingestion of exogenous testosterone will result in small differences in the carbon isotopic ratio of the endogenous anabolic, androgenic steroids comprising the steroid profile to the carbon isotopic ratio of an endogenous reference compound which is not implicated in the testosterone metabolic pathway. These differences can be determined by the GC/C/IRMS technique [5]. However, considerable sample preparation is required so that GC/C/IRMS is normally used as a confirmatory assay when there is an atypical result in the steroid profile. This technique is now systematically applied, in addition to urinary steroid profiling, before reaching a conclusion on an athlete's sample.

Recently, it has been reported that preparations containing nandrolone or testosterone with carbon isotope ratios which are close to those to be found naturally in populations in some regions of the world are available, which, if used for doping, would complicate interpretation of the results obtained from testing.

The technique is not restricted to testosterone and its metabolites but is also used to confirm the exogenous administration of other prohibited substances which may be generated endogenously or through microbial degradation of other urinary steroids, e.g., norandrosterone (the metabolite of nandrolone), boldenone, formestane, prednisone, and prednisolone.

Blood Doping
For many years, particularly for endurance sports, various forms of blood doping have been practiced to increase oxygen capacity of athletes and consequently their endurance. Initially, blood transfusion was the method of choice of the athlete using the blood either of a donor (homologous blood transfusion) or stored blood of the athlete (autologous blood transfusion). Testing blood samples using flow cytometry is successful in detecting homologous blood transfusion by differences in the antigens associated with the donor and the recipient. However, the technique cannot detect the use of autologous blood transfusion.

A complementary approach, now being applied, is monitoring of the hematological parameters of athletes at different times (at rest, before competition, and during training), the results of which are included in the blood doping module of the athlete biological passport. The presence of the doping agent or the doping method used may not be detectable, but the effects produced on the hematological profile will remain for a much longer period. The values of hemoglobin and the percentage of reticulocytes are used to calculate the "off score," the result of which may reveal blood doping. The profiles are monitored, and atypical variations may trigger a test in blood or urine for synthetic erythropoiesis-stimulating agents (ESAs) or be considered as sufficiently abnormal to be consistent with blood doping. Several athletes have now been sanctioned on the sole basis of their abnormal blood profile.

Erythropoietin (EPO) is a naturally occurring glycoprotein essential in the regulation of hematopoiesis (red blood cell formation). In the

1980s, recombinant human EPO became available for the treatment of anemia but was quickly abused by some athletes to increase their blood levels. The detection of recombinant EPO is extremely difficult due to its very similar structure and composition to naturally occurring EPO and to the very low levels found in blood and particularly in urine. In 2000, the elegant approach combining ultrafiltration, isoelectric focusing, and double blotting with chemiluminescent detection permitted the direct detection of the recombinant human EPO by differentiating its isoforms from those of human urinary EPO [6]. The advent of other ESAs, which prolong the biological half-life of the drug, prompted the development of a complementary test, including SDS-PAGE and SAR-PAGE [7]. These electrophoretic methods are used to identify forms of EPO, including those where the peptide backbone of EPO has been modified and is hyperglycosylated or has been conjugated with polyethylene glycol.

Despite efforts to improve the analytical testing methods to detect blood doping, the efficacy of anti-doping tests has been criticized. The success rate in catching blood doping has been considered modest, as a relatively low number of cases have been reported annually (<50). Unfortunately, the microdosage of ESAs now often utilized by the athletes, the short detection window for recombinant EPO, and insufficient sensitivity of the analytical methods presently available, may result in the inability to detect doping in some instances when it has occurred. Presently, there is not a validated method to detect directly autologous blood transfusions. Nonetheless, the introduction of the blood module of the athlete biological passport greatly assists in detecting doping cases.

Growth Hormone
Commercially available recombinant human growth hormone (rhGH), a polypeptide, differs slightly from its human analog of pituitary origin. It is produced by recombinant biotechnology as the monomeric 22-kDa isoform, whereas endogenous hGH consists of a mixture of isoforms, including dimers and oligomers, the most predominant of which is the 22-kDa isoform. It is secreted in a pulsatile manner, and the concentration present in urines is low. In contrast to EPO and testosterone, no physicochemical or analytical technique such as isoelectric focusing, PAGE, or IRMS has yet been found to be capable of differentiating the drug from its natural analogue. However, a test referred to as the "differential isoform test" has been developed, which requires the use of a dual monoclonal antibody, sandwich-type immunoassay [8]. In order to meet the high specificity requirements, 2 kits, each containing one "recombinant" and one "pituitary" assay, must be used for confirmation purposes. The "recombinant" assays bind preferentially to the 22-kDa isoform, while several isoforms of naturally occurring hGH, including the 22-kDa isoform, are bound in the "pituitary" assays but with less affinity. The administration of exogenous rhGH leads to an increase in the concentration of the 22-kDa isoform and of its ratio to all other forms bound by the pituitary antibody. A ratio of the determined concentrations is made for each pair ("recombinant"/"pituitary"), and only when the values exceed the preestablished gender-specific decision limits established from a cohort of volunteers and athletes can an adverse finding be reported [9]. This approach is, however, only effective when the blood sample is taken within a few hours of administration of the rhGH.

The differential isoform test has been complemented by a "biomarker" approach (indirect method) by which the administration of rhGH is indicated [10] by measuring the dose-dependent increase in the concentrations of both insulin-like growth factor I (IGF-I) and the N-terminal peptide of procollagen type III (P-III-NP). The advantage of this test is that the doping with hGH can be detected over a longer time span, potentially days rather than hours.

In order to perform the test, an assay pairing formed by an IGF-I and a P-III-NP assay is utilized for the initial testing procedure, whereas two different IGF-I/P-III-NP assay pairings are used for the confirmation procedures. One IGF-I/P-III-NP assay pairing may be the same as that used in the initial testing procedure. It is recommended that the LC-MS/MS assay for IGF-I be applied as part of the confirmation procedure where possible. The results of each assay pairing are then used to calculate the GH-2000 score. The discriminant function formulae are sex specific, based on the natural logarithm of IGF-I and P-III-NP serum concentrations (required to normalize the data distribution) and include an adjustment for age to reflect the age-related decline in hGH and marker concentrations.

A score is calculated applying the applicable discriminant function formula for the pairing: when it exceeds the established decision limits, it indicates the use of rhGH.

New Therapeutic and Designer Drugs

Expanding the spectrum of analytes tested in routine doping controls is a demanding task, especially when data on drug metabolism, disposition, and elimination are unavailable for nonlicensed drugs, including those discontinued or illicitly produced (designer drugs). For instance, a large number of illicit designer stimulants (e.g., methylhexanamine or N-ethyl-1-phenyl-2-butamine) and anabolic, androgenic steroids [11], including (e.g., norbolethone, tetrahydrogestrinone, desoxymethyltestosterone, or methyldrostanolone) can be easily synthesized and distributed via the Internet as the substance itself or as an ingredient of sport hormonal supplements. These are intended for doping athletes hoping to enhance their performances in the belief that they are undetectable. Since 2002, many of these prohibited substances have been found in products offered on the Internet and detected in athletes' samples.

Similarly, the drug candidate GW1516, which was discontinued from clinical development in 2006 due to substantial undesirable side effects, has been detected in a few doping control urine samples since 2012 [12]. Moreover, new anabolic agents, not yet approved for marketing by the competent authorities, such as selective androgen receptor modulators [13], are frequently detected in routine sports drug testing samples. Lately, the emergence of peptidic drugs such as GH-releasing peptides (e.g. GHRP-2, GHRP-6, hexarelin, or ipamorelin) has further contributed to the analytical challenges to the anti-doping testing laboratories [14]. Many of the above examples often necessitate research into the metabolism and pharmacokinetics of such substances by the anti-doping laboratories. However, human administration studies may be impractical due to ethical and health concerns. Thus, in vitro, electrochemical, and animal models have often served as surrogates to provide the information required to detect the drug and/or its metabolites in (usually) urine [15].

Recent additions to the doping arsenal are inorganic compounds and gases, such as cobalt and xenon [16, 17]. Whilst obsolete in modern anemia therapy, cobalt chloride is an ESA administered for the treatment of anemia in veterinary and human medicine. Due to a variety of undesirable side effects, this treatment was abandoned for humans. However, it is used, in high dosage, as a doping agent for racehorses to increase their "staying power." Cobalt-based treatments do not exist in today's medical armamentarium. Nevertheless, there is a growing market of dietary supplements containing substantial amounts of ionic cobalt so that it may be recommended by the committee to include cobalt salts in the WADA list of prohibited substances and methods based on evidence of abuse by athletes. Since cobalt is naturally present in the body, it will be necessary to set a threshold above which doping is deemed to have occurred. The anti-doping testing laboratories will also be obliged to introduce new procedures and a suitable instrumental technique to determine this element at considerable costs.

There is anecdotal evidence to suggest that, during the Sochi Olympic Games, some athletes used inhalers containing the gas xenon. As a result, xenon was rapidly added to the list of prohibited substances by WADA [18]. Notably, xenon has not been banned from sports due to its narcotic anesthetic properties but rather for its activating effect on the hypoxia-inducible factor-α, a protein produced and operating upstream of EPO and ultimately increasing red blood cells. Headspace GC-MS may be the method of choice to detect xenon in whole blood, serum/plasma, and urine, as demonstrated by testing authentic patient samples having undergone anesthesia. However, the applicability to nontherapeutic drug use regimens (e.g., shorter exposure and lower inhaled concentrations) and routinely applied doping control protocols (sample collection, transport, and storage) remains to be demonstrated.

Consumption of Contaminated Food and Ailments

Modern analytical instrumentation is so sensitive that anti-doping laboratories are capable of detecting growth promoters which are employed in the cattle industry in the urine of athletes who have consumed meat contaminated with their residues. Since adequate sanitary controls are not applied evenly throughout the world, athletes traveling in certain countries may, on eating meat, produce urine samples in the following days in which prohibited substances may be detected [19]. Clenbuterol is a β$_2$-agonist employed illegally in stock farming to hasten maturity in the animal and to produce leaner meat, and it may still be present not only in offal, as it was initially reported, but also in flesh. Several cases have been reported regularly since 2010, where clenbuterol has been found in urine samples collected from athletes present in or returning from these countries.

In the summer of 2014, zilpaterol, another growth promoter, which had been prohibited for several years, was detected in several samples from a group of athletes tested. Subsequently, 3 other isolated cases were reported in the following months in the same country [unpubl. results]. These were the first-ever cases to be reported. The nature of the substance, the low levels at which it was detected in these samples, and the circumstances strongly suggested that the consumption of meat containing residues of the growth promoter was the explanation for the finding but not doping. Similarly, the ingestion of the mycotoxin zearalenone, which is not a prohibited substance, may result in a false-positive finding as it has been shown to lead to the formation of zeranol, a prohibited anabolic agent [20].

Conclusion

Presently, in 2017, there are 34 anti-doping laboratories accredited by WADA, located unevenly around the world, mostly in Europe. The number of blood and urine samples analyzed annually by each is highly variable, ranging from a minimum of 3,000 to several tens of thousands. Although the financial and professional resources differ, all accredited laboratories must provide the full range of tests required to detect and confirm the presence of prohibited substances and methods according to the quality criteria enshrined in the ISL. However, with the advent of more sophisticated methods requiring a considerable investment in more advanced and novel instrumental techniques and the employment of specialized analysts for their operation, in the future, it may be necessary to foresee a situation where only a limited number of laboratories would be able to perform some types of analyses to confirm determinations of a presumptive AAF.

References

1 Hemmersbach P: History of mass spectrometry at the Olympic Games. J Mass Spectrom 2008;43:839–853.
2 World Anti-Doping Agency: What Is Prohibited. 2017 List of Prohibited Substances and Methods. Montreal, WADA, 2017, http://www.wada-ama.org/en/prohibited-list.
3 Thevis M: Mass Spectrometry in Sports Drug Testing – Characterization of Prohibited Substances and Doping Control Analytical Assays. Hoboken, Wiley, 2010.
4 Ayotte C: Detecting the administration of endogenous anabolic androgenic steroids. Handb Exp Pharmacol 2010;195:77–98.
5 Becchi M, Aguilera R, Farizon Y, Flament MM, Casabianca H, James P: Gas chromatography/combustion/isotope-ratio mass spectrometry analysis of urinary steroids to detect misuse of testosterone in sport. Rapid Commun Mass Spectrom 1994;8:304–308.
6 Lasne F, de Ceaurriz J: Recombinant erythropoietin in urine. Nature 2000; 405:635.
7 Reichel C: SARCOSYL-PAGE: a new electrophoretic method for the separation and immunological detection of PEGylated proteins. Methods Mol Biol 2012;869:65–79.
8 Wu Z, Bidlingmaier M, Dall R, Strasburger CJ: Detection of doping with human growth hormone. Lancet 1999;353: 895.
9 Hanley JA, Saarela O, Stephens DA, Thalabard JC: hGH isoform differential immunoassays applied to blood samples from athletes: decision limits for anti-doping testing. Growth Horm IGF Res 2014;24:205–215.
10 Holt RI: Detecting growth hormone abuse in athletes. Anal Bioanal Chem 2011;401:449–462.
11 Catlin DH, Ahrens BD, Kucherova Y: Detection of norbolethone, an anabolic steroid never marketed, in athletes' urine. Rapid Commun Mass Spectrom 2002;16:1273–1275.
12 Thevis M, Möller I, Beuck S, Schänzer W: Synthesis, mass spectrometric characterization, and analysis of the PPARδ agonist GW1516 and its major human metabolites: targets in sports drug testing. Methods Mol Biol 2013;952:301–312.
13 Mohler ML, Bohl CE, Jones A, et al: Nonsteroidal selective androgen receptor modulators (SARMs): dissociating the anabolic and androgenic activities of the androgen receptor for therapeutic benefit. J Med Chem 2009;52:3597–3617.
14 Thomas A, Delahaut P, Krug O, Schänzer W, Thevis M: Metabolism of growth hormone releasing peptides. Anal Chem 2012;84:10252–10259.
15 Gauthier J, Poirier D, Ayotte C: Characterization of desoxymethyltestosterone main urinary metabolite produced from cultures of human fresh hepatocytes. Steroids 2012;77:635–643.
16 Jelkmann W: The disparate roles of cobalt in erythropoiesis, and doping relevance. Open J Hematol 2012;3:6.
17 Ma D, Lim T, Xu J, et al: Xenon preconditioning protects against renal ischemic-reperfusion injury via HIF-1α activation. J Am Soc Nephrol 2009;20:713–720.
18 Breathe it in. The Economist, February 8, 2014.
19 Hemmersbach P, Tomten S, Nilsson S, et al: Illegal use of anabolic agents in animal fattening – consequences for doping analysis; in Donike M, Geyer H, Gotzmann A, Mareck-Engelke U (eds): Recent Advances in Doping Analysis. Cologne, Sportverlag Strauss, 1995, pp 185–191.
20 Baldwin RS, Williams RD, Terry MK: Zeranol: a review of the metabolism, toxicology, and analytical methods for detection of tissue residues. Regul Toxicol Pharmacol 1983;3:9–25.

Prof. Christiane Ayotte, PhD
Directrice du laboratoire de contrôle du dopage
INRS-Institut Armand-Frappier
531, Boulevard des Prairies
Laval, QC H7V 1B7 (Canada)
E-Mail Christiane.Ayotte@iaf.inrs.ca

Achievements and Challenges in Anti-Doping Research

Larry D. Bowers[a] · Xavier Bigard[b]

[a]US Anti-Doping Agency (USADA), Colorado Springs, CO, USA; [b]French Anti-Doping Agency (AFLD), Paris, France

Abstract

The most important element in achieving athlete compliance with anti-doping rules is the certainty of detection. Thus, scientific research plays a mission critical role in achieving clean competition. Many factors contribute to the advances in detection. Incremental advances in the ability to detect prohibited substances and methods, and identification of long-lived metabolites continue to lengthen detection windows. While the athlete biological passport hematological and steroidal modules hold great promise, experience shows that new research is needed to improve the sensitivity and specificity of the approach for current doping techniques. Indirect detection strategies using biomarkers or transcriptomic techniques have been increasingly investigated. The incorporation of more cost-effective sampling strategies using dried blood and plasma spots, oral fluid, and breath analysis show great promise toward increasing the number of tests while remaining within testing budget constraints. Despite the importance of research to ensuring rule compliance, a major challenge for anti-doping research is achieving and maintaining sufficient funding in the reality of the myriad of new substances introduced for disease treatment but abused for performance enhancement. In addition, obtaining metabolism and population reference range data, particularly for new drugs or designer drugs that have not obtained approval for administration to human subjects, remains a significant problem. Nevertheless, research continues to contribute important data to support anti-doping efforts.

© 2017 S. Karger AG, Basel

Introduction

The goal of an anti-doping program is to deter athletes from using prohibited performance-enhancing drugs. One model of deterrence involves the athlete (and/or their advisors) weighing the risks and rewards of doping before making his or her rational choice [1, 2]. The certainty of detection and punishment is one of the most important factors in determining whether an individual will choose to comply with the rules. Risk perceptions of sanctions imposed by authorities appear to be less important in determining behaviors than indirect sanction risk perceptions or reward perceptions. Indirect sanctions are those that involve significant others and include shame and embarrassment. Studies have consistently shown that the certainty of punishment is more important for decision making than the severity of the punishment [3, 4]. The ability of the testing program to detect prohibited substances and methods, which is dependent on both the timing and unpredictability of collections and the analytical capability of the laboratory, is critical to establishing that certainty.

It has been clearly demonstrated through interviews with athletes who have admitted doping and through analysis of blood test results [5] that athletes change their doping behaviors based on their perception of the risk of being detected by testing. Unfortunately, the behavior changes frequently involve engaging in new doping practices that the athletes and their scientific advisors perceive as undetectable. An example is the change of the route of administration of erythropoietin (EPO) from subcutaneous to intravenous and the dose from a therapeutic dose to a microdose. The deterrent effects of risk perceptions are also impacted negatively by experiential learning with respect to whether they or others engage in doping behaviors that are detected or not. Thus, continued development of tests that are effective in detecting doping behaviors is mission critical. The remainder of this chapter will provide an overview of the research done in anti-doping, its importance, and some of the unique challenges faced in anti-doping research.

In addition to the need for additional research to detect drug use when athletes alter their doping behaviors, there is also the reality of a seemingly ever-expanding list of classes of prohibited substances. Although the classes of prohibited substances have changed only slightly between 2004 and 2016, the composition of the list within each class has dramatically changed [6, 7]. For example, a new S0 class entitled non-approved substances was added to deal with any pharmacological substance that is not currently approved for human use. In the category of anabolic agents, the number of listed endogenous substances has increased from 5 to 28, and a new class was added to prohibit selective androgen receptor modulators. The peptide hormone class from the 2004 List – which listed 6 subclasses/substances – has been transformed into the class of peptide hormones, growth factors, related substances, and mimetics, and some substances in the peptide hormone class from 2004 have moved to the class of hormones and metabolic modulators in 2016. The expansion of the list requires research both to understand the metabolism of the substances as well as the development of new methods for detection of those substances and/or metabolites.

The purpose of anti-doping testing is to produce evidentiary data that will establish a violation of the anti-doping rules to the comfortable satisfaction of a panel of arbitrators [8, 9]. The information content of a set of measurements is thus very important. For example, the finding of 2 or more metabolites formed from a prohibited anabolic steroid contains more information about the probability of doping than detecting one metabolite. One of the challenges facing researchers in anti-doping is that in addition to an appreciation for forensic science, they must have expertise in a number of analytical techniques, including gas chromatography (GC) and liquid chromatography (LC), electrophoresis, flow cytometry, immunoassay, and mass spectrometry (MS), as well as the disciplines of clinical chemistry, endocrinology, hematology, genetics, physiology, and pharmacology. Many of the research problems in anti-doping also require the ability to organize clinical trial studies.

Achievements in Anti-Doping Research

In essentially every discipline of science, new advances and understanding are preceded by improvements in measurement technology. Anti-doping science is no different. Recent advances in commercial MS, such as the development of mass analyzers with greatly improved ion storage and scanning capabilities and increased mass resolution, have revolutionized the organization of routine testing and empowered research into detection of prohibited substances. Lower limits of detection using techniques such as tandem and high mass resolution MS have opened new avenues of detection. Advances in interface efficiency between gas and liquid chromatographs and mass spectrometers have decreased limits of detection. Finally, advances in chromatographic techniques themselves, including improved high-performance LC column technology (e.g., ultrahigh performance LC) and two-dimensional GC [10] and LC [11], can be used to optimize separation speed and resolution.

Improved Methodology for the Detection of Prohibited Substances
Synthetic Anabolic Steroids
In late 2015, about 14% of samples collected at a world championship competition had adverse analytical findings for anabolic steroids, peptide hormones, and other prohibited substances. The reason for this 10-fold greater than normal rate of detection was primarily due to advances in initial and confirmation testing strategies. The development of "dilute and shoot" approaches to urine analysis has not only increased laboratory efficiency, but also provided a means to rapidly detect an unprecedented range of compounds in a single instrumental run [12, 13]. Advances in MS such as field asymmetric (FAIMS) and classical drift tube ion mobility spectrometry have the potential to improve sample throughput and increase structural specificity of the MS technique [14].

The certainty of detection is improved not only when limits of detection are lowered, but also when the window of detection is large. The instability of sulfate metabolites of 17-alkylated steroids in urine [15] has resulted in the discovery of a number of long-lived metabolites that are the result of the elimination of the sulfate group and rearrangement and further metabolism of the resulting nonphysiological structure (Fig. 1). For example, a metabolite of methandienone, 18-nor-17β-hydroxymethyl-17α-methyl-androst-1,4,13-trien-3-one, can be detected in urine for 19 days after a single ingestion, almost quadrupling the detection window [16]. Studies involving similar compounds derived from other 17-alkylated anabolic steroids have also been reported, some extending the detection window to 30 days [17–19]. The advances in LC-MS and LC-MS/MS have also facilitated the direct detection of glucuronide and sulfate conjugates of steroids. A long-lived metabolite of stanozolol, 17-epistanozolol-N-glucuronide (Fig. 1), has been reported to be observed for 28 days after ingestion [20]. Detection of the conjugates of other steroids has also been reported [21, 22]. While LC-MS(/MS) and LC-high-resolution MS have been used for many of these studies, the application of GC-chemical ionization-MS/MS has also resulted in expanded detection window opportunities [23]. This dramatic increase in the certainty of detection for a longer period of time has the potential for significantly impacting doping control practice and illustrates the importance of research in facilitating deterrence.

Improving the limits of detection and increasing the detection window, however, does not necessarily result in a panacea. Detection of small quantities of clenbuterol in doping control samples, for example, has exposed a significant issue regarding meat contamination in some countries [24]. Understanding the long-term urinary elimination of steroids encountered in the environment will pose a challenge for anti-doping research in the future.

Naturally Occurring Anabolic Steroids
Donike et al. [25] proposed the testosterone-epitestosterone (T/E) ratio for the detection of the abuse of testosterone in 1986 based on the observation that intramuscular doses of testosterone

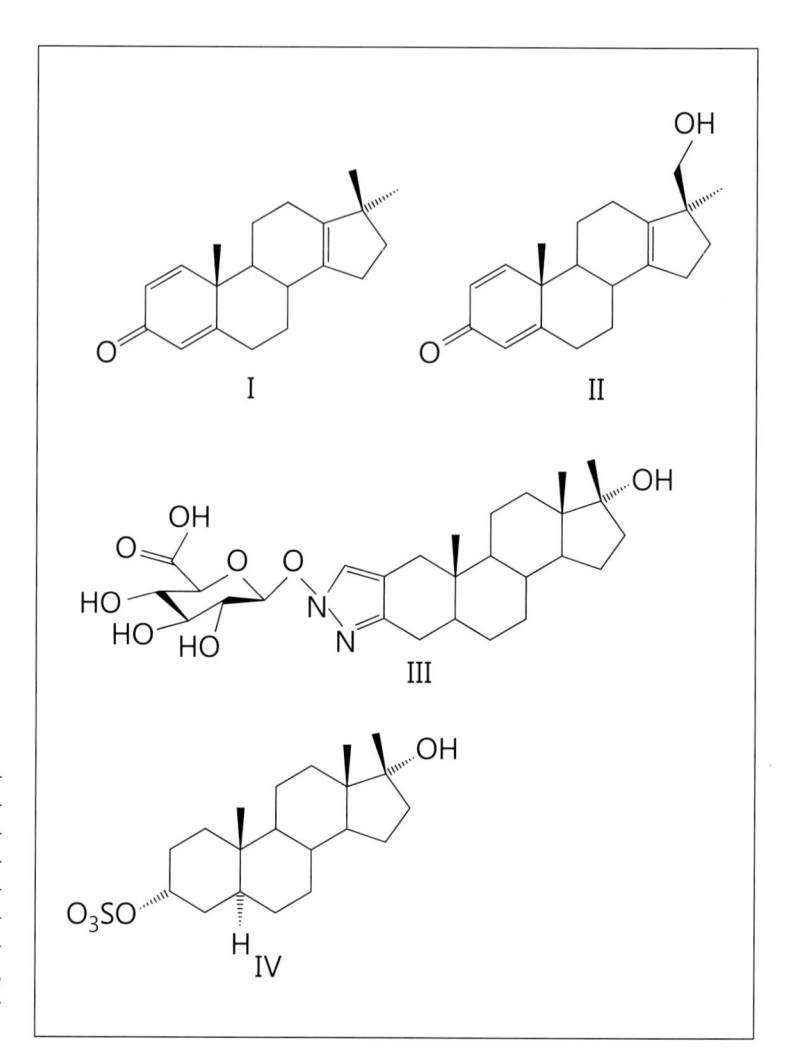

Fig. 1. The structures of the long-lived metabolites of several 17-alkylated anabolic steroids. I, 18-nor-17,17-dimethyl-androst-1,4,13-trien-3-one [13]; II, 18-nor-17β-hydroxymethyl-17α-methyl-androst-1,4,13-trien-3-one [14]; III, 17-epi-stanozolol-N-glucuronide [18]; IV, 17β-methyl-5α-androstan-3α,17α-diol 3α-sulfate [20].

were excreted primarily in the urine as testosterone glucuronide. By the early 1990s, the steroid profile had been developed [26], and longitudinal monitoring using individuals as their own reference range had been described [27, 28]. Sottas et al. [29] gave longitudinal monitoring a more robust mathematical basis by using a bayesian network to incorporate confounding factors and a means to transition from population-based statistics to individual-based statistics. Nevertheless, the use of oral, transdermal, and intranasal routes of administration have decreased the detection capability of the athlete biological passport (ABP) steroidal module (SM). New research opportunities utilizing minor metabolites of endogenous steroids have been pursued. The response of minor metabolites of testosterone and dehydroepiandrosterone (DHEA) such as 4-hydroxy-androstenedione, 6α-hydroxy-androstenedione, 16α-hydroxy-androstenedione, 3α5-cyclo-5α-androstane-6β-ol-17-one, 7β-hydroxy-DHEA, and 16α-hydroxy-DHEA to testosterone and DHEA administration has also been investigated and shown to be more sensitive to administration than the current steroid profile [30, 31]. Base-labile cysteine conjugates of minor testosterone metabolites such as 1,4- and 4,6-androstadiene-3,17-dione, 4,6-androstadiene-3β-ol-17-one, and 15-androstene-3,17-dione have also shown improved sensitivity to detection of endogenous steroid administration [32]. Further research into testosterone metabolism will increase certainty of detection of steroid doping and probably cause athletes to seek new doping agents.

Since steroid metabolism plays a role in the detection of endogenous steroids, genetic polymorphisms, such as in the UDP-glucuronosyltransferase enzyme (UGT2B17) most responsible for making testosterone glucuronide, have been shown to result in individuals who excrete low amounts of testosterone glucuronide resulting in a physiological T/E ratio of about 0.1 and for whom administration of testosterone has little effect on the T/E ratio [33]. Metabolic effectors, such as ethanol [34] and oral contraceptives [35], can also have a significant effect on the T/E ratio, as can the ovulatory cycle and conditions such as the polycystic ovary syndrome.

As a result, a direct method of detecting exogenous testosterone was sought. GC/combustion (C)/isotope ratio MS (IRMS) was first used for anti-doping purposes in 1994. Detecting exogenous administration relies on the difference in the ^{13}C versus ^{12}C content of the natural and exogenous testosterone molecules and their mole fraction in the metabolic pool. While finding an altered carbon isotope ratio is indicative of a doping violation, a negative finding is not informative. As a result, detection of the carbon isotope ratio in smaller steroid metabolic pools (e.g., testosterone vs. androsterone) is transitioning from research studies to routine testing. Both comprehensive GCxGC/C/IRMS [36] and heart-cutting two-dimensional GC/C/IRMS [37] have been reported. Comprehensive GCxGC/C/IRMS has demonstrated 40-fold increases in limits of detection for testosterone due to peak trapping in the second dimension, but instrumental and data handling issues have prevented adoption of the technique for routine testing illustrating the challenge of translating research to routine testing. Hydrogen isotope ratios have also been investigated as potential markers for doping [38].

Indicators of Hematological Manipulation

Increasing oxygen transport to the tissues and generating energy is the most effective way of increasing performance. Thus, detection of EPO-stimulating agents (ESAs) and allogeneic and autologous blood transfusions is an important task for anti-doping. As part of the legacy of the 2000 Sydney Olympic Games, the Australian government supported research to develop a biomarker test for EPO abuse. The initial research measured a large number of biomarkers of hematopoiesis and iron metabolism after subcutaneous recombinant human EPO (rhEPO) administration, including reticulocyte hematocrit, serum EPO, soluble transferrin receptor, hematocrit, hemoglobin concentration, and percent macrocytes, and the results were analyzed by logistic regression to develop 2 models for the detection of exogenous EPO use (ON and OFF model) [39]. Probably the most important conclusion arising from this work was that it is necessary to collect blood and serum/plasma samples in order to truly impact the fight against doping. The group later developed a simpler OFF model using only hemoglobin concentration, percent reticulocytes (OFF_{hr}), and serum erythropoietin (OFF_{hre}). The OFF_{hre} performed better than OFF_{hr}, detecting about 40% of individuals using about 20 IU/kg of rhEPO as opposed to 25% 14 days after cessation of administration, but required the collection of a blood and a serum sample [40]. Sharpe et al. [41] showed that intra-individual longitudinal monitoring of the OFF_{hr} score eliminated between-individual variability and increased detection capability to about 65% in the 20 IU/kg group (1 in 1,000 false-positive probability). Robinson et al. [42] used the predictive bayesian network model

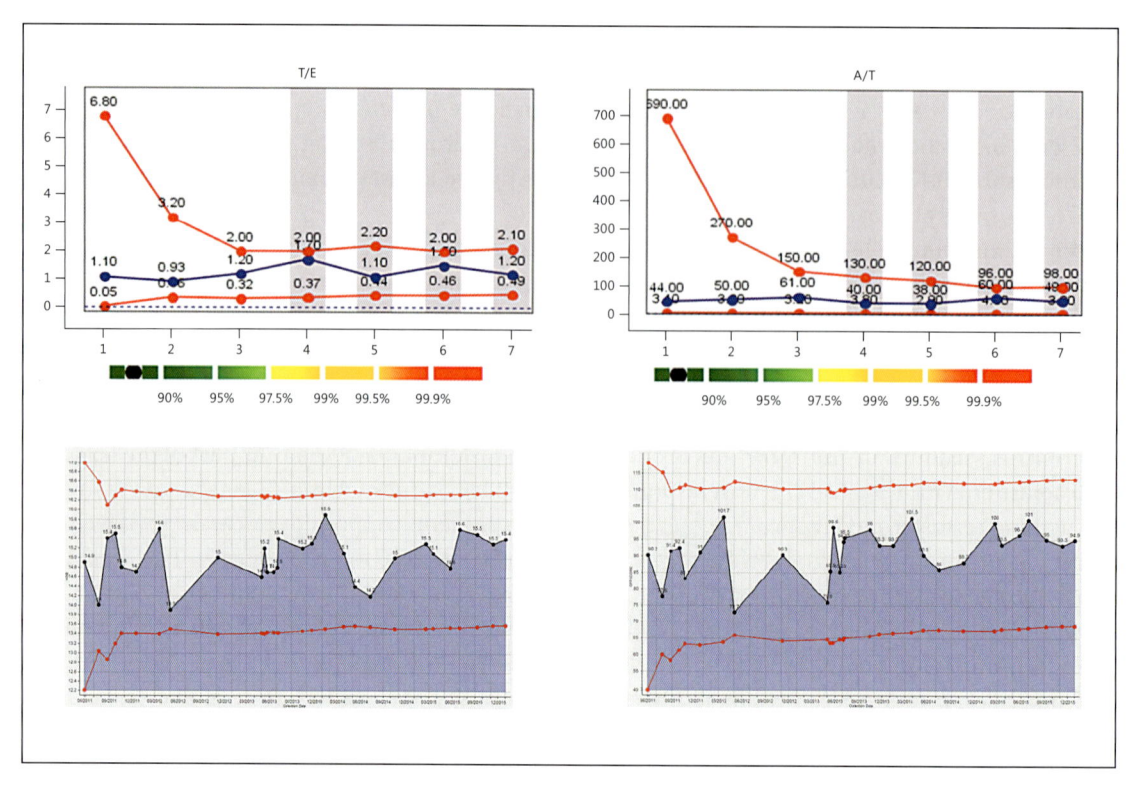

Fig. 2. Examples of the "Athlete Biological Passport" intra-individual reference range approach applied to urinary steroid (top) and hematological (bottom) data. The top two panels show the sequential ratios in an individual athlete for testosterone (T), epitestosterone (E), and androsterone (A) using the WADA ADAMS predictive model software. The bottom two panels show the individual variations in hemoglobin concentration (left) and the "OFF score" (right) using the USADA CHRONOS program. In both cases, the red lines show the individually based limits of variability for the parameter and the blue (top) and black (bottom) lines show the actual data from sequential collections.

to further refine individual longitudinal monitoring (Fig. 2). Confounding factors, such as altitude exposure, require expert evaluation of individual profiles. Nevertheless, the modest sensitivity of the ABP hematological module (HM) to low-dose rhEPO administration suggests that research opportunities into other markers of the hematopoiesis and iron metabolism, such as serum iron, serum transferrin receptor, ferritin, hepcidin [43], and erythroferrone, and incorporating the concepts of neocytolysis [44] and variation in red blood cell dynamics [45] could add significantly to certainty of detection. With the introduction of new therapeutic hematopoiesis-stimulating agents, such as the EPO-Fc fusion protein and stabilizers of the hypoxia-inducible factors (HIFs), improved sensitivity of the ABP-HM will be needed.

Also, in 2000, Lasne and de Ceaurriz [46] reported on an isoelectric focusing method for the direct detection of rhEPO in urine based on the double blotting technique reported by Lasne [47]. Isoelectric focusing separates the various glycoforms of native and rhEPO. Polyacrylamide gel electrophoresis has also been used for the detection of rhEPO and related ESAs [48] and is currently the preferred method of detection. The differences in rhEPO and native EPO involve the glycosylation sites [49], and with the increasing sensitivity of mass spectrometers, the ultimate direct detection approach for ESAs could be isolation from blood or urine with the EPO receptor binding protein and analysis by LC-MS/MS [50].

The development of a test for autologous blood transfusion has thus far been elusive. A flow-cytometric test for allogeneic blood transfusion based on red blood cell surface markers has been reported [51] and used as evidence in establishing a doping violation. The difficulty in incorporating flow cytometry into the testing routine will be discussed further below.

A number of pharmaceutical companies have developed therapeutic agents based on the inhibition of the prolyl hydroxylase that regulates the oxygen-sensing system in cells. These compounds are in phase II and phase III clinical trials, and thus they are not readily available from the manufacturer. Athletes are apparently obtaining the drugs from other sources making compounds "for research use only." Thus, individuals are taking a drug, assuming the structure is correct and purity standards are maintained, whose long-term health effects may not be known. The metabolic fate of the drugs has not been published, but clearly has been studied by the drug company. Unfortunately, the pharmaceutical company may not be in a position to share reference materials or information with anti-doping agencies. In the case of HIF stabilizers, agencies received tips that the compounds were being used. In the absence of cooperation and with evidence of potential use, the anti-doping laboratories were required to develop methods and conduct in vitro metabolism studies to detect the drug in urine. Recently, FG4592 was detected in the urine of 2 athletes using LC-MS/MS [52]. The above discussion illustrates a number of challenges for the anti-doping community when confronting new doping agents. It also demonstrates some athlete's disregard for potential health risks when the "win-at-all-costs" attitude dominates.

Peptide Hormones

GH Variants and Biomarkers. Sönksen proposed development of a test for growth hormone (GH) in the mid-1990s and assembled a group of expert scientists with funding from the European Union and the IOC with the goal of developing a test for the 2000 Olympic Games in Sidney. Two test strategies emerged from the research: a direct measurement of GH variants and an indirect measurement of GH through detection of biomarkers of bioactivity. The variant approach has been well described by Bidlingmaier et al. [53]. The main drawback of any test based on the direct measurement of GH is the relatively short detection window. The biomarker test is based on the measurement of insulin-like growth factor 1 (IGF-1) and the N-terminal peptide of the prohormone of type III collagen (P-III-NP). There have been numerous publications supporting the calculation of a score from these 2 parameters and the athlete's age and from which detection limits have been established [54]. While early stages of the research relied totally on immunoassay technology, an LC-MS/MS method for IGF-1 was developed for anti-doping purposes [55]. In addition to providing both identification and concentration data, the LC-MS/MS method is not subject to the stability and availability of commercial immunoassay kits. Work continues on the development of an LC-MS/MS method for P-III-NP as well, again illustrating the importance of improvements in mass spectrometer limits of detection.

Other Peptide Hormones. The prohibited list contains a large number of other peptide and protein hormones under classes S0 Non-Approved Substances, S2 Peptide Hormones, Growth Factors, Related Substances, and Mimetics, and S4 Hormone and Metabolic Modulators. Since the primary matrix currently used for anti-doping is urine, a very important contribution of anti-doping research was the discovery of peptide metabolites that would be encountered in urine [56–59], including metabolism at the site of administration [60]. Other research on human chorionic gonadotrophin using LC-MS/MS detection has provided insight into the time course of urinary excretion of both intact human chorionic gonadotropin and its metabolites (e.g., β core fragment) [61]. While much of this research is necessary for a clear understanding of pharmacokinetics and excretion for anti-doping, the results of the research apply to laboratory medicine and pharmacology as well.

Genomic, Transcriptomic, Proteomic, and Metabolomic Approaches to Detection

The recent advances in gene therapy and stem cell technology pose a real and tangible threat to its abuse for performance gain by athletes. The nontherapeutic misuse of gene transfer technology requires reliable and sensitive analytical techniques to detect gene doping. The technique must have the potential to be used in a readily available biological fluid, not tissue biopsy. Recombinant adeno-associated viral (rAAV) vectors and naked plasmid are 2 different gene transfer systems used for intramuscular delivery in animal models and in humans [62]. It has been shown that rAAV vectors, which were administered intramuscularly in nonhuman primates, can be detected for several months in white blood cells [63]. The long-term persistence of rAAV sequences in circulating blood cells provides the basis for detecting vector sequences in blood a long time after vector-transferred exogenous DNA within skeletal muscle. Recent transgene detection strategies have been developed, and nested quantitative polymerase chain reaction (PCR) assays were shown to be extremely sensitive and reliable strategies for the detection of exogenous cDNA [64]. These assays were, therefore, shown be suitable for the detection of gene doping with circular or linear vectors that harbor target cDNA sequences. Baoutina et al. [65] developed real-time PCR assays that target sequences within the transgene complementary DNA corresponding to exon/exon junctions. Since these junctions are not present in the endogenous gene due to the presence of introns, this approach allows detection of trace amounts of a transgene in a large background of the endogenous gene.

Varlet-Marie et al. [66] suggested that changes in specific gene expression could be used as markers of ESA misuse. Five genes remained overexpressed about 1 week after the end of rhEPO administration at doses of approximately 20 IU/kg, while the direct urine method failed to detect the presence of rhEPO. Significant interindividual variation was observed between both subjects. The authors of the study point out that the confounding effects of training at altitude and permitted methods such as hypoxic normobaric chambers will have to be understood before a gene expression test could be put into practice. Using different quantitative gene expression technologies, additional recent results confirmed that rhEPO administration led to a signature pattern of several genes first upregulated and subsequently downregulated 4 weeks after the administration of 50 IU/kg of rhEPO [67]. The challenge for the use of gene expression markers is the same as that for biomarkers – the gene response to a drug must be sufficiently different than the response to permitted training regimens and pathological conditions to differentiate doping from confounding factors.

Another promising area of research is the use of circulating microRNA (miRNA), small single-stranded noncoding, regulatory segments of RNA, for doping detection. Leuenberger et al. [68] demonstrated that plasma miR-144, associated with erythropoiesis, was elevated for up to 27 days after treatment with the ESA Mircera. Several plasma miRNAs associated with liver and pulmonary toxicity were elevated after autologous transfusion, and the combination of miR-30b with serum EPO concentration was reasonably diagnostic [69]. Improvements in the day-to-day repeatability of real-time quantitative PCR technology and the development of better normalization and control procedures should make miRNA more appealing in the future. As with the other indirect markers of doping methods, demonstrating the specificity of the miRNA technique may require time-consuming studies of disease states and medical conditions.

While proteomics has yet to be used in anti-doping, metabolomics has been explored and in principle could be used to detect classes of drugs during an initial test should it demonstrate sufficient specificity. The basic idea is that drug interventions lead to changes in the total low-molecular weight or metabolite content of body fluids that can be considered as metabolic signatures detectable using metabolomic technologies. For example, hypoxanthine has been shown to be elevated after application of salbutamol [70]. A number of studies using untargeted metabolic profiling have also resulted in the identification of new metabolites useful for doping control analyses [71, 72]. Taken together, these studies provided the initial proof of concept for omic-based strategies for the detection of new doping substances and potentially opened a new field of research for the anti-doping application of "omic" technologies [see chapter by Wang et al., this vol., pp. 119–128].

Special Challenges in Anti-Doping Research

While some of the successes of anti-doping science research are provided above, the field also faces significant challenges. High on the list for scientific anti-doping research is funding. The importance of certainty of detection and the recalibration of athlete perceptions regarding anti-doping sample collection and testing in deterrence are discussed above, which makes anti-doping science research mission critical. This critical need, however, vies with an ever-increasing programmatic expansion in the areas of social science and education as well as the development of investigational resources for an essentially constant pool of money within WADA. The situation seems to require either a significant change in research projects and fund management or an infusion of new funds.

A second significant problem is the increasing breadth of technology used for research in anti-doping and the transference of that technology to the WADA-accredited laboratories. The introduction of flow cytometry into the laboratories for the purpose of detecting allogeneic blood transfusion through the use of immunological detection of red blood cell surface markers is but one example. Initial studies in a research laboratory of an expert in flow cytometry clearly demonstrated the power of the technology [51]. The cost of technology transference, however, includes not only the cost of a flow cytometer but also requires significant resources for personnel training and validation of each of the assays in an area where the WADA-accredited laboratories had little previous expertise. Other than one very important anti-doping rule violation case in 2004, no additional cases have been detected to support the expense of blood collections and routine testing with flow cytometry.

Population Reference Range and Metabolism Studies

Many of the studies that need to be conducted for anti-doping advances include either administration studies in healthy, trained individuals or population studies to establish thresholds and decision limits for naturally occurring compounds. Studies involving either administration of drugs or removal of blood samples require human subjects' approval, and while subjecting individuals to a treatment with the goal of diagnosing or curing a disease is considered an ethically acceptable tradeoff, concern has been expressed in some countries about subjecting healthy individuals to a treatment that has no perceived benefit but does involve risks, however small. In addition, a recent project to study the efficacy and safety of exposure to xenon gas required an application for an investigational new drug exemption from the Food and Drug Administration prior to obtaining human subjects' approval because the use of xenon for this purpose was not approved. Such bureaucratic necessities can cause significant delays in developing new approaches to doping detection. Finally, some groups of athletes have expressed concern that population reference range studies do not apply to highly trained, elite athletes. At the same time, given the opportunity to donate their samples for research after routine testing, only slightly more than half of athletes have agreed. Similarly, when opportunities are presented to participate in research studies, the response is modest. A means must be found to bridge this gap because the purpose of anti-doping testing is to protect the clean athlete. All of the above argue for a centralized storage and sharing of samples whenever possible to facilitate research studies involving human subjects.

Designer Drugs
Since the detection of norbolethone in 2002, the potential for designer drugs has been a serious concern in anti-doping. In recent years, a variety of previously unreported stimulants and anabolic steroids have been sold on the Internet, some as dietary supplements. In the past, selected ion monitoring and selected reaction monitoring were used employing specific mass and retention time windows, and the potential for avoiding detection was significant. The use of high-resolution full-scanning mass spectrometers (such as quadrupole time of flight) with either LC or GC raises the potential for retrospectively searching acquired spectra for designer drugs rather than storing samples that are reanalyzed at a later date with a method that includes the correct acquisition parameters. It should be noted, however, that the efficiency of ion production for various molecular structures with, for example, electrospray ionization can vary nearly 5,000-fold. Thus, it appears that for the present, storage of samples will be required in order to potentially detect designer drugs.

Reference Materials
A significant challenge for the anti-doping field is the development of reference materials to be used in the identification and quantification of prohibited substances. The synthesis of the long-lived 17α-methyl anabolic steroid metabolites may be facilitated by the use of the fungus *Cunninghamella elegans* that forms the 17-sulfate conjugate of many steroids [73]. Traditional chemical synthesis has also been used to prepare metabolites of anabolic steroids and other prohibited substances. Financial support for the production of these compounds has come from research funding, but in the future this enterprise needs to be supported by routine testing revenues.

Alternative Matrices
As indicated earlier, urine was historically the only specimen used in anti-doping, primarily because the initial classes of doping substances (stimulants and anabolic steroids) were easily detected in the urine. Further, it was perceived as less invasive than taking a blood sample. In 2000, it was recognized that blood doping and some peptide and hormone agents could only be detected in blood. One significant drawback to blood is the expense of collection and shipping. A variety of other possible specimen matrices exist that could significantly alter testing strategies, including dried blood spots [74, 75], dried plasma spots, oral fluid [76], and breath [77]. Each matrix has its own strengths and weaknesses, but many of these alternative matrices could significantly reduce collection and shipping costs, and allow the collection of a significantly greater number of samples, thus impacting the athlete's perception of the certainty of detection.

Summary and Conclusions

Research plays a critical role in achieving deterrence, the goal of anti-doping. The perceived certainty of being detected is the most important contributor to the decision to comply with anti-doping rules. If there are no methods to detect abused substances, whether new agents or methods or changes in the method of administration of agents, deterrence is diminished. While investigations have resolved a number of cases and can provide valuable assistance in guiding research into new methods, it is difficult to envision investigations replacing testing because of limitations imposed by the lack of ability to compel testimony or to subpoena documents and records, which greatly lengthens the time to resolve cases. While value-based education is an important contributor to diminishing drug use, there is little evidence to show that it inhibits doping behaviors in situations where temptation or peer pressure weakens resolve.

There is a compelling rationale for the funding of scientific research, which is central to the mission of anti-doping. Given the inadequate resources available in anti-doping, it is important to balance the research portfolio between innovative approaches that have maximal impact (high risk/high reward) and the stepwise advances required to maintain detection capabilities. It is also important to ensure that a large proportion of research results are translated into the routine testing capabilities and strategies. Anti-doping research has a number of unique challenges that will not be easily addressed. It is imperative, however, that the community continues and enhances its commitment to the best science.

References

1 Weiss DB, Loughran TA, Ray Paternoster R: Deterrence; in Piquero AR (ed): The Handbook of Criminological Theory. Chichester, Wiley, 2015, pp 50–74.
2 Jalleh G, Donovan RJ, Jobling I: Predicting attitude towards performance enhancing substance use: a comprehensive test of the Sport Drug Control Module with elite Australian athletes. J Sci Med Sport 2013;17:574–579.
3 Apel R: Sanctions, perceptions, and crime: implications for criminal deterrence. Quant Criminol 2013;29:67–101.
4 Paternoster R: How much do we really know about criminal deterrence? J Crim Law Criminol 2010;10:765–823.
5 Zorzoli M, Rossi F: Implementation of the biological passport: the experience of the International Cycling Union. Drug Test Anal 2010;2:542–547.
6 World Anti-Doping Agency: The World Anti-Doping Code. The 2004 Prohibited List International Standard. Montreal, WADA, 2004, https://wada-main-prod.s3.amazonaws.com/resources/files/WADA_Prohibited_ List_2004_EN.pdf (accessed February 10, 2016).
7 World Anti-Doping Agency: World Anti-Doping Code International Standard Prohibited List. Montreal, WADA, 2016, https://wada-main-prod.s3.amazonaws.com/resources/files/wada-2016-prohibited-list-en.pdf (accessed February 10, 2016).
8 World Anti-Doping Agency: The World Anti-Doping Code International Standard for Laboratories (2015). Montreal, WADA, https://wada-main-prod.s3.amazonaws.com/resources/files/WADA-ISL-2015-Final-v8.0-EN.pdf (accessed February 10, 2016).
9 World Anti-Doping Agency: World Anti-Doping Code 2015. Montreal, WADA, https://wada-main-prod.s3.amazonaws.com/resources/files/ wada-2015-world-anti-doping-code.pdf (accessed February 10, 2016.
10 Murray JA: Qualitative and quantitative approaches in comprehensive two-dimensional gas chromatography. J Chromatogr A 2012;1261:58–68.
11 Carr PW, Stoll DR, Wang X: Perspectives on recent advances in the speed of high-performance liquid chromatography. Anal Chem 2011;83:1890–1900.
12 Guddat S, Solymos E, Orlovius A, Thomas A, Sigmund G, Geyer H, Thevis M, Schänzer W: High-throughput screening for various classes of doping agents using a new 'dilute-and-shoot' liquid chromatography-tandem mass spectrometry multi-target approach. Drug Test Anal 2011;3:836–850.
13 Guddat S, Thevis M, Kapron J, Thomas A, Schanzer W: Application of FAIMS to anabolic androgenic steroids in sport drug testing. Drug Test Anal 2009;1: 545–553.
14 Thomas A, Görgens C, Guddat S, Thieme D, Dellanna F, Schänzer W, Thevis M: Simplifying and expanding the screening for peptides <2 kDa by direct urine injection, liquid chromatography, and ion mobility mass spectrometry. J Sep Sci 2016;39:333–341.
15 Edlund PO, Bowers LD, Henion JD: Determination of methandrostenolone and its metabolites in equine plasma and urine by coupled-column liquid chromatography with ultraviolet detection and confirmation by tandem mass spectrometry. J Chromatogr 1989;487:341–356.

16 Schänzer W, Geyer H, Fusshöller G, Halatcheva N, Kohler M, Parr MK, Guddat S, Thomas A, Thevis M: Mass spectrometric identification and characterization of a new long-term metabolite of metandienone in human urine. Rapid Commun Mass Spectrom 2006;20:2252–2258.

17 Sobolevsky T, Rodchenkov G: Detection and mass spectrometric characterization of novel long-term dehydrochloromethyltestosterone metabolites in human urine. J Steroid Biochem Mol Biol 2012;128:121–127.

18 Sobolevsky T, Rodchenkov G: Mass spectrometric description of novel oxymetholone and desoxymethyltestosterone metabolites identified in human urine and their importance for doping control. Drug Test Anal 2012;4:682–691.

19 Guddat S, Fußhöller G, Beuck S, Thomas A, Geyer H, Rydevik A, Bondesson U, Hedeland M, Lagojda A, Schänzer W, Thevis M: Synthesis, characterization, and detection of new oxandrolone metabolites as long-term markers in sports drug testing. Anal Bioanal Chem 2013; 405:8285–8294.

20 Schänzer W, Guddat S, Thomas A, Opfermann G, Geyer H, Thevis M: Expanding analytical possibilities concerning the detection of stanozolol misuse by means of high resolution/high accuracy mass spectrometric detection of stanozolol glucuronides in human sports drug testing. Drug Test Anal 2013;5:810–818.

21 Lu J, Fernández-Álvarez M, Yang S, He G, Xu Y, Aguilera R: New clostebol metabolites in human urine by liquid chromatography time-of-flight tandem mass spectrometry and their application for doping control. J Mass Spectrom 2015; 50:191–197.

22 Gómez C, Pozo OJ, Marcos J, Segura J, Ventura R: Alternative long-term markers for the detection of methyltestosterone misuse. Steroids 2013;78:44–52.

23 Polet M, Van Gansbeke W, Van Eenoo P, Deventer K: Gas chromatography/chemical ionization triple quadrupole mass spectrometry analysis of anabolic steroids: ionization and collision-induced dissociation behavior. Rapid Commun Mass Spectrom 2016;30:511–522.

24 Guddat S, Fußhöller G, Geyer H, Thomas A, Braun H, Haenelt N, Schwenke A, Klose C, Thevis M, Schänzer W: Clenbuterol – regional food contamination a possible source for inadvertent doping in sports. Drug Test Anal 2012;4:534–538.

25 Donike M, Bärwald K-R, Klostermann K, Schänzer W, Zimmermann J: Nachweis von exogenem Testosteron; in Heck H, Hollman W, Liesen H, Rost R (eds): Sport: Leistung und Gesundheit – Deutscher Sportärztekongress '82 Köln. Cologne, Deutscher Ärzte Verlag, 1983, pp 293–298.

26 Donike M: Steroid profiling in Cologne; in Donike M, Geyer H, Gotzmann A, Mareck-Engelke U, Rauth S (eds): Proceedings of the 10th Cologne Workshop on Dope Analysis. Cologne, Sport & Buch Straus, 1993, pp 47–68.

27 Baenziger J, Bowers LD: Variability of T/E ratios in athletes; in Donike M, Geyer H, Gotzmann A, Mareck-Engelke U, Rauth S (eds): Proceedings of the 11th Cologne Workshop on Dope Analysis. Cologne, Sport & Buch Straus, 1994, pp 41–51.

28 Donike M, Rauth S, Mareck-Engelke U, Geyer H, Nitschke R: Evaluation of longitudinal studies, the determination of subject-based reference ranges of the testosterone/epitestosterone ratio; in Donike M, Geyer H, Gotzmann A, Mareck-Engelke U, Rauth S (eds): Proceedings of the 11th Cologne Workshop on Dope Analysis. Cologne, Sport & Buch Straus, 1994, pp 33–39.

29 Sottas PE, Saudan C, Schweizer C, Baume N, Mangin P, Saugy M: From population- to subject-based limits of T/E ratio to detect testosterone abuse in elite sports. Forensic Sci Int 2008;174:166–172.

30 Van Renterghem P, Van Eenoo P, Delbeke FT: Population based evaluation of a multi-parametric steroid profiling on administered endogenous steroids in single low dose. Steroids 2010;75:1047–1057.

31 Van Renterghem P, Sottas PE, Saugy M, Van Eenoo P: Statistical discrimination of steroid profiles in doping control with support vector machines. Anal Chim Acta 2013;768:41–48.

32 Fabregat A, Marcos J, Segura J, Ventura R, Pozo OJ: Factors affecting urinary excretion of testosterone metabolites conjugated with cysteine. Drug Test Anal 2016;8:110–119.

33 Schulze JJ, Lundmark J, Garle M, Skilving I, Ekström L, Rane A: Doping test results dependent on genotype of uridine diphospho-glucuronosyl transferase 2B17, the major enzyme for testosterone glucuronidation. J Clin Endocrinol Metab 2008;93:2500–2506.

34 Thieme D, Grosse J, Keller L, Graw M: Urinary concentrations of ethyl glucuronide and ethyl sulfate as thresholds to determine potential ethanol-induced alteration of steroid profiles. Drug Test Anal 2011;3:851–856.

35 Schulze JJ, Mullen JE, Berglund Lindgren E, Ericsson M, Ekström L, Hirschberg AL: The impact of genetics and hormonal contraceptives on the steroid profile in female athletes. Front Endocrinol (Lausanne) 2014;5:50.

36 Tobias HJ, Zhang Y, Auchus RJ, Brenna JT: Detection of synthetic testosterone use by novel comprehensive two-dimensional gas chromatography combustion-isotope ratio mass spectrometry. Anal Chem 2011;83:7158–7165.

37 Brailsford AD, Gavrilović I, Ansell RJ, Cowan DA, Kicman AT: Two-dimensional gas chromatography with heart-cutting for isotope ratio mass spectrometry analysis of steroids in doping control. Drug Test Anal 2012;4:962–969.

38 Piper T, Emery C, Thomas A, Saugy M, Thevis M: Combination of carbon isotope ratio with hydrogen isotope ratio determinations in sports drug testing. Anal Bioanal Chem 2013;405:5455–5466.

39 Parisotto R, Gore CJ, Emslie KR, Ashenden MJ, Brugnara C, Howe C, Martin DT, Trout GJ, Hahn AG: A novel method utilising markers of altered erythropoiesis for the detection of recombinant human erythropoietin abuse in athletes. Haematologica 2000;85:564–572.

40 Gore CJ, Parisotto R, Ashenden MJ, Stray-Gundersen J, Sharpe K, Hopkins W, Emslie KR, Howe C, Trout GJ, Kazlauskas R, Hahn AG: Second-generation blood tests to detect erythropoietin abuse by athletes. Haematologica 2003; 88:333–344.

41 Sharpe K, Ashenden MJ, Schumacher YO: A third generation approach to detect erythropoietin abuse in athletes. Haematologica 2006;91:356–363.

42 Robinson N, Sottas PE, Mangin P, Saugy M: Bayesian detection of abnormal hematological values to introduce a no-start rule for heterogeneous populations of athletes. Haematologica 2007;92: 1143–1144.
43 Leuenberger N, Barras L, Nicoli R, Robinson N, Baume N, Lion N, Barelli S, Tissot JD, Saugy M: Hepcidin as a new biomarker for detecting autologous blood transfusion. Am J Hematol 2016; 91:467–472.
44 Song J, Yoon D, Christensen RD, Horvathova M, Thiagarajan P, Prchal JT: HIF-mediated increased ROS from reduced mitophagy and decreased catalase causes neocytolysis. J Mol Med (Berl) 2015;93:857–866.
45 Higgins JM: Red blood cell population dynamics. Clin Lab Med 2015;35:43–57.
46 Lasne F, de Ceaurriz J: Recombinant erythropoietin in urine. Nature 2000; 405:635.
47 Lasne F: Double-blotting: a solution to the problem of nonspecific binding of secondary antibodies in immunoblotting procedures. Methods Mol Biol 2015;1312:277–283.
48 Reichel C, Abzieher F, Geisendorfer T: SARCOSYL-PAGE: a new method for the detection of MIRCERA- and EPO-doping in blood. Drug Test Anal 2009;1: 494–504.
49 Reichel C: Differences in sialic acid O-acetylation between human urinary and recombinant erythropoietins: a possible mass spectrometric marker for doping control. Drug Test Anal 2013;5:877–889.
50 Vogel M, Blobel M, Thomas A, Walpurgis K, Schänzer W, Reichel C, Thevis M: Isolation, enrichment, and analysis of erythropoietins in anti-doping analysis by receptor-coated magnetic beads and liquid chromatography-mass spectrometry. Anal Chem 2014;86:12014–12021.
51 Nelson M, Popp H, Sharpe K, Ashenden M: Proof of homologous blood transfusion through quantification of blood group antigens. Haematologica 2003;88: 1284–1295.
52 Buisson C, Marchand A, Bailloux I, Lahaussois A, Martin L, Molina A: Detection by LC-MS/MS of HIF stabilizer FG-4592 used as a new doping agent: Investigation on a positive case. J Pharm Biomed Anal 2016;121:181–187.

53 Bidlingmaier M, Suhr J, Ernst A, Wu Z, Keller A, Strasburger CJ, Bergmann A: High-sensitivity chemiluminescence immunoassays for detection of growth hormone doping in sports. Clin Chem 2009;55:445–453.
54 Holt RI, Böhning W, Guha N, Bartlett C, Cowan DA, Giraud S, Bassett EE, Sönksen PH, Böhning D: The development of decision limits for the GH-2000 detection methodology using additional insulin-like growth factor-I and amino-terminal pro-peptide of type III collagen assays. Drug Test Anal 2015;7:745–755.
55 Cox HD, Lopes F, Woldemariam GA, Becker JO, Parkin MC, Thomas A, Butch AW, Cowan DA, Thevis M, Bowers LD, Hoofnagle AN: Inter-laboratory agreement of insulin-like growth factor 1 concentrations measured by mass spectrometry. Clin Chem 2014;60:541–548.
56 Thomas A, Höppner S, Geyer H, Schänzer W, Petrou M, Kwiatkowska D, Pokrywka A, Thevis M: Determination of growth hormone releasing peptides (GHRP) and their major metabolites in human urine for doping controls by means of liquid chromatography mass spectrometry. Anal Bioanal Chem 2011; 401:507–516.
57 Semenistaya E, Zvereva I, Thomas A, Thevis M, Krotov G, Rodchenkov G: Determination of growth hormone releasing peptides metabolites in human urine after nasal administration of GHRP-1, GHRP-2, GHRP-6, hexarelin, and ipamorelin. Drug Test Anal 2015;7: 919–925.
58 Thomas A, Schänzer W, Thevis M: Determination of human insulin and its analogues in human blood using liquid chromatography coupled to ion mobility mass spectrometry (LC-IM-MS). Drug Test Anal 2014;6:1125–1132.
59 Thomas A, Geyer H, Kamber M, Schänzer W, Thevis M: Mass spectrometric determination of gonadotrophin-releasing hormone (GnRH) in human urine for doping control purposes by means of LC-ESI-MS/MS. J Mass Spectrom 2008; 43:908–915.
60 Thomas A, Brinkkötter P, Schänzer W, Thevis M: Metabolism of human insulin after subcutaneous administration: a possible means to uncover insulin misuse. Anal Chim Acta 2015;897:53–61.

61 Woldemariam GA, Butch AW: Immunoextraction-tandem mass spectrometry method for measuring intact human chorionic gonadotropin, free β-subunit, and β-subunit core fragment in urine. Clin Chem 2014;60:1089–1097.
62 Wu Z, Asokan A, Samulski RJ: Adeno-associated virus serotypes: vector toolkit for human gene therapy. Mol Ther 2006; 14:316–327.
63 Ni W, Le Guiner C, Gernoux G, Penaud-Budloo M, Moullier P, Snyder RO: Longevity of rAAV vector and plasmid DNA in blood after intramuscular injection in nonhuman primates: implications for gene doping. Gene Ther 2011;18:709–718.
64 Neuberger EW, Perez I, Le Guiner C, Moser D, Ehlert T, Allais M, Moullier P, Simon P, Snyder RO: Establishment of two quantitative nested qPCR assays targeting the human EPO transgene. Gene Ther 2016;23:330–339.
65 Baoutina A, Coldham T, Bains GS, Emslie KR: Gene doping detection: evaluation of approach for direct detection of gene transfer using erythropoietin as a model system. Gene Ther 2010;17: 1022–1032.
66 Varlet-Marie E, Audran M, Ashenden M, Sicart MT, Piquemal D: Modification of gene expression: help to detect doping with erythropoiesis-stimulating agents. Am J Hematol 2009;84:755–759.
67 Durussel J, Haile DW, Mooses K, Daskalaki E, Beattie W, Mooses M, Mekonen W, Ongaro N, Anjila E, Patel RK, Padmanabhan N, McBride MW, McClure JD, Pitsiladis YP: Blood transcriptional signature of recombinant human erythropoietin administration and implications for antidoping strategies. Physiol Genomics 2016;48:202–209.
68 Leuenberger N, Jan N, Pradervand S, Robinson N, Saugy M: Circulating microRNAs as long-term biomarkers for the detection of erythropoiesis-stimulating agent abuse. Drug Test Anal 2011;3: 771–776.
69 Leuenberger N, Schumacher YO, Pradervand S, Sander T, Saugy M, Pottgiesser T: Circulating microRNAs as biomarkers for detection of autologous blood transfusion. PLoS One 2013; 8:e66309.

70 Wang Y, Caldwell R, Cowan DA, Legido-Quigley C: LC-MS-based metabolomics discovers purine endogenous associations with low-dose salbutamol in urine collected for antidoping tests. Anal Chem 2016;88:2243–2249.

71 Van Renterghem P, Van Eenoo P, Delbeke FT: Population based evaluation of a multi-parametric steroid profiling on administered endogenous steroids in single low dose. Steroids 2010;75:1047–1057.

72 Raro M, Ibáñez M, Gil R, Fabregat A, Tudela E, Deventer K, Ventura R, Segura J, Marcos J, Kotronoulas A, Joglar J, Farré M, Yang S, Xing Y, Van Eenoo P, Pitarch E, Hernández F, Sancho JV, Pozo ÓJ: Untargeted metabolomics in doping control: detection of new markers of testosterone misuse by ultrahigh performance liquid chromatography coupled to high-resolution mass spectrometry. Anal Chem 2015;87:8373–8380.

73 Rydevik A, Bondesson U, Thevis M, Hedeland M: Mass spectrometric characterization of glucuronides formed by a new concept, combining *Cunninghamella elegans* with TEMPO. J Pharm Biomed Anal 2013;84:278–284.

74 Thomas A, Geyer H, Schänzer W, Crone C, Kellmann M, Moehring T, Thevis M: Sensitive determination of prohibited drugs in dried blood spots (DBS) for doping controls by means of a benchtop quadrupole/Orbitrap mass spectrometer. Anal Bioanal Chem 2012;403:1279–1289.

75 Verplaetse R, Henion JD: Quantitative determination of opioids in whole blood using fully automated dried blood spot desorption coupled to on-line SPE-LC-MS/MS. Drug Test Anal 2016;8:30–38.

76 Anizan S, Huestis MA: The potential role of oral fluid in antidoping testing. Clin Chem 2014;60:307–322.

77 Stephanson N, Sandqvist S, Lambert MS, Beck O: Method validation and application of a liquid chromatography-tandem mass spectrometry method for drugs of abuse testing in exhaled breath. J Chromatogr B Analyt Technol Biomed Life Sci 2015;985:189–196.

78 Görgens C, Guddat S, Dib J, Geyer H, Schanzer W, Thevis M: Mildronate (meldonium) in professional sports – monitoring doping control urine samples using hydrophilic interaction liquid chromatography – high resolution/high accuracy mass spectrometry. Drug Test Anal 2015;7:973–979.

Larry D. Bowers, PhD
Chief Science Officer
US Anti-Doping Agency (USADA)
5555 Tech Center Drive, Suite 200
Colorado Springs, CO 80919 (USA)
E-Mail lbowers@usada.org

Xavier Bigard, MD, PhD
Scientific Adviser
Agence Française de Lutte contre le Dopage (AFLD)
229 Boulevard Saint Germain
FR–75007 Paris (France)
E-Mail x.bigard@afld.fr

Gene and Cell Doping: The New Frontier – Beyond Myth or Reality

Elmo W.I. Neuberger · Perikles Simon

Department of Sports Medicine, Rehabilitation, and Disease Prevention, Johannes Gutenberg University Mainz, Mainz, Germany

Abstract

The advent of gene transfer technologies in clinical studies aroused concerns that these technologies will be misused for performance-enhancing purposes in sports. However, during the last 2 decades, the field of gene therapy has taken a long and winding road with just a few gene therapeutic drugs demonstrating clinical benefits in humans. The current state of gene therapy is that viral vector-mediated gene transfer shows the now long-awaited initial success for safe, and in some cases efficient, gene transfer in clinical trials. Additionally, the use of small interfering RNA promises an efficient therapy through gene silencing, even though a number of safety concerns remain. More recently, the development of the molecular biological CRISPR/Cas9 system opened new possibilities for efficient and highly targeted genome editing. This chapter aims to define and consequently demystify the term "gene doping" and discuss the current reality concerning gene- and cell-based physical enhancement strategies. The technological progress in the field of gene therapy will be illustrated, and the recent clinical progress as well as technological difficulties will be highlighted. Comparing the attractiveness of these technologies with conventional doping practices reveals that current gene therapy technologies remain unattractive for doping purposes and unlikely to outperform conventional doping. However, future technological advances may raise the attractiveness of gene doping, thus making it easier to develop detection strategies. Currently available detection strategies are introduced in this chapter showing that many forms of genetic manipulation can already be detected in principle.

© 2017 S. Karger AG, Basel

Introduction

Experts in gene therapy indicated the possible applications of gene transfer technology and genetic manipulation for performance-enhancing purposes for the first time in 2001 [1]. Since that time, it has been speculated at every Olympic Games that genetic manipulation could push human performance to new extremes with genetically modified "super humans" [2, 3]. In the public eye, it is expected that gene doping holds the potential for extraordinary performance enhancement, exceeding the natural physiological boundaries. However, this perception is challenged by 2 main reasons. Human performance is a highly complex phenotypical trait with an unknown number of genetic elements that interact in highly complex and coordinated ways. Secondly, the research progress in the field of gene therapy underlines the difficulties for successful addition or manipulation of even single genes. About 2 decades ago, it was believed that a small number of "sports genes" determine the phenotype of high-level performance [4]. This rather deterministic concept has been challenged during recent years. Firstly, geneticists and molecular biologists gained a deeper understanding of how genetic factors contribute to the makeup of phenotypic traits that are of sports practical relevance such as body size [5], body weight [6], or maximal aerobic capacity ($\dot{V}O_{2\,max}$) [7] to mention only a few. The idea that a handful of genes can determine these phenotypic traits has now been discredited [8]. It became obvious that a large number of genes interact in a highly complex way. For example, it is estimated that approximately 200,000 gene locations contribute to the phenotype height each with small single effects [5]. Moreover, genes or genetic elements do not act together in a simple independent and additive way but can interact at different levels, including the genome, the transcriptome, and the epigenome [9]. It seems obvious that high-level sporting performance will depend on a complex network of hundreds or thousands of genetic elements that can act together to create a loose and open framework limiting a phenotypic trait [10]. This complexity restricts the scope of genetic manipulation. Two examples can be presented of how genes can have major effects on physiological traits and can affect human performance. These are rare mutations in the gene myostatin (*MSTN*) that lead to extraordinary muscle growth [11, 12], as well as a rare mutation in the erythropoietin (EPO) receptor gene (*EPOR*) that was discovered in the world class cross-country skier Eero Mäntyranta [13]. The latter mutation led to stably increased hematocrit levels (approx. 68%) and hemoglobin mass >200 g/L, and consequently to an increased oxygen transport to skeletal muscles [13]. Similar to doping with recombinant human EPO, such a mutation could theoretically give an athlete an advantage in endurance sport disciplines [14]. While this advantage alone cannot explain elite performance per se, induction of such a beneficial genetic makeup in an athlete that is already elite may provide a notable advantage. Gene doping targets that could have reasonable performance-enhancing effects are *EPO*, *EPOR*, insulin-like growth-factor-I (*IGF-I*), *MSTN*, vascular endothelial growth factor (*VEGF*), and follistatin (*FST*) [15–18].

This chapter provides not only an overview of the latest clinical and technological progress in gene therapy in medicine, but also possible applications of gene therapeutic technologies to doping in sport. Additionally, the current progress in the field of gene doping detection is described. The chapter ends by comparing the applicability of gene doping versus classical doping with prohibited substances.

The Historical Development of the Content of "M3 Gene Doping"

In anticipation of the misuse of gene therapeutic technology, the World Anti-Doping Agency (WADA) sponsored a meeting with representatives of the scientific and athletic community to discuss the impending possibility of gene doping in sport. The meeting was held at the Banbury Center at the Cold Spring Harbor Laboratory (Long Island, NY, USA) in March 2002 [19]. In 2003 the International Olympic Committee (IOC) and in 2004 WADA included gene doping in the list of prohibited substances and methods [20]. Despite this inclusion more than a decade ago, not a single athlete has been convicted of gene doping. The first recorded expression of in-

Table 1. Changes in the wording of "M3 Gene Doping" by WADA

Year	Definition of M3 Gene Doping
2003/2004	Gene or cell doping is defined as the nontherapeutic use of genes, genetic elements, and/or cells that have the capacity to enhance athletic performance
2005–2008	The nontherapeutic use of cells, genes, genetic elements, *or of the modulation of gene expression,* having the capacity to enhance athletic performance, is prohibited
2009	Transfer of cells or genetic elements or the use of cells, genetic elements, or pharmacological agents to modulating expression of endogenous genes, having the capacity to enhance athletic performance, is prohibited *PPARδ agonists (e.g., GW1516) and AMPK axis agonists (e.g., AICAR) are prohibited*
2010	The following, with the potential to enhance athletic performance, are prohibited: 1 The transfer of cells or genetic elements *(e.g., DNA, RNA)* 2 The use of pharmacological or biological agents that alter gene expression PPARδ agonists (e.g., GW1516) and AMPK axis agonists (e.g., AICAR) are prohibited
2011	The following, with the potential to enhance sport performance, are prohibited: 1 *The transfer of nucleic acids or nucleic acid sequences* 2 The use of *normal or genetically modified* cells 3 **The use of agents that directly or indirectly affect functions known to influence performance by altering gene expression** **PPARδ agonists (e.g., GW1516) and AMPK axis agonists (e.g., AICAR) are prohibited**
2012–2017	The following, with the potential to enhance sport performance, are prohibited: 1 The transfer of nucleic acids or nucleic acid sequences 2 The use of normal or genetically modified cells

Parts that were added are italicized. Deleted parts are highlighted in bold (modified from Thieme [24]). PPARδ, peroxisome proliferator-activated receptor δ; AMPK, PPARδ-AMP-activated protein kinase.

terest to misuse gene therapy arose from an email correspondence of a German athletic coach with his drug dealer [21]. Reportedly, the trainer asked for a drug (Repoxygen; Oxford BioMedical), which comprised of an adeno-associated virus (AAV) vector system containing the *EPO* gene. After intramuscular injection, the muscle cells of the recipient would be expected to produce EPO endogenously. The safety of the drug was not approved, and the production of the drug was stopped before it reached clinical trials in humans [14]. At this time, the gene doping procedure was principally undetectable and was considered as a threat to elite sports.

In order to deal with the threat of gene doping, WADA included a section M3 [20]. The historical development of the wording of this section is presented in Table 1. Comparing the first version in 2003/2004 with the current version, 2 slight differences exist. One relates to the purpose of the use, which was in the very first version described as merely nontherapeutic in nature, while it has now been rendered more precisely to the performance-enhancing capacity of the procedure. The other aspect that has changed over the last few years is that not only delivery of genes or genetic elements is prohibited but also delivery of nucleic acids (Table 1). As will be discussed in this chapter, this change now relates to doping procedures that may use short stretches of nucleic acids, for instance small interfering ribonucleic acids (siRNAs) that will not alter the genome permanently, but theoretically have the capacity to modify our genetic activity for a limited amount of time [22]. However, considering the mechanism of action, siRNAs could also be listed in section S4 that relates to pharmaceuticals that do not alter the genome but act on the activity of our genes for performance-enhancing purposes. There are previous precedents, such as a shift of 2 pharmaceuticals from M3 to S4 covered in the 2009 and 2010 versions of the list. Amongst these are AICAR, which is a ribonucleotide present in our body, and GW1516. The justification for such a reclassification is simply that these substances do not act more profoundly on modulating our genetic activity than other long-known doping substances like testosterone. Looking at the history of M3 development, one can see that the "modulation of gene expression" as a conceptual term was prohibited in the second version (Table 1). This term has been removed, since it would basically include almost all conventional doping substances along with the techniques of RNA interference (RNAi) using the siRNAs mentioned above [23].

The present definition is now more closely related to the definitions of different gene and cell therapy societies. It still covers all known molecular biological techniques that are applied to treat diseases including somatic gene therapy, ex vivo gene therapy, stem cell therapy, and various kinds of RNA-related therapies. However, the wording "use of normal cells" without further specification lacks unique certainty. As described later, the use of normal cells, such as stem cells, is unlikely to have a performance-enhancing effect per se. Furthermore, the wording normal cells would also refer to other doping practices such as blood doping. In the future, it is foreseeable that with the advances in the field of gene and cell transfer technology, there will be concrete procedures that could be used for gene doping purposes, and those concrete procedures could be listed in M3.

The Clinical Equivalent of M3 Gene Doping and Possible Gene Doping Scenarios

The classical concept of gene therapy emerged in the 1970s with the goal to replace a defective gene or introduce a new gene into the cells of an individual to cure or favorably modify the condition of a disease. Since the first approved gene therapy trial in 1990, more than 2,400 clinical trials have been conducted to treat cancer, inherited diseases, and chronic infections [25].

Classical Gene Therapy

For the delivery of genetic material, viral and nonviral vectors can be used. Viruses are highly evolved biological machines that efficiently introduce genetic material into cell nuclei. Different kinds of replication-deficient viral vector systems were developed, and their efficacy, specificity, and safety were tested in clinical trials [26]. Two main groups of viruses can be differentiated according to whether they integrate their genome into the cellular genome of the host (oncoretroviruses and lentiviruses) or the genome persists mainly as extrachromosomal episome in the cell nucleus (herpes simplex virus, adeno virus, or AAV). Depending on the type of gene therapy, different vector systems are used. For in vivo gene therapy, for example, the direct injection of viral vectors into the body, typically nonintegrating vectors, are used. The transgene of nonintegrating vectors remains episomal, reducing the risk of disrupting the host genome (Fig. 1). For ex vivo gene transfer, when cells are taken from a donor, manipulated, and expanded out of the body, integrating vectors are required. Without an integrating vector system, the transgene would gradually get lost with each cell division. Viral vector systems have advantages and disadvantages as they differ with respect to transduction efficacy for different cells and the immuno- or genotoxicity [27]. In recent years, especially the groups of recombinant AAV (rAAV) and lentiviral vector systems demonstrated their ex-

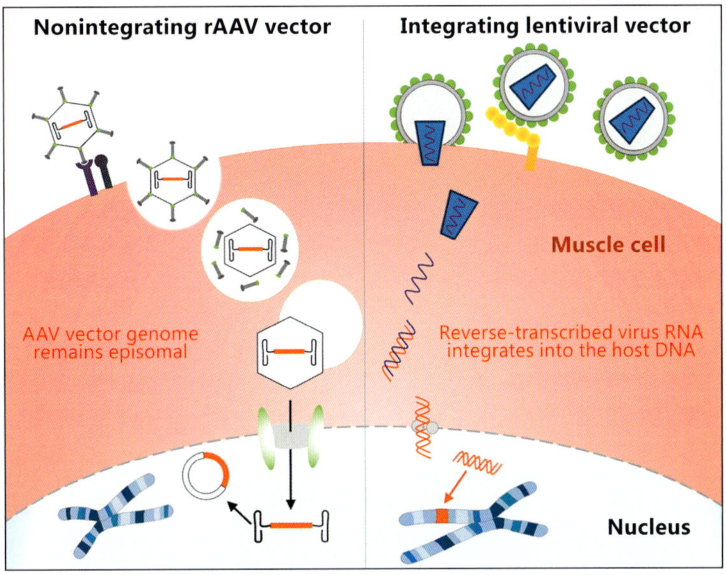

Fig. 1. Illustration of the cellular uptake and genome integration of recombinant adeno-associated virus (rAAV) and lentiviral vectors. The transgene of nonintegrating rAAV vectors remains episomal, reducing the risk of genotoxicity. For applications that require stable genetic modifications, lentiviral vectors can be used. Upon cell entry, the viral RNA genome (purple) is converted into double-stranded DNA (red) and is integrated into the host genome.

cellent transduction efficacy and safety in a number of clinical trials [28, 29].

It is notable that nonviral vectors such as naked plasmids or plasmids complexed in liposomes are not efficient enough for in vivo gene addition purposes due to limited uptake of the transgenic DNA in the nucleus [26]. The major antagonist against successful viral gene transfer in vivo is the immune system of the host that can be activated in response to the viral protein, the transgene, or the expressed protein [28]. The importance of the host's immune reaction was painfully realized in 1999. After the systemic injection of a highly immunogenic adenoviral vector, an 18-year-old patient died from organ failure in a gene therapy trial. It was discovered that the patient died due to an immune response against the vector capsid [30]. rAAV vectors showed low immunogenicity and became the vector system of choice for in vivo gene transfer [28]. In 2012, the first rAAV vector-based gene therapeutic drug was granted market approval by the European Commission and the American Food and Drug Administration [31]. The drug named Glybera® (uniQure) is an AAV-based vector that is injected intramuscularly for the treatment of patients with a rare inherited mutation that leads to lipoprotein lipase deficiency. The final market authorization was registered as a clear signal and paved the way for more gene therapeutic drugs [31]. Some of these gene therapeutic drugs could potentially have performance-enhancing effects. A promising candidate would be rAAV vector-mediated *FST* gene therapy. *FST* is a naturally occurring inhibitor of *MSTN*, which in turn inhibits muscle growth. After promising preclinical animal studies demonstrated a strength-increasing effect of *FST*, a preclinical study and clinical phase 1/2a trial was conducted for Becker muscular dystrophy patients [32]. As reported in 2015, intramuscular injections of the rAAV vector led to performance improvements in a 6-min walk test in 4 out of 6 patients, while no adverse events were reported [32]. The use of other unapproved gene doping candidates such as *IGF-1* or *EPO* would be high risk. In a number of studies, *EPO* gene transfer caused serious side effects requiring several animals to be euthanized [33, 34]. *IGF-1* gene therapy has not been tested in humans, and its efficacy remains speculative. The production of viral vectors can be handled in a typical molecular biological laboratory [35]. However, good manufacturing practices that guarantee the purity of the vector system are necessary to avoid adverse effects and to guarantee transduction efficacy. Despite extensive experience in the field of gene therapy, the use of viral vectors for in vivo gene therapy is facing a number of hurdles. This includes uncertain dose-response relationships with respect to interindividual differences. For gene doping purposes in athletes, no dosing regimen exists, and the outcome remains uncertain. Therefore, athletes would be guinea pigs, and the choice of the vector system, vector doses, and route of application would rely on experimental data which currently show conflicting results. In this context, it is notable that a unique viral vector system can only be used once as a result of an adapted immune system. Currently, these technical barriers, the restricted accessibility of the technology, as well as the lack of knowledge about biological dose-response relationships make gene therapeutic drugs unattractive for gene doping purposes. An attempt to use unapproved vector systems and transgenes bears a high risk of failure.

The Hurdles of Stem Cell Therapy
Stem cells can be divided into 3 main cell types: adult stem cells, human embryonic stem cells (ESCs), and induced pluripotent stem cells (iPSC). ESCs have the capacity for self-renewal and can develop into virtually any cell type. Adult stem cells have the capacity for self-renewal, but their division is restricted to a specialized cell type like muscle tissue. Stem cell therapy has the potential to treat or prevent diseases [36]. The conventional hematopoietic stem cell (HSC) therapy, without genetic modification of the cells, is the most relevant and clinically validated therapy. According to the World Health Organization, more than 50,000 transplantations are carried out annually to treat patients with hematological diseases, and the clinical benefit of this therapy has been validated comprehensively [37]. Since the early 1990s, HSCs were used for stem cell gene therapy. After initial drawbacks related to insertional oncogenesis [38], the improvement in vector design led to impressive clinical benefit of HSC gene therapy for a number of hematological diseases [29]. In 2016, the second gene therapeutic drug was granted market approval by the European Medicines Agency (EMA) [39]. It was developed for the treatment of adenosine deaminase-deficient severe combined immunodeficiency. However, this kind of therapy is very invasive and would be unfavorable for gene doping purposes. After the isolation of autologous HSCs from bone marrow or blood, the cells could be genetically modified to produce performance-relevant cytokines or growth factors. However, the ex vivo approach bears the risk of insertional oncogenesis. Moreover, reinfusion of the genetically modified HSCs needs cytoreductive conditioning using chemotherapy [40]. Without this treatment, only minimal or no cells engraft [40], making this gene doping approach most likely unacceptable for athletes.

Another promising and successful kind of cell-based gene therapy is the chimeric antigen receptor (CAR) T-cell therapy. In this fast growing field, a large number of clinical trials are ongoing to target hematopoietic malignancies and solid cancers [41]. After isolation of endogenous T cells and ex vivo reengineering via viral vector, the cells carry CARs on their surface. These CARs enable T cells to recognize cancer-specific antigens. After multiplication and reinfusion into the patient, the CAR T cells recognize and kill the tumor cells that would otherwise escape immune detection [41]. However, there is no direct applicability for gene doping purposes.

As already mentioned, for diseased individuals, the classical HSC therapy has substantial clinical benefits. It was hoped that these benefits would apply to other kinds of stem cell therapy like mesenchymal stem cell (MSC) therapy [36]. MSCs are multipotent adult stem cells present in multiple tissues and can differentiate into bone, cartilage, muscle, and adipose cells. MSCs can be easily isolated and grown in high numbers in culture [36]. However, typical problems include the limited survival, homing, proliferation, and differentiation of the cells. As reviewed by Dimmeler et al. [42], typically only a small number of cells incorporate into the target tissue after transplantation and survive for long periods of time. This limitation profoundly restricts the clinical benefits, while the nonincorporated dying cells could cause side effects [42].

There is some evidence that MSCs can be used in sports in order to accelerate wound healing. According to their function to produce anti-inflammatory factors, angiogenic factors, and other factors stimulating tissue-specific stem cells, MSCs have been studied for the treatment of cartilage damage, tendinopathy, and bone repair [43]. However, stem cell therapy without genetic modification of the cells seems to have no performance-enhancing effect. The same applies to iPSCs. In 2006, it became possible to transform adult, differentiated cells into pluripotent stem cells, which have properties comparable to ESCs [44]. However, for clinical application in humans, more research is required to ensure the long-term safety and efficacy of stem cell therapy using reprogrammed iPSCs [36]. The challenges with iPSCs include poor initial cell survival and long-term engraftment, as well as impaired function due to senescence, imprecision in controlling cell fate, and mutations [42, 45]. In summary, in its present form, stem cell therapy and stem cell gene therapy is of little value for performance enhancement, and the cost-benefit ratio is unfavorable for athletes.

Therapeutic Oligonucleotides: RNAi Rebooted
The large field of therapeutic oligonucleotides comprises molecules that bind to RNA (antisense oligonucleotides, siRNA, antagomirs, and mRNAs itself), oligonucleotides that bind to DNA (antigene oligonucleotides), as well as protein-binding oligonucleotides (aptamers, decoys, and CpG oligonucleotides) [46]. As reviewed by Lundin et al. [23], a number of therapeutic oligonucleotides found their way into clinical applications. Given their clinical relevance, and the applicability for doping purposes, siRNAs are the most relevant candidates [47]. siRNAs are small double-stranded RNAs that lead to an efficient knockdown of genes. The so-called RNAi was discovered in 1998, and in just 8 years the gene silencing technique resulted in the award of the Nobel Prize to A.Z. Fire and C.C. Mello in Physiology or Medicine in 2006 [22].

RNAi describes the naturally occurring biological process in which small RNA molecules, called siRNAs, or naturally occurring microRNAs (miRNAs) modulate the expression of genes (Fig. 2). After processing, the molecules regulate protein expression by triggering mRNA degradation or inhibiting its translation into protein. Typically, miRNAs bind to the 3′-untranslated region of an mRNA.

During the last 20 years, more than 2,500 mature miRNAs were predicted in the human genome [48], and it is estimated that more than 60% of protein-coding genes are regulated by miRNAs [49]. Each miRNA can regulate a larger number of mRNAs, and 1 mRNA can be regulated by a large number of miRNAs; illustrating one of the major difficulties of siRNAs. Because siRNAs do not only target one mRNA specifically, off-target effects such as cytotoxicity can occur. Despite immense potential and owing primarily to the off-target effects of siRNA, numerous biotech companies have halted RNAi research and drug development despite having invested large amounts of money. For example, the Swiss company Roche ended the RNAi research in 2010 after 3 years and a USD 500-million investment. Additionally, Merck and Novartis stopped most RNAi research [22]. Next to the off-target effect, the delivery of siRNAs is still a large hurdle, and the transfer of siRNA to other organs than the liver is still inefficient [50]. Re-

Fig. 2. RNA interference (RNAi) describes the naturally occurring process that small double-stranded RNAs regulate the expression of protein-coding genes. These small RNAs can be naturally occurring microRNAs (miRNAs) or small interfering RNA (siRNA) that can be produced synthetically. Naturally occurring miRNAs are transcribed from DNA and form double-stranded hairpin structures (1). After enzymatic restriction, the mature miRNA is exported into the nucleus. Mature miRNAs and exogenous siRNAs share the same pathway (3, 4). After processing by dicer (4), the small RNAs bind to the RNA-induced silencing complex (RISC) (5) and regulate the protein expression posttranscriptionally.

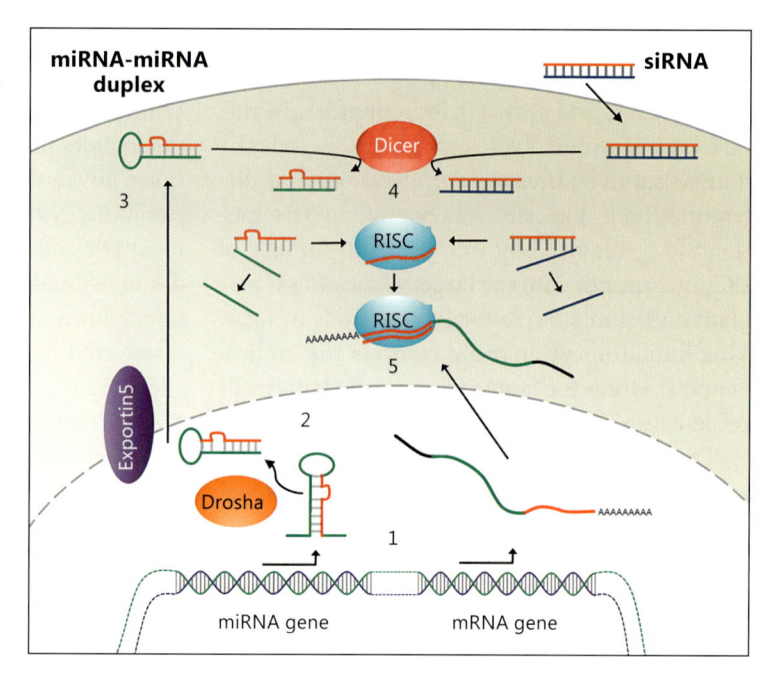

cently, siRNAs were developed that have neutral phosphotriester groups along their phosphate backbone (so-called siRNNs) [51]. The neutral phosphotriester groups prevent the molecules from degradation by nucleases. Additionally, the ability to cross a cellular membrane is increased. In a liver-directed in vivo experiment in mice, the siRNAs decreased the expression of a target gene by up to 60% compared to an siRNA that inhibited the expression by about 20% [51]. Modifications like this could pave the way for the systemic delivery of siRNAs and thus a targeted use of oligonucleotides in disease treatment. A putative performance-enhancing siRNA could target EgIN prolyl hydroxylases. Systemic administration to murine liver cells led to a significant improvement in red blood cell production [52]. The effect of these siRNAs after systemic administration in humans is not yet known and could mediate off-target effects and cytotoxicity-reducing sports performance.

New Techniques on the Horizon: Gene Editing

In 2012, the field of molecular biology was once again revolutionized with the discovery of gene-editing technology CRISPR/Cas9 [53]. Briefly, bacteria use this enzyme to cut the DNA of parasites such as viruses. After an infection, the bacteria retain DNA of the viruses and store them in the bacterium's own genome called the CRISPR locus. After transcription into RNA, Cas9 uses this CRISPR RNA (crRNA) as a guiding RNA. If there is a match between crRNA and DNA, the Cas9 enzyme cuts the DNA [54]. In 2012, Jinek et al. [53] showed that it was possible to cut DNA in vitro using the Cas9 with a single guide RNA that can be programmed with custom-designed crRNAs. This development has led to a flurry of investigations and the use of CRISPR for targeted deletion of DNA as well as DNA replacement. Compared to former genome-editing methods, including zinc finger nucleases and TALEN-mediated gene editing, the CRISPR system is easy to produce and enables precise genome modifications [55]. CRISPR/Cas9 has enormous potential within the different fields of gene therapy. These include ex vivo cell therapies using HSCs and iPSCs. In 2015, the CRISPR system was used to modify human nonviable embryos (triponuclear zygotes) [56]. The study included 86 embryos aiming to edit the human β-globin gene. After 48 h, 71 embryos survived, and 54 were genetically tested. Of these, 28 were spliced successfully while only 4 embryos showed the introduction of the desired genetic material. Importantly, large amounts of off-target mutations were also introduced by unspecific restriction of the CRISPR/Cas9 system. Recently, Kleinstiver et al. [57] engineered a so-called high-fidelity CRISPR/Cas9 nuclease that has improved specificity and, therefore, less induction of off-target effects. After manipulating human cancer cells with the engineered CRISPR system, GUIDE-seq experiments and targeted next generation sequencing (NGS) revealed that the off-target effects could be eliminated almost entirely [57]. However, the off-target effects are still a major safety concern [58]. As CRISPR technology could lead to successful modification of the DNA in embryos or the germline, this raises significant ethical concerns [59, 60]. Most notably, the germline modifications could be inherited to the next generation.

In principle, CRISPR could be used to design babies with the intention to produce a high-performance athlete. However, the possibility that designer babies become a reality in the world of sport in the next few decades is unlikely. Relevant candidates are, for example, *MSTN*, *EPOR*, *IGF1*, and *FST* [17]. However, due to the complexity of the genome and the tightly regulated orchestration during embryo development, even small changes can have large unknown effects [61]. It remains to be determined if these effects are replicated in humans. The most relevant targets for genetic manipulation would be the naturally occurring mutations, including *MSTN* and *EPOR*. As summarized by Lee [62], different naturally occurring mutations in the *MSTN* gene were discovered in animals, including whippet dogs [11] and humans [12]. In 2007, Mosher et al. [11] quantitatively linked the MSTN mutation with sprinting performance among 85 whippets that were homozygote or heterozygote for a *MSTN* loss-of-function mutation. Dogs with the homozygous mutation in the *MSTN* gene were over-muscled. The heterozygote dogs were among the fastest, but not all of the dogs were faster than the dogs without the mutation [11]. On the one hand, this highlights the need for optimization instead of maximization in sports to reach maximal performance. Secondly, even with the favorable genotype for a single gene, high-level performance is not guaranteed. In addition to greater muscle size, superior sprinting performance is envisaged to require a certain muscle fiber type distribution, tendon flexibility and stability, as well as an optimized metabolism. Sports performance is highly complex, and the modification of a small number of genes does not guarantee high-level performance [63]. In addition to the genetic manipulation of embryos, CRISPR could be used for somatic gene therapy, e.g., the use of CRISPR-guided cell modifications in a grown organism. However, it remains questionable if the efficacy is high enough to yield therapeutic effects. A major limitation is the difficulty to target sufficient amounts of tissue, e.g., muscle tissue [64].

Development of a Gene Doping Test

Despite the difficulties and limitations previously described, a number of examples underline that members of the athlete's entourage in elite sports are prepared to exploit pharmaceutical and biotechnological drug inventions [65]. Currently, there is no evidence that gene doping is being used to enhance sporting performance. However, further advances might render gene therapeutic approaches more attractive for doping purposes. Hence, it is important that the anti-doping authorities continue to respond in a proactive rather than reactive way. Reliable and legally defensible gene doping detection assays are critical to discourage athletes from using gene transfer technologies.

Indirect and Direct Detection of Gene Doping
Since the introduction of doping tests at the Olympic Games in 1968, a large number of sophisticated direct and indirect doping detection approaches have been introduced. The direct detection approaches aim to identify prohibited substances or their metabolites in biological fluids like urine or blood. The use of chromatography coupled with mass spectrometry revolutionized the detectability of a large number of exogenous substances [see chapter by Bowers and Bigard, this vol., pp. 77–90]. However, in some cases, direct detectability is difficult or impossible, especially for substances that are identical to endogenously produced substances [66]. With the implementation of indirect detection strategies, some of the difficulties of direct testing could potentially be overcome. The idea is to screen for biological markers that are indicative for doping. Since the introduction of an athlete biological passport (ABP), a hematological module and a steroidal module are used to analyze the data of athletes longitudinally [67]. For example, the application of *EPO* gene doping could potentially be detected with the hematological module of the ABP. This would require an "abnormal" variation in the approved ABP markers such as reticulocytes and hemoglobin mass. While the sensitivity of detection can be hampered by applying strategies such as microdosing to increase serum EPO levels only slightly over time, or instigating blood draws and making infusions to minimize the EPO effects on the ABP parameters, there are approaches specifically aimed at identifying these manipulations Arguably, a more substantive problem of all the indirect tests is the lack of potential to demonstrate specificity of the test for doping. Nevertheless, it is widely acknowledged that the introduction of the ABP has been a valuable tool in the fight against doping in sports [68] [see chapter by Robinson et al., this vol., pp. 107–118].

An alternative indirect method to detect doping is the so-called "omic" approach [69]. The idea is that doping leads to distinct expression patterns in omic measures such as in the transcriptome, the proteome, or the metabolome. Intra-individual variations in these omic measures when implemented in the ABP would lead to improved detection [67]. Some support for this idea is beginning to emerge. For example, the transcriptional profiling of the whole blood transcriptome in European and Kenyan endurance-trained athletes before, during, and after high-dose injections of recombinant human EPO revealed 34 significantly expressed transcripts [70]. Further research is ongoing to validate these biomarkers against internal and external influences to protect against false positives. A major limitation of this and all other indirect detection strategies is that these methods do not identify the manipulation per se (e.g., drug or gene doping) but are an indication of doping albeit with a high level of probability [see chapter by Wang et al., this vol., pp. 119–128].

Detection of Transgenic Proteins
A test for the detection of transgenic proteins was first proposed in 2004 [71]. Lasne et al. [71] transduced a macaque with an AAV vector intramuscularly containing macaque *EPO* cDNA and subsequently analyzed the isoelectric focusing patterns of EPO isoforms in serum before and after gene transfer. Intriguingly, the authors discovered that the isoelectric patterns of serum EPO differed after intramuscular gene transfer. This was a result of different posttranscriptional glycosylation of the EPO molecules that can vary between cells and tissues [71]. While the application of these EPO results to humans can only be assumed, a human growth hormone (hGH) isoform test was successfully applied in humans to detect hGH doping. The hGH test depends on the detection of the different isoforms of hGH (22- vs. 20-kDa forms) in plasma [72]. Theoretically, if gene doping is ap-

plied with the 22-kDa variant, a shift in the ratio could be detected. It is not clear, however, if the ratio would be distinguishable from naturally occurring ratios. The detection of transgenic protein is further hampered by the fact that these assumptions cannot be generalized to all possible gene doping candidates. For its direct detection, a transgenic protein would need to undergo posttranscriptional modification, and it needs to be detectable in the blood. Furthermore, transcriptional modification may differ depending on the gene transfer protocol, the route of vector administration, the vector used, and the target tissue. These many unknowns remain to be resolved in humans.

The Present Stage of Direct Detection of Gene Doping including siRNA and Transgene Molecules

Kohler et al. [73] and Thomas et al. [74] established a mass-spectrometric assay for the detection of siRNA oligonucleotides with and without common molecule modifications. In a proof-of-concept study, 6 rats received high doses of siRNA with the intention to interfere with *MSTN* mRNA [74]. The detection of the RNA was possible for up to 24 h in urine but was undetectable after 33 h. This detection window of approximately 0–30 h [74] may suffice as RNAi therapeutics need to be used more frequently depending on their stability. These results provide evidence that siRNA-mediated gene doping and also other siRNAs including different kinds of modifications are detectable. The assays need to be established for relevant siRNA molecules. Therefore, it is mandatory to follow up siRNAs that are used in clinical trials and might induce performance-enhancing effects.

An approach designed to detect transgenic DNA (tDNA) molecules that serve as a template for the production of potentially performance-enhancing transgenic proteins was published in 2008 [75]. Naturally occurring genomic DNA (gDNA) contains exonic and intronic sequences. As a result of posttranslational modifications, only exonic regions are translated into protein. Due to safety concerns and packaging constraints of vector systems, tDNA contains only exons. To distinguish between gDNA and tDNA, specific PCR assays can be developed using primers or probes that exclusively bind at exon-exon junctions. In recent years, different PCR-based approaches have been developed, including quantitative PCR (qPCR) [76, 77], nested PCR [78], nested qPCR [79], and digital droplet PCR [80].

Currently, the nested qPCR approach represents the most relevant strategy for low copy number transgene detection. Compared to other PCR-based approaches, especially one-round PCR approaches, this method has the highest sensitivity, thus favoring long-term detection, and has a limit of quantification established by in vivo testing warranting a high enough specificity to objectively control for and avoid false positives, if such a technique is introduced into sports [79].

The ability to detect transgene molecules in relevant gene doping scenarios has been validated in a number of animal models. After intramuscular injection of rAAV vector systems containing the *EPO* gene, the transgene molecules could be detected for up to 57 weeks in blood cells of nonhuman primates [77]. It is noteworthy that the period of possible transgene detection goes along with the transduction efficiency. Higher transduction efficacies and less immune reaction against the gene transfer procedure lead to longer cell survival and hence to longer detectability of the transgene in principle. A unique advantage of the PCR-based detection approach is that it can be adapted for all tDNA targets that might be misused for performance-enhancing purposes. In contrast to classical pharmaceuticals, however, our expectation is that successful abuse of this technology will be restricted primarily to those procedures that have an approval for clinical use, given the high risk of serious side effects of nonestablished approaches.

During the last decade, NGS technology became widely available and offers a rapid and cost-effective technology for whole genome sequencing [81]. Especially in the field of personalized medicine, NGS shows clinical relevance [82]. Furthermore, the technology can be used effectively to monitor genetically modified organisms [83]. For the detection of gene doping, the NGS technology sounds very appealing because all different kinds of gene doping would be detectable in principle. However, a number of pitfalls hamper its direct applicability, especially for viral vector-mediated gene doping detection. Biodistribution studies in animals and humans show that the detectability of transgenic molecules in serum are restricted to several days or weeks [84, 85], whereas the transgene can be detected in blood cells for months up to years [77, 85]. According to the high level of gDNA background in whole blood, the required sequencing coverage is prohibitive for NGS. Consequently, targeted sequencing or more relevantly PCR-based pre-amplification is required, and relevant assays need to be established, increasing costs and handling time.

Gene Doping: The Future of Doping?

A careful examination of the recent history of doping in elite sports reveals that athletes seem to have a preference for doping procedures that are timely and not detectable. Such procedures can involve drugs and methods with more or less unknown side effects, such as the designer steroid THG (tetrahydrogestrinone) or the use of artificial oxygen carriers. Furthermore, evidence from doping cases such as BALCO (Bay Area Laboratory Co-Operative) [86] and the Lance Armstrong scandals [87] demonstrates that athletes are willing to take all kinds of combinations of drugs and methods in the quest for performance enhancement with minimal risk of detection [87]. If and when gene doping could become a method of choice for athletes remains impossible to determine. However, the timing is likely to depend on the risk-benefit perception of the doping athlete and their entourage. Potential health risks might be accepted within certain limits, whereas potential decreases in physical performance as a result of gene therapeutic intervention is unlikely to be accepted.

The so-called Goldman dilemma assumes that about half of the elite athletes would accept death in 5 years for a doping procedure that would warrant victory [88]. However, this concept may not be universally accepted. More recently, an Australian working group surveyed 212 track and field athletes for the Goldman dilemma [89]. They reported that only approximately 1% of athletes would accept death after 5 years according to the original question of the Goldman dilemma. Between 5.5 and 6.8% would accept the death after 5 years if the method (the "magic drug") would be legal [89]. Despite the percentage of 1–7% is considerably less than 52%, this is still an alarmingly high number of athletes who would accept death after 5 years for Olympic success.

As stated previously, clinically approved gene or stem cell therapeutic procedures will most likely not be an attractive option for doping purposes in elite athletes. This issue is primary driven by possible side effects that outweigh the potential for performance enhancement. Most of the gene transfer technology has been developed to treat fatally ill patients. These approaches are primarily disease specific and not designed to evoke a performance-enhancing effect in healthy athletes. At present, there are only two 2 therapeutic procedures that are clinically approved in Western countries targeting rare diseases [31, 90]. A single treatment with the gene therapeutic drug Glybera costs about EUR 1 million [29] and does not offer any performance-enhancing effect. However, other medications may follow, which may have the potential to enhance performance but will come at about the same price and with similar recommendations to ensure effectiveness and safety of treatment. Of course, the drug should only be applied by experienced gene therapists and will require emergency medical monitoring as well as immunosuppressive treatment. Anticipated frequent side effects of the treatment include headaches, fatigue, pain in the extremities, and fever [91]. Moreover, the effectiveness of the drug is still a matter of debate. We can envision that even if a potential gene therapeutic drug hits the market, dopers will not be very enthusiastic about it.

While gene doping procedures appear to be a rather unlikely choice for a person that is searching for the ultimate doping endeavor, there is a plethora of nondetectable conventional pharmaceuticals that include a number of peptide hormones. Moreover, there is some evidence of performance enhancement with conventional pharmaceuticals while maintaining the perception that potential short- and medium-term side effects are within an acceptable range, allowing the athlete to train and finally compete with an increased performance [92]. Today, attempts to escape doping tests can be achieved by organizing the doping and the dosing in a sophisticated way. This includes the use of doping substances with microdoses, making the detection more difficult [93]. Moreover, use of substances like recombinant human IGF-1, human insulin, and testosterone synthesized with a close to human carbon isotope ratio can be misused [87, 94] to favor doping escape strategies.

Conclusion

Just like the clinical introduction of gene therapy took roughly 40 years, it may now take another 20 years before gene therapeutic technology is a real option for doping in sport. One of the most crucial factors arguing against the application of gene transfer or stem cell therapy in healthy athletes for performance enhancement is that these therapies are designed to treat severely diseased individuals, and currently these methods are accompanied by serious side effects that could reduce physical performance. For classical, viral vector-mediated gene therapeutic approaches, the dose-response effects are still unknown, and the efficacy of the treatment remains questionable in healthy humans and especially in trained athletes. Typically, the field of virus-mediated gene therapy is struggling with inefficient gene transfer in humans. This reduces the attraction of this technology for gene doping. Future advances in vector designs may improve the efficacy of gene transfer technology, making it reasonable to develop detection strategies that can be adapted for reasonable targets. The recent success in siRNA therapy, especially in targeting the liver, makes it worthwhile to further develop strategies for the detection of different kinds of siRNA molecules. Stem cell therapy without genetic modifications in the cells appears unlikely to enhance performance capacity. The risk-benefit ratio to genetically modify these cells is unfavorable, especially because the number of cells that integrate is low. Stem cell doping may be able to modify the regenerative capacity after injury. However, once this is demonstrated in a clinical context, it would simply become a standard therapy. Indisputably, the breakthrough of the CRISPR/Cas9 system in 2012 was an enormous step into the direction of targeted and precise gene editing that may be misused for germline editing. However, sports performance is a very complex phenotypic trait, and the modification of a small number of genes does not guarantee high-level performance. The most concerning aspect is that CRISPR/Cas9 is a cheap, easily accessible, and usable method. At this time, the most important issue that renders gene doping scenarios less feasible is the fact that the expected positive effects of the treatment will most likely not outperform the typical effects that can be achieved with conventional doping strategies. Therefore, a major challenge facing antidoping in the future will be the use of modern molecular therapies along with unique ways to produce drugs, and especially human hormones, in a manner that renders them undetectable by direct detection approaches. Gene doping will not lead to the situation of "super humans" entering and disturbing the field of elite sports. The magnitude of gene doping effects may not even reach the levels that have already been achieved by potent natural doping substances like testosterone. The aspects that should worry us the most when it comes to gene or cell doping procedures are simply ethical as well as safety- and health-related issues. It is, therefore, advisable that the sports world is seeking the help of gene and cell therapeutic communities to make sure that the abuse of this technology remains an unlikely scenario.

References

1 Friedmann T, Koss JO: Gene transfer and athletics – an impending problem. Mol Ther 2001;3:819–820.
2 Friedmann T: How close are we to gene doping? Hastings Cent Rep 2010;40:20–22.
3 Thompson H: Performance enhancement: superhuman athletes. Nature 2012;487:287–289.
4 Montgomery HE, Marshall R, Hemingway H, Myerson S, Clarkson P, Dollery C, Hayward M, Holliman DE, Jubb M, World M, Thomas EL, Brynes AE, Saeed N, Barnard M, Bell JD, Prasad K, Rayson M, Talmud PJ, Humphries SE: Human gene for physical performance. Nature 1998;393:221–222.
5 Wood AR, Esko T, Yang J, Vedantam S, Pers TH, Gustafsson S, Chu AY, Estrada K, Luan J, Kutalik Z, Amin N, Buchkovich ML, Croteau-Chonka DC, Day FR, Duan Y, Fall T, Fehrmann R, Ferreira T, Jackson AU, Karjalainen J, et al: Defining the role of common variation in the genomic and biological architecture of adult human height. Nat Genet 2014;46:1173–1186.
6 Locke AE, Kahali B, Berndt SI, Justice AE, Pers TH, Day FR, Powell C, Vedantam S, Buchkovich ML, Yang J, Croteau-Chonka DC, Esko T, Fall T, Ferreira T, Gustafsson S, Kutalik Z, Luan J, Magi R, Randall JC, Winkler TW, et al: Genetic studies of body mass index yield new insights for obesity biology. Nature 2015;518:197–206.
7 Rankinen T, Fuku N, Wolfarth B, Wang G, Sarzynski MA, Alexeev DG, Ahmetov II, Boulay MR, Cieszczyk P, Eynon N, Filipenko ML, Garton FC, Generozov EV, Govorun VM, Houweling PJ, Kawahara T, Kostryukova ES, Kulemin NA, Larin AK, Maciejewska-Karlowska A, et al: No evidence of a common DNA variant profile specific to world class endurance athletes. PLoS One 2016;11:e0147330.
8 Bouchard C: Exercise genomics – a paradigm shift is needed: a commentary. Br J Sports Med 2015;49:1492–1496.
9 Ritchie MD, Holzinger ER, Li R, Pendergrass SA, Kim D: Methods of integrating data to uncover genotype-phenotype interactions. Nat Rev Genet 2015;16:85–97.
10 Ehlert T, Simon P, Moser DA: Epigenetics in sports. Sports Med 2013;43:93–110.
11 Mosher DS, Quignon P, Bustamante CD, Sutter NB, Mellersh CS, Parker HG, Ostrander EA: A mutation in the myostatin gene increases muscle mass and enhances racing performance in heterozygote dogs. PLoS Genet 2007;3:e79.
12 Schuelke M, Wagner KR, Stolz LE, Hubner C, Riebel T, Komen W, Braun T, Tobin JF, Lee SJ: Myostatin mutation associated with gross muscle hypertrophy in a child. N Engl J Med 2004;350:2682–2688.
13 Juvonen E, Ikkala E, Fyhrquist F, Ruutu T: Autosomal dominant erythrocytosis caused by increased sensitivity to erythropoietin. Blood 1991;78:3066–3069.
14 Jelkmann W, Lundby C: Blood doping and its detection. Blood 2011;118:2395–2404.
15 Baoutina A, Alexander IE, Rasko JE, Emslie KR: Developing strategies for detection of gene doping. J Gene Med 2008;10:3–20.
16 Haisma HJ, de Hon O: Gene doping. Int J Sports Med 2006;27:257–266.
17 van der Gronde T, de Hon O, Haisma HJ, Pieters T: Gene doping: an overview and current implications for athletes. Br J Sports Med 2013;47:670–678.
18 Wells DJ: Gene doping: the hype and the reality. Br J Pharmacol 2008;154:623–631.
19 Schneider AJ, Friedmann T: Gene doping in sports: the science and ethics of genetically modified athletes. Adv Genet 2006;51:1–110.
20 World Anti-Doping Agency: WADA Prohibited List. Montreal, WADA, 2004, https://wada-main-prod.s3.amazonaws.com/resources/files/WADA_Prohibited_List_2004_EN.pdf (accessed February 21, 2017).
21 Reynolds G: Outlaw DNA. The New York Times, June 3, 2007, http://www.nytimes.com/2007/06/03/sports/playmagazine/0603play-hot.html (accessed February 21, 2017).
22 Hayden EC: RNA interference rebooted. Nature 2014;508:443.
23 Lundin KE, Gissberg O, Smith CI: Oligonucleotide therapies: the past and the present. Hum Gene Ther 2015;26:475–485.
24 Thieme D: Labordiagnostische Ansätze zum Nachweis von Gendoping; in Körner S, Erber-Schropp JM (eds): Gendoping. Wiesbaden, Springer Spektrum, 2016.
25 Gene Therapy Clinical Trials Worldwide. J Gene Med, 2016, http://www.abedia.com/wiley/years.php (accessed February 21, 2017).
26 Kay MA: State-of-the-art gene-based therapies: the road ahead. Nat Rev Genet 2011;12:316–328.
27 Nayerossadat N, Maedeh T, Ali PA: Viral and nonviral delivery systems for gene delivery. Adv Biomed Res 2012;1:27.
28 Mingozzi F, Buning H: Adeno-associated viral vectors at the frontier between tolerance and immunity. Front Immunol 2015;6:120.
29 Naldini L: Gene therapy returns to centre stage. Nature 2015;526:351–360.
30 Raper SE, Chirmule N, Lee FS, Wivel NA, Bagg A, Gao GP, Wilson JM, Batshaw ML: Fatal systemic inflammatory response syndrome in a ornithine transcarbamylase deficient patient following adenoviral gene transfer. Mol Genet Metab 2003;80:148–158.

31 Bryant LM, Christopher DM, Giles AR, Hinderer C, Rodriguez JL, Smith JB, Traxler EA, Tycko J, Wojno AP, Wilson JM: Lessons learned from the clinical development and market authorization of Glybera. Hum Gene Ther Clin Dev 2013;24:55–64.

32 Mendell JR, Sahenk Z, Malik V, Gomez AM, Flanigan KM, Lowes LP, Alfano LN, Berry K, Meadows E, Lewis S, Braun L, Shontz K, Rouhana M, Clark KR, Rosales XQ, Al-Zaidy S, Govoni A, Rodino-Klapac LR, Hogan MJ, Kaspar BK: A phase 1/2a follistatin gene therapy trial for Becker muscular dystrophy. Mol Ther 2015;23:192–201.

33 Chenuaud P, Larcher T, Rabinowitz JE, Provost N, Cherel Y, Casadevall N, Samulski RJ, Moullier P: Autoimmune anemia in macaques following erythropoietin gene therapy. Blood 2004;103: 3303–3304.

34 Gao G, Lebherz C, Weiner DJ, Grant R, Calcedo R, McCullough B, Bagg A, Zhang Y, Wilson JM: Erythropoietin gene therapy leads to autoimmune anemia in macaques. Blood 2004;103:3300–3302.

35 Snyder RO, Flotte TR: Production of clinical-grade recombinant adeno-associated virus vectors. Curr Opin Biotechnol 2002;13:418–423.

36 Trounson A, McDonald C: Stem cell therapies in clinical trials: progress and challenges. Cell Stem Cell 2015;17:11–22.

37 World Health Organization: Haematopoietic Stem Cell Transplantation HSCtx. Geneva, WHO, 2016, http://www.who.int/transplantation/hsctx/en/ (accessed February 21, 2017).

38 Biasco L, Baricordi C, Aiuti A: Retroviral integrations in gene therapy trials. Mol Ther 2012;20:709–716.

39 Mullard A: EMA greenlights second gene therapy. Nat Rev Drug Discov 2016;15:299.

40 Gaspar HB: Gene therapy for ADA-SCID: defining the factors for successful outcome. Blood 2012;120:3628–3629.

41 Holzinger A, Barden M, Abken H: The growing world of CAR T cell trials: a systematic review. Cancer Immunol Immunother 2016;65:1433–1450.

42 Dimmeler S, Ding S, Rando TA, Trounson A: Translational strategies and challenges in regenerative medicine. Nat Med 2014;20:814–821.

43 Osborne H, Anderson L, Burt P, Young M, Gerrard D: Australasian College of Sports Physicians-position statement: the place of mesenchymal stem/stromal cell therapies in sport and exercise medicine. Br J Sports Med 2016;50:1237–1244.

44 Takahashi K, Yamanaka S: Induction of pluripotent stem cells from mouse embryonic and adult fibroblast cultures by defined factors. Cell 2006;126:663–676.

45 Matsu-Ura T, Sasaki H, Okada M, Mikoshiba K, Ashraf M: Attenuation of teratoma formation by p27 overexpression in induced pluripotent stem cells. Stem Cell Res Ther 2016;7:30.

46 Goodchild J: Therapeutic oligonucleotides. Methods Mol Biol 2011;764:1–15.

47 Kohler M, Schanzer W, Thevis M: RNA interference for performance enhancement and detection in doping control. Drug Test Anal 2011;3:661–667.

48 Kozomara A, Griffiths-Jones S: miRBase: integrating microRNA annotation and deep-sequencing data. Nucleic Acids Res 2011;39:D152–D157.

49 Friedman RC, Farh KKH, Burge CB, Bartel DP: Most mammalian mRNAs are conserved targets of microRNAs. Genome Res 2009;19:92–105.

50 Kanasty R, Dorkin JR, Vegas A, Anderson D: Delivery materials for siRNA therapeutics. Nat Mater 2013;12:967–977.

51 Meade BR, Gogoi K, Hamil AS, Palm-Apergi C, van den Berg A, Hagopian JC, Springer AD, Eguchi A, Kacsinta AD, Dowdy CF, Presente A, Lonn P, Kaulich M, Yoshioka N, Gros E, Cui XS, Dowdy SF: Efficient delivery of RNAi prodrugs containing reversible charge-neutralizing phosphotriester backbone modifications. Nat Biotechnol 2014;32:1256–1261.

52 Querbes W, Bogorad RL, Moslehi J, Wong J, Chan AY, Bulgakova E, Kuchimanchi S, Akinc A, Fitzgerald K, Koteliansky V, William GW: Treatment of erythropoietin deficiency in mice with systemically administered siRNA. Blood 2012;120:1916–1922.

53 Jinek M, Chylinski K, Fonfara I, Hauer M, Doudna JA, Charpentier E: A programmable dual-RNA-guided DNA endonuclease in adaptive bacterial immunity. Science 2012;337:816–821.

54 Urnov F: The domestication of Cas9. Nature 2016;529:468–469.

55 Gaj T, Gersbach CA, Barbas CF 3rd: ZFN, TALEN, and CRISPR/Cas-based methods for genome engineering. Trends Biotechnol 2013;31:397–405.

56 Liang P, Xu Y, Zhang X, Ding C, Huang R, Zhang Z, Lv J, Xie X, Chen Y, Li Y, Sun Y, Bai Y, Songyang Z, Ma W, Zhou C, Huang J: CRISPR/Cas9-mediated gene editing in human tripronuclear zygotes. Protein Cell 2015;6:363–372.

57 Kleinstiver BP, Pattanayak V, Prew MS, Tsai SQ, Nguyen NT, Zheng ZL, Joung JK: High-fidelity CRISPR-Cas9 nucleases with no detectable genome-wide off-target effects. Nature 2016;529:490–495.

58 Tsai SQ, Joung JK: Defining and improving the genome-wide specificities of CRISPR-Cas9 nucleases. Nat Rev Genet 2016;17:300–312.

59 Caplan AL, Parent B, Shen M, Plunkett C: No time to waste – the ethical challenges created by CRISPR: CRISPR/Cas, being an efficient, simple, and cheap technology to edit the genome of any organism, raises many ethical and regulatory issues beyond the use to manipulate human germ line cells. EMBO Rep 2015;16:1421–1426.

60 Bosley KS, Botchan M, Bredenoord AL, Carroll D, Charo RA, Charpentier E, Cohen R, Corn J, Doudna J, Feng GP, Greely HT, Isasi R, Ji WZ, Kim JS, Knoppers B, Lanphier E, Li JS, Lovell-Badge R, Martin GS, Moreno J, et al: CRISPR germline engineering – the community speaks. Nat Biotechnol 2015;33:478–486.

61 Baltimore D, Berg P, Botchan M, Carroll D, Charo RA, Church G, Corn JE, Daley GQ, Doudna JA, Fenner M, Greely HT, Jinek M, Martin GS, Penhoet E, Puck J, Sternberg SH, Weissman JS, Yamamoto KR: A prudent path forward for genomic engineering and germline gene modification. Science 2015;348:36–38.

62 Lee SJ: Sprinting without myostatin: a genetic determinant of athletic prowess. Trends Genet 2007;23:475–477.

63 Mattsson CM, Wheeler MT, Waggott D, Caleshu C, Ashley EA: Sports genetics moving forward: lessons learned from medical research. Physiol Genomics 2016;48:175–182.

64 High K, Gregory PD, Gersbach C: CRISPR technology for gene therapy. Nat Med 2014;20:476–477.

65 Camporesi S, McNamee MJ: Performance enhancement, elite athletes and anti doping governance: comparing human guinea pigs in pharmaceutical research and professional sports. Philos Ethics Humanit Med 2014;9:4.

66 Robinson N, Saugy M, Vernec A, Pierre-Edouard S: The athlete biological passport: an effective tool in the fight against doping. Clin Chem 2011;57:830–832.

67 Pitsiladis YP, Durussel J, Rabin O: An integrative "omics" solution to the detection of recombinant human erythropoietin and blood doping. Br J Sports Med 2014;48:856–861.

68 Zorzoli M, Pipe A, Garnier PY, Vouillamoz M, Dvorak J: Practical experience with the implementation of an athlete's biological profile in athletics, cycling, football and swimming. Br J Sports Med 2014;48:862–866.

69 Friedmann T, Rabin O, Frankel MS: Ethics. Gene doping and sport. Science 2010;327:647–648.

70 Durussel J, Haile DW, Mooses K, Daskalaki E, Beattie W, Mooses M, Mekonen W, Ongaro N, Anjila E, Patel RK, Padmanabhan N, McBride MW, McClure JD, Pitsiladis YP: The blood transcriptional signature of recombinant human erythropoietin administration and implications for anti-doping strategies. Physiol Genomics 2016;48:202–209.

71 Lasne F, Martin L, de Ceaurriz J, Larcher T, Moullier P, Chenuaud P: "Genetic doping" with erythropoietin cDNA in primate muscle is detectable. Mol Ther 2004;10:409–410.

72 Bidlingmaier M, Suhr J, Ernst A, Wu Z, Keller A, Strasburger CJ, Bergmann A: High-sensitivity chemiluminescence immunoassays for detection of growth hormone doping in sports. Clin Chem 2009;55:445–453.

73 Kohler M, Thomas A, Walpurgis K, Schanzer W, Thevis M: Mass spectrometric detection of siRNA in plasma samples for doping control purposes. Anal Bioanal Chem 2010;398:1305–1312.

74 Thomas A, Walpurgis K, Delahaut P, Kohler M, Schanzer W, Thevis M: Detection of small interfering RNA (siRNA) by mass spectrometry procedures in doping controls. Drug Test Anal 2013;5:853–860.

75 Beiter T, Zimmermann M, Fragasso A, Armeanu S, Lauer UM, Bitzer M, Su H, Young WL, Niess AM, Simon P: Establishing a novel single-copy primer-internal intron-spanning PCR (spiPCR) procedure for the direct detection of gene doping. Exerc Immunol Rev 2008;14:73–85.

76 Baoutina A, Coldham T, Fuller B, Emslie KR: Improved detection of transgene and nonviral vectors in blood. Hum Gene Ther Methods 2013;24:345–354.

77 Ni W, Le Guiner C, Gernoux G, Penaud-Budloo M, Moullier P, Snyder RO: Longevity of rAAV vector and plasmid DNA in blood after intramuscular injection in nonhuman primates: implications for gene doping. Gene Ther 2011;18:709–718.

78 Beiter T, Zimmermann M, Fragasso A, Hudemann J, Niess AM, Bitzer M, Lauer UM, Simon P: Direct and long-term detection of gene doping in conventional blood samples. Gene Ther 2011;18:225–231.

79 Neuberger EW, Perez I, Le Guiner C, Moser D, Ehlert T, Allais M, Moullier P, Simon P, Snyder RO: Establishment of two quantitative nested qPCR assays targeting the human EPO transgene. Gene Ther 2016;23:330–339.

80 Moser DA, Braga L, Raso A, Zacchigna S, Giacca M, Simon P: Transgene detection by digital droplet PCR. PLoS One 2014;9:e111781.

81 Goodwin S, McPherson JD, McCombie WR: Coming of age: ten years of next-generation sequencing technologies. Nat Rev Genet 2016;17:333–351.

82 Rabbani B, Nakaoka H, Akhondzadeh S, Tekin M, Mahdieh N: Next generation sequencing: implications in personalized medicine and pharmacogenomics. Mol BioSyst 2016;12:1818–1830.

83 Willems S, Fraiture MA, Deforce D, De Keersmaecker SC, De Loose M, Ruttink T, Herman P, Van Nieuwerburgh F, Roosens N: Statistical framework for detection of genetically modified organisms based on next generation sequencing. Food Chem 2016;192:788–798.

84 Favre D, Provost N, Blouin V, Blacho G, Cherel Y, Salvetti A, Moullier P: Immediate and long-term safety of recombinant adeno-associated virus injection into the nonhuman primate muscle. Mol Ther 2001;4:559–566.

85 Manno CS, Pierce GF, Arruda VR, Glader B, Ragni M, Rasko JJ, Ozelo MC, Hoots K, Blatt P, Konkle B, Dake M, Kaye R, Razavi M, Zajko A, Zehnder J, Rustagi PK, Nakai H, Chew A, Leonard D, Wright JF, et al: Successful transduction of liver in hemophilia by AAV-factor IX and limitations imposed by the host immune response. Nat Med 2006;12:342–347.

86 Vogel G: A race to the starting line. Science 2004;305:632–635.

87 Report on Proceedings under the World Anti-Doping Code and the USADA Protocol. Colorado Springs, USADA, 2012, https://d3epuodzu3wuis.cloudfront.net/ReasonedDecision.pdf (accessed February 21, 2017).

88 Goldman B, Bush PJ, Klatz R: Death in the Locker Room: Steroids & Sports. South Bend, Icarus Press, 1984.

89 Connor J, Woolf J, Mazanov J: Would they dope? Revisiting the Goldman dilemma. Br J Sports Med 2013;47:697–700.

90 Scott CT, DeFrancesco L: Gene therapy's out-of-body experience. Nat Biotechnol 2016;34:600–607.

91 EMA: Glybera Summary of Product Characteristics. 2016, http://www.ema.europa.eu/docs/en_GB/document_library/EPAR_-_Product_Information/human/002145/WC500135472.pdf (accessed February 21, 2017).

92 Tentori L, Graziani G: Doping with growth hormone/IGF-1, anabolic steroids or erythropoietin: is there a cancer risk? Pharmacol Res 2007;55:359–369.

93 Morkeberg J: Blood manipulation: current challenges from an anti-doping perspective. Hematology Am Soc Hematol Educ Program 2013;2013:627–631.

94 Thevis M, Kuuranne T, Walpurgis K, Geyer H, Schanzer W: Annual banned-substance review: analytical approaches in human sports drug testing. Drug Test Anal 2016;8:7–29.

Prof. P. Simon
Department of Sports Medicine, Rehabilitation and Disease Prevention
Johannes Gutenberg University Mainz
Albert Schweitzer Street 22
DE–55128 Mainz (Germany)
E-Mail simonpe@uni-mainz.de

Next Generation Anti-Doping Approaches

The Athlete Biological Passport: How to Personalize Anti-Doping Testing across an Athlete's Career?

Neil Robinson[a] · Pierre-Edouard Sottas[b] · Yorck Olaf Schumacher[c]

[a]Swiss Laboratory for Doping Analyses, University Center of Legal Medicine, Geneva and Lausanne, Epalinges, and
[b]World Anti-Doping Agency, Lausanne, Switzerland; [c]Aspetar Orthopedic and Sports Medicine Hospital, Doha, Qatar

Abstract

For decades, drug testing has been the main instrument at the disposal of anti-doping authorities. The availability in the 1980s of substances identical to those produced by the human body, including the "big 3" (erythropoietin, testosterone, and growth hormone), necessitated a new paradigm in anti-doping. The athlete biological passport (ABP) is a new paradigm, complementary to traditional drug testing, based on the personalized monitoring of doping biomarkers. Athletes who abuse doping substances do so to trigger physiological changes that provide performance enhancement. The ABP aims to detect these changes through its 3 hematological, steroidal, and endocrine modules. Any deviation of a biomarker from what is expected in a healthy physiological condition can be attributable to doping or a medical condition, which, interestingly, is also the criterion used to define a banned substance. Recent advances in proteomics and metabolomics offer immense opportunities to enhance the ABP. The ABP shares multiple aspects with the present customization of health care and personalized medicine.

© 2017 S. Karger AG, Basel

The Concept of the Athlete Biological Passport

Given the constant development of new technologies and substances in medicine in general, it was inevitable that the conventional doping tests would require upgrading and modernization to become fit for purpose. Athletes were abusing substances that were near identical to endogenous constituents (e.g., autologous blood and recombinant human erythropoietin), which made direct detection difficult if not impossible (Table 1). However, it was clear that the effect of such doping substances would still be discernable as any effect on performance will most likely also cause variations in key biomarkers. The concept of the "athlete biological passport" (ABP) is therefore to detect such variations caused by doping through the longitudinal monitoring of such biomarkers.

To determine whether a variation in the ABP is normal for an athlete or not, each result is

Table 1. Various doping scandals and important milestones during the last 20–30 years in the fight against doping

When?	What?	Who?	How?
1984–1985	During the 1984 Summer Olympic Games in Los Angeles, many athletes were doped with blood transfusion; in 1985, the IOC banned transfusions (Eichner [1], 2007)	Apparently, 30% of all American cyclists got transfusions before competing; none of the athletes were banned as blood transfusions were not forbidden and could not be detected	Rumors indicating blood doping at the 1984 Summer Olympic Games appeared; Patrick McDonough admitted later to blood doping in 1984 and revealed that the US team was doing the same
1988	Doping scandal during the 1988 Summer Olympic Games in Seoul (Boudreau and Konzak [2], 1991)	Ben Johnson, a 100-m runner, was tested positive for stanozolol, a powerful anabolic agent	State-of-the-art technology was applied to detect anabolic agents in urine
1996–1997	To fight indirectly EPO abuse in sports, a very common drug used especially in endurance disciplines, some federations introduced a "no start" rule to prevent doped athletes to take part to sports events (Saugy et al. [3], 2009; Schumacher et al. [4], 2000)	FIS and UCI implemented the famous 17.0 g/dL hemoglobin and 50% hematocrit cutoff values	Unannounced blood tests were conducted prior to sports events to determine those athletes allowed to take part to the event or not
1998	Doping scandal during the 1998 Tour de France	The cycling team Festina medically doped its athletes	A medical team member was arrested by French customs officers while crossing the border with many banned products; 3 days later, he explained the doping habits set up by the team physician and supported by the team
1999	WADA is set up	IOC and intergovernmental organizations, governments, and public authorities put in place WADA	A World Conference on Doping was held in Lausanne in 1999; the basis of an independent agency was accepted by all stakeholders
2000–2001	One year after the scientific publication of the EPO urine test based on IEF, the first positive cases are declared (Lasne and de Ceaurriz [5], 2000)	The French anti-doping laboratory developed and validated the urine EPO test; UCI was the first federation to accept the test, and in 2001 the first positive cases were declared by the Lausanne anti-doping laboratory	Athletes with abnormal hematological data were selected for the EPO urine test; some urine samples tested positive for EPO using the IEF method
2002	The pharmaceutical industry and the US anti-doping laboratory worked together to fight second generation EPO	During the 2002 Winter Olympic Games in Salt Lake City, a top level cross-country skier was disqualified due to the abuse of darbepoetin α	During the Winter Games, an athlete had an isoelectric profile compared to data obtained by the US anti-doping laboratory and the pharmaceutical company Amgen; his urine was declared positive
2003	An undetectable anabolic designer steroid was produced and sold to top level athletes (Catlin et al. [6], 2004)	BALCO, a Californian company, was producing and selling THG to various top level athletes in athletics, baseball, boxing, football, and cycling	A whistle-blower gave the information to US authorities; then, the enquiry began, and the US anti-doping laboratory performed some urine reanalyses, and some samples tested positive for THG
2002–2004	Two years after the first publication of the flow cytometry approach to detect homologous blood transfusion, the first positive cases were declared (Nelson et al. [7], 2002)	The Australian research team developed and published the homologous blood transfusion test in 2002 and 2003; 1 year later, the Lausanne anti-doping laboratory validated, implemented, and declared the first anti-doping test in blood for homologous blood transfusion	Blood data were showing that athletes were not doping with EPO anymore, but with blood transfusion; a few positive cases were declared; this was very deterrent as homologous blood transfusion can be detected for a very long time
2004	The IOC decided to store all anti-doping samples collected during Olympic venues for future retrospective analyses	In collaboration with WADA, the IOC decided to set up this strategy as an additional anti-doping tool to prevent doping in the future	The IOC financed the shipment and the storage of all anti-doping samples for a period of 8 years

Table 1 (continued)

When?	What?	Who?	How?
2004–2008	Setup and implementation of the blood passport to fight blood doping (EPO and transfusion) (Sottas et al. [8], 2011; Robinson et al. [9], 2011; Zorzoli and Rossi [10], 2012)	WADA supported and helped to implement the blood passport	WADA and various stakeholders put their knowledge together and set up a frame for the blood passport; the official passport guidelines were then released
2004–2008	In agreement with WADA, the pharmaceutical industry worked hand by hand with anti-doping laboratories to set up an anti-doping test to detect third generation EPO (Lamon et al. [11]; Leuenberger et al. [12], 2011)	WADA, Roche, and the Lausanne anti-doping laboratory put resources together to have a test ready before CERA (a third generation EPO) was on the market	End of autumn 2008, the anti-doping test was ready and was applied retrospectively on all blood samples collected during the Summer Olympic Games in Beijing and the 2008 Tour de France; a few athletes were tested positive
2011	The first blood sample tested positive for hGH abuse was reported using the isoform test (Bidlingmaier et al. [13], 2009)	The London anti-doping laboratory performed the hGH test according to the rules in force settled by WADA	The London anti-doping laboratory applied the test as described by the manufacturer and found out that 1 athlete had his hGH ratio well above the cutoff limit
2012	The IOC launched the first batch of retrospective analyses of urine samples collected during the Summer Olympic Games in Athens	Some targeted samples were analyzed in the Lausanne anti-doping laboratory; specific methods were applied to these samples	An innovative long-term metabolite detection approach was developed jointly by the Moscow and Cologne laboratories; this method was applied and a few positive cases were reported
2012	The indirect biomarker approach was applied to fight hGH abuse; some athletes were tested positive with this new method	The London anti-doping laboratory performed the indirect approach hGH analyses	This method was applied on serum samples collected during the 2012 Summer Olympic Games in London; 2 athletes were tested positive
2014	In January 2014, the urine steroidal passport is launched to fight especially anabolic steroid abuse	All athletes with urine samples tested have their individual passport; athletes taking anabolic agents are identified immediately	All national and international federations as well as national anti-doping organizations using ADAMS have a passport implemented

ADAMS, anti-doping administration and management system; BALCO, Bay Area Laboratory Co-Operative; EPO, erythropoietin; FIS, International Skiing Federation; hGH, human growth hormone; IEF, isoelectric focusing; IOC, International Olympic Committee; THG, tetrahydrogestrinone; UCI, International Cycling Federation; WADA, World Anti-Doping Agency.

mathematically compared to the previous values of the same athlete. For this purpose, bayesian statistics are used [14]. Individual reference ranges for each athlete are calculated based on the athlete's own previous results (Fig. 1). These reference ranges are usually adjusted to indicate a 99 or 99.9% specificity for abnormality of a given result, i.e., if an athlete has a result beyond his individual limits ("atypical passport finding") set at 99%, the likelihood for this abnormality to occur assuming pure chance is 100:1, at 99.9%, it is 1,000:1. The calculations are performed automatically by a software system integrated into the anti-doping administration and management system (ADAMS) and provide an objective first identification of abnormal blood profiles. This is the first step of the ABP process illustrated in Figure 2.

In the next step, the blood profiles flagged as abnormal by the software are anonymously evaluated by experts (see below) who have to determine if:

- The values are an extreme of natural variation and are thus considered as normal.
- The values are suspicious, but no clear doping-specific pattern can be identified at this stage (further data are required).
- The values may be the result of the use of a prohibited substance or prohibited method (in this case, 2 further experts will anonymously

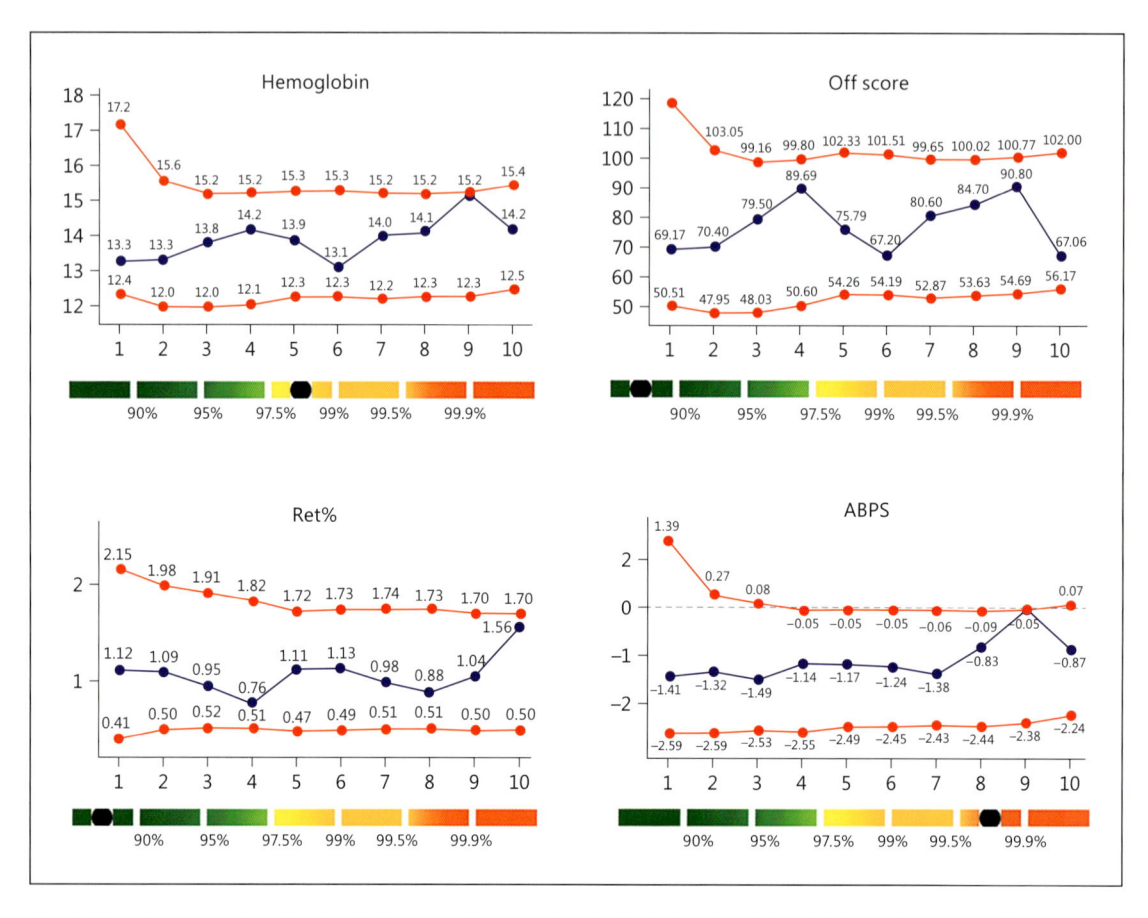

Fig. 1. Blood passport: longitudinal follow-up of the markers included in the athlete biological passport. The numbers on the horizontal axis represent the samples in chronological order, and the blue line shows the respective results. The red lines represent the individually calculated upper and lower reference limits for each marker. ABPS, abnormal blood profile score.

and independently review the data without access to the first expert's comment).
- The values might be a sign of a pathology.

If a profile is flagged as abnormal by the software and subsequently evaluated independently by 3 experts as possibly being caused by doping considering all aspects (including a detailed review of the sample quality together with the evaluation of the documentation packages for each sample), an "adverse passport finding" is declared, and the sporting body responsible for the athlete is informed [15, 16].

Ideally, these two first steps are performed independently from the sporting governing bodies by so-called "athlete passport management units (APMU)", which are responsible for managing the results of each athlete and the expert evaluation of the data. A second function of the ABP central to the APMU is the use of the results for improved conventional doping tests. Based on the results of the ABP tests and the evaluations of the experts for each profile, the APMU can recommend specific target testing schemes using conventional anti-doping tests to directly detect

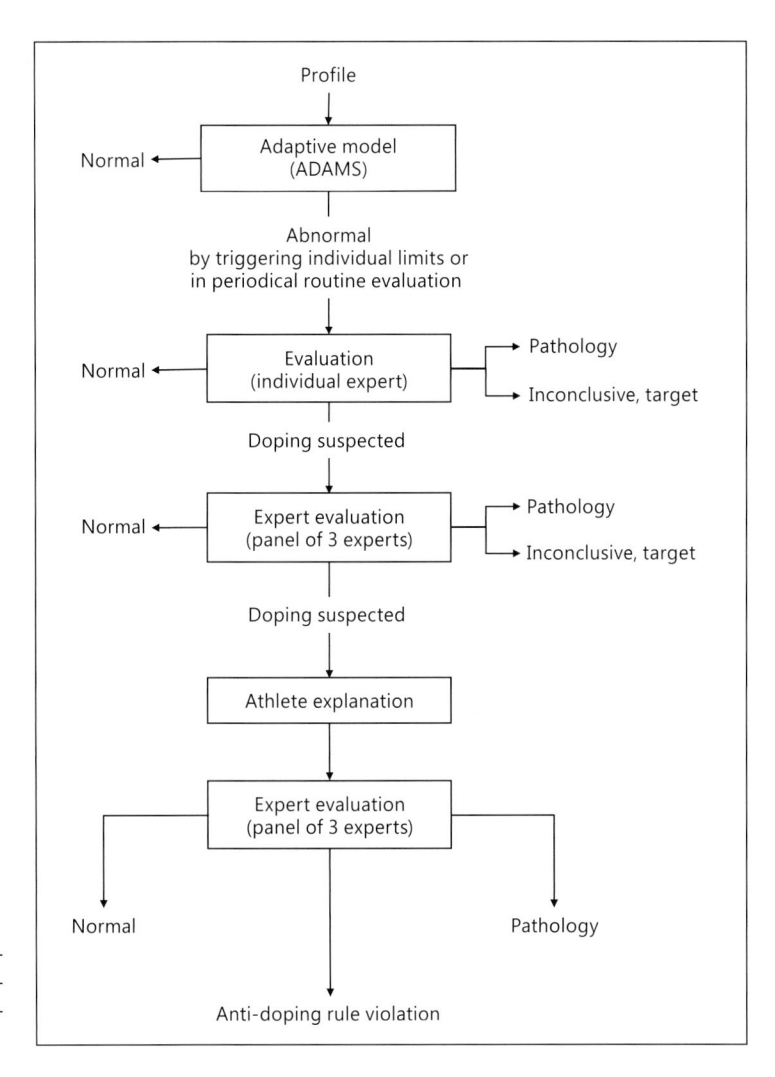

Fig. 2. Flowchart to detect anti-doping rule violation. ADAMS, anti-doping administration and management system.

forbidden substances in athletes displaying suspicious constellations in their profile. In recent years, such ABP-based target testing has led to a number of positive findings with conventional tests. This application constitutes another major strength of the passport approach. It can be expected that for the sophisticated doping athletes, this latter approach will be more relevant than the direct declaration of an anti-doping rule violation, which might be difficult when advanced doping schemes and strategies to avoid large variations in the profile are used.

The Hematological Module

For the purpose of detecting blood manipulations with erythropoietic stimulants such as erythropoietin (EPO) or blood transfusions, hemoglobin (Hb) concentration and reticulocyte levels were identified as potential biomarkers [17].

Markers and Analytics

Hb is the oxygen-carrying protein of the body. Increasing the amount of Hb allows an increase in oxygen transport capacity and ultimately an increase in performance. Thus, the ultimate aim of blood doping is to increase the body's Hb content.

Reticulocytes are young red blood cells that are in the last stage of their maturation, after being expelled from the bone marrow into peripheral blood. The life span of reticulocytes is only 1–2 days before they become mature erythrocytes. Reticulocyte percentage (Ret%) in peripheral blood will typically give an indication of the productive activity of the bone marrow. A high reticulocyte content indicates an increased red cell production of the marrow (for example stimulated by EPO, blood loss, or hypoxia), while a low reticulocyte content indicates reduced activity (when total red cell mass is increased above physiological levels and no red cell production is required).

From an analytical point of view, Hb is the most measured biochemical variable worldwide, and thus great efforts have been made to standardize its measurement. In contrast, reticulocyte analysis is not as standardized, and different analyzers might produce slightly different results. This fact has been circumvented by implementing a standardized hematology analyzer for all ABP analysis, which are only conducted in WADA-accredited and -approved laboratories. Stringent rules for blood sampling, sample processing, and evaluation of the results have been established to guarantee reliable results across all analyzing institutions [9]. Furthermore, all laboratories participate in a centralized monthly quality control scheme which guarantees the comparability of results between different analyzers.

Information obtained from Hb concentration and Ret% are supported by other blood measures such as mean corpuscular volume, mean corpuscular Hb (MCH), and MCH concentration of the red cell. Other variables are derived from these measured markers, i.e., the so-called "off score" (a combination of Hb and reticulocytes [18]) and the so-called "abnormal blood profile score" (a combination of hematocrit, Hb, red blood cell count, Ret%, mean corpuscular volume, MCH, and MCH concentration [19]) is also calculated to help with the evaluation.

Expert Evaluation
Every profile flagged as abnormal by the software algorithm will anonymously be submitted to independent experts for review to determine the cause of the abnormality. The experts ideally come from different, complementary fields of expertise to cover the different angles necessary to fully investigate an abnormal profile.

It is important that the experts provide a probability for each of the 4 causes of abnormality mentioned previously, while considering that one unlikely option does not make the other options more likely (so-called "prosecutor fallacy"). If the experts identify a profile as typical for doping, they should provide a so-called doping scenario, i.e., an example how the athlete has doped to display the data visible in the profile.

Critical Challenges
The main confounding factor for any biological marker measured as a concentration in blood (e.g., Hb) is the potential impact of plasma volume variations. Indeed, Hb cannot only change due to doping through the increase in the number of Hb molecules in the circulation through doping, but also through the variation in the liquid part of the blood, namely plasma volume. Such plasma volume shifts are triggered by exercise or environmental conditions, such as heat or altitude, stressors to which high performance athletes are often exposed. A critical challenge in the future will be to correct passport markers for these variations.

Another challenge is the integration of new markers into the hematological module. Given the stringent criteria for the inclusion of a marker for longitudinal monitoring, only a few variables are currently conceivable. Most of these are related to iron metabolism, and therefore blood production. However, more research is needed before any of these markers of iron metabolism can be introduced in practice.

The Steroidal Module

For many years, anabolic androgenic steroids were the most frequently banned substances reported by anti-doping laboratories [20]. To prevent testosterone misuse, Manfred Donike proposed in the early 1980s the T/E value, a ratio of glucuroconjugated testosterone (T) to epitestosterone (E). Unless this ratio was abnormally elevated due to physiological or pathological conditions, a ratio higher than 6 was highly likely due to an abuse of testosterone. The abuse of different testosterone formulations as well as the supplementary intake of various testosterone precursors questioned the validity of the T/E ratio [21]. For that reason, it was decided to include other inactive metabolites (androsterone, etiocholanolone, androstanediols [5αAdiol or 5βAdiol]) to constitute what is called the steroid profile. At that time (beginning 2000), indirect multiparametric approaches were not fully accepted by the scientific community involved in anti-doping analyses probably because gas chromatography/combustion/isotopic ratio mass spectrometry (GC/C/IRMS) analyses were supposed to be the ultimate direct detection tool to determine if testosterone was from endogenous or exogenous origin [22]. From 2004, a GC/C/IRMS analysis was performed on all samples presenting a T/E ratio greater than 4 or an abnormal metabolite concentration. It was found that indeed most healthy elite male Caucasian athletes have a T/E ratio close to 1.0, with a 95% cutoff value close to 4 [21]. It appeared that some healthy subjects had a T/E ratio well below 1.0 mainly due to a lower concentration of testosterone glucuronide. This phenotype is regularly observed in Asian populations, which has been explained by a deletion polymorphism (UGT2B17) decreasing significantly the activity of a specific enzyme (uridine diphosphoglucuronosyl transferase) [23]. With the support of scientists, anti-doping organizations decided to store steroidal profiles in simple databases such as Excel sheets to follow individual endogenous steroid data over time [24]. Except for a few cases (e.g., menstrual cycle and oral contraceptives), the individual T/E values did not deviate by more than 30% from the mean value. Steroid profiles were mainly used as a targeting tool to identify those athletes probably manipulating and requiring additional urine tests or specific GC/C/IRMS analyses. Table 2 shows the inadequacy of T/E values to detect some doping agents commonly used in sports, such as dehydroepiandrosterone and dihydrotestosterone.

Scientific research and the initial follow-up of steroid profiles enabled the identification of parameters that identified the abuse of testosterone and related compounds. This in-depth analysis revealed that some abnormal data were due to heterogeneous (e.g., sex, age, and genotype) and confounding factors [25]. Furthermore, steroid analyses conducted in different anti-doping laboratories also revealed that in some cases, the steroidal passports were flagged due to nonstandardized analytical procedures. For this reason, it was necessary to introduce protocols, such as the WADA Technical Documents (TD2016EAAS; https://www.wada-ama.org/sites/default/files/resources/files/wada-td2016eaas-eaas-measurement-and-reporting-en.pdf).

Currently, ADAMS sorts all information and integrates the urine steroid profile data from an athlete to generate the so-called steroidal passport, and the adaptive model is then used to calculate individual limits. If steroidal profile data fall outside individual limits, then the sample is flagged, and additional analyses are requested.

Figure 3 shows the steroidal profile of a male athlete tested 8 times. With the number of tests increasing, the adaptive model creates the steroidal passport and adapts the individual limits. Without much background information about

Table 2. Behavior of urine biomarkers following the intake of testosterone, dehydroepiandrosterone (DHEA), or dihydrotestosterone (DHT)

	A	Etio.	A/Etio.	E	T	T/E	A/T	5αAdiol	5βAdiol	5αAdiol/5β	5αAdiol/E
Oral/injection of T	+++	++	++		+++	+++	---	++	++		
Transdermal T	+++	++	++	--		++	++	++		++	+
DHEA	--	+++	--		+++	+++	---	+	+++		
DHT	+++		+++				++	++		++	++
Contraceptive pill				--		++					+
Ethanol	--	-			++	++	---				

Common confounding factors such as contraceptive pills and ethanol are shown to modify some of these biomarkers. A, androsterone; E, epitestosterone; Etio., etiocholanolone; T, testosterone.

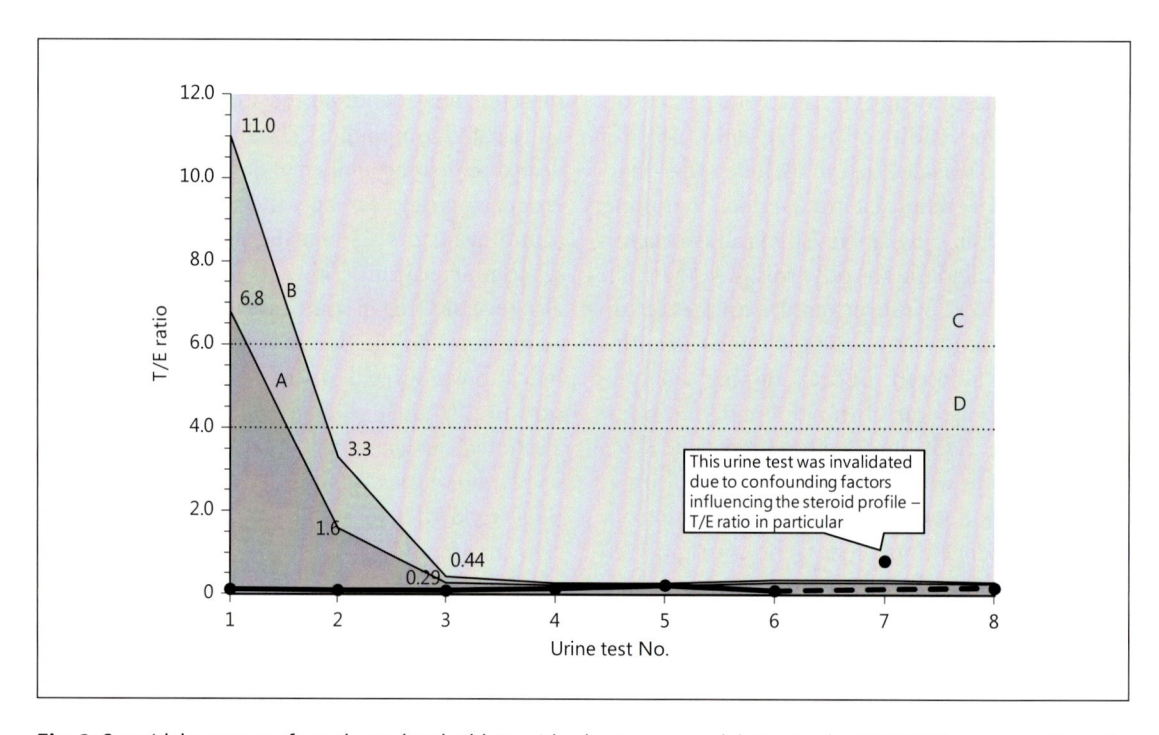

Fig. 3. Steroidal passport of a male top level athlete with a homozygous deletion in the UGT2B17 genotype. The athlete was tested 8 times with 1 invalid sample (sample 7 was invalidated: presence of ethanol, a confounding factor known to increase the testosterone/epitestosterone, T/E, ratio). Lines A and B correspond to the upper individual limits with a specificity of 99 and 99.9%, respectively. The T/E ratio for this subject should be within the dark gray zone taking into account pre-analytical, analytical (within- and between-laboratory variations), and biological variations. Horizontal lines C and D correspond to historical limits established at the time by Manfred Donike and WADA.

the athlete, initial limits (see test 1) are set on a population base with an upper limit of 6.8 and a lower limit of 0.05 (specificity of 99%; 11.0 and 0.02 for a specificity of 99.9%). This athlete has a mean T/E ratio of 0.12 (coefficient of variation = 37%). Prior reliance only on the Donike threshold (T/E = 6), which was adapted later on in 2004 (T/E = 4), this athlete could have doped with testosterone or related compounds without the possibility of being detected. Currently, the adaptive model would flag this athlete as suspicious. Any T/E ratio above 0.44 would lead first to a confirmation procedure (reanalysis of the sample) and then to a detailed examination of confounding factors. GC/C/IRMS analysis is conducted only if the confirmation procedure returns similar results as the initial testing.

Future

Endocrine Module

The steroidal module of the ABP is able to detect many forms of steroidal doping, direct or indirect, but it fails to detect other growth factors, such as growth hormone (GH), which is the goal of the more general endocrine module of the ABP. GH is a peptide hormone that presents several isoforms and whose main function is to stimulate cell growth and cell regeneration. GH has been abused in sports at least from the beginning of the 1980s, at a time where "cadaver GH" was extracted and purified from pituitary glands withdrawn from human cadavers. In 1985, GH was one of the first hormones to be produced by recombinant DNA technology. It was only in the mid-2000s that an anti-doping test based on the degenerated isoform pattern of recombinant GH was first introduced [13]. At the same time, interesting biomarkers of GH doping were discovered, including markers of GH action on the liver, such as insulin-like growth factor (IGF)-1 and IGF-binding protein (IGFBP-3) and markers of GH action on soft tissue collagen turnover, such as procollagen III peptide [26]. A detection method based on such biomarkers represents a great advantage in terms of sensitivity not only to all forms of direct GH doping but also to all stimulators of GH secretion, including ghrelin, GH-releasing hormone, and other popular GH secretagogues such as ipamorelin, CJC-1295, GH-releasing peptides (GRPH-2 and GRPH-6), and even to GH gene doping.

IGF-1 and procollagen III peptide form the basis of the so-called GH-2000 test that was first applied during the 2012 Olympic Games. These markers have been evaluated for several confounding factors, including age, sex, ethnicity, exercise, bony and soft tissue injury, and sporting discipline [27]. Interestingly, all these biomarkers are known to present low intraindividual variations [28, 29], so that the use of the athlete as his own reference can significantly increase the sensitivity to direct and indirect GH doping. However, since intraindividual variations comprise both analytical [30] and biological components and since a precise knowledge of these variations following the strict procedures of the ABP is still lacking today, additional longitudinal studies are required to implement these biomarkers in an endocrine module of the ABP.

As is the case with all modules of the ABP, the endocrine module can be used for both target testing (to GH using the isoform immunoassay and to all stimulators of GH secretion by chromatography-mass spectrometry [31]) and pursuing an anti-doping rule violation. The knowledge accrued in the application of the hematological and steroidal modules will facilitate the implementation of the endocrine module and any future "omics" module of the ABP.

Omics

Genome-wide association studies including the latest next generation sequencing examinations have up to now generated outcomes with small effect size in the clinics [32]. On the other hand, functional phenotypic intermediates, such as RNAs, proteins, and metabolites, have the advantage to be affected not only by genetic changes but also by external factors coming from the environment [33], including the administration of an exogenous substance. In the ABP, genetic information is not directly associated to the cause (here doping) but rather used to personalize the concentrations of phenotypic biomarkers to improve the detection of doping.

The transcriptome, proteome, and metabolome represent a treasure trove of biomarkers of doping that can be integrated in the ABP. High-throughput omics techniques, mainly by liquid chromatography high-resolution mass spectrometry, are able today to robustly quantify up to 50,000 biomolecules in a single drop of blood. In order to fully take advantage of this technological progress, clinical trials involving both doped and control subjects following rigorous protocols of sample collection and analysis are required to discover and validate new biomarkers. Panels of biomarkers validated following an untargeted approach, such as multiparametric scores obtained using pattern classification tools without a good understanding of the underlying pathways, are best candidates for efficient and low-cost target testing to traditional drug tests, while only a panel of biomarkers validated following a targeted approach can be used to pursue an anti-doping rule infraction following the principles of the ABP [34].

The ability of the ABP to protect sports from doping with current and future drugs depends on the magnitude of biomarker discovery for the ABP. In this context, it is naïve at best to believe that the administration of a doping substance would affect a single protein or metabolite while leaving all other biomolecules unaffected. In biological systems, information is known to be distributed, and the recognition of patterns induced by doping in the high-dimensional omic profiles should be preferred over the detection of a single biomarker. Multiparametric markers such as "off scores" and abnormal blood profile scores are already routinely used in the ABP. More recently, it has been shown that the personalization of a large panel of urinary steroid metabolites by removing interindividual variations and their combination to define multiparametric biomarkers significantly improved the detection of multiple steroid preparations [35].

All these recent advances in state-of-the-art technologies demonstrate the large deterrent potential of the ABP. In the future, it is foreseen that the ABP as the longitudinal record of snapshots of an athlete's physiology, consisting of large panels of phenotypic biomarkers of doping measured from multiplex assays personalized according to genetic differences, would be able to detect the physiological signature of most doping substances and methods.

Application to Personalized Medicine

The expertise acquired for the development and validation of the ABP can be applied to the concept of personalized medicine [8]. Today, a paradox exists between the rapid development of personalized medicine and the outdated but still most prevalent use of population-based reference ranges to interpret biological data. This situation is particularly problematic since most biomarkers present significantly higher inter- than intraindividual variations. A longitudinal record of biological data is an invaluable tool to tailor medical decisions to an individual patient.

In drug development, safety and efficacy assessment can benefit from a personalized evaluation of biological data. For example, the use of longitudinal personalized laboratory data improves the cost-effectiveness of drug development resulting in earlier decisions in the trial and better treatment to patients. Similarly, the ability to identify a drug effect on an individual-participant basis in early-phase studies permits drug developers to recognize issues early in development and rapidly engage in risk-benefit analysis [36].

The concept of a biological passport in which longitudinal records of large panels of phenotypic biomarkers individualized based on the knowledge of metabolic pathways and previous readings is particularly interesting when the early detection of a disease is critical to patient outcome. An obvious application is the early detection of cancer. Another application is the early detection of kidney dysfunction using biomarkers as common as serum creatinine and urea [37].

The ABP shares similarities not only with personalized medicine but also with fields as popular as patient monitoring (ordering of biological data over time), big data (collation and evaluation of large omic profiles), and the management of electronic health records (entire patient history available electronically), which makes the biological passport a promising approach not only in anti-doping but in medicine as well.

References

1 Eichner ER: Blood Doping. Sports Med 2007;37:389–391.
2 Boudreau F, Konzak B: Ben Johnson and the use of steroids in sport: sociological and ethical considerations. Can J Sport Sci 1991;16:88–98.
3 Saugy M, Robinson N, Saudan C: The fight against doping: back on track with blood. Drug Test Anal 2009;1:474–478.
4 Schumacher YO, Grathwohl D, Barturen JM, Wollenweber M, Heinrich L, Schmid A, Huber G, Keul J: Haemoglobin, haematocrit and red blood cell indices in elite cyclists. Are the control values for blood testing valid? Int J Sports Med 2000;21:380–385.
5 Lasne F, de Ceaurriz J: Recombinant erythropoietin in urine. Nature 2000;405:635–635.
6 Catlin DH, Sekera MH, Ahrens BD, Starcevic B, Chang YC, Hatton CK: Tetrahydrogestrinone: discovery, synthesis, and detection in urine. Rapid Commun Mass Spectrom 2004;18:1245–1049.
7 Nelson M, Ashenden M, Langshaw M, Popp H: Detection of homologous blood transfusion by flow cytometry: a deterrent against blood doping. Haematologica 2002;87:881–882.
8 Sottas PE, Robinson N, Rabin O, Saugy M: The athlete biological passport. Clin Chem 2011;57:969–976.
9 Robinson N, Sottas PE, Pottgiesser T, Schumacher YO, Saugy M: Stability and robustness of blood variables in an anti-doping context. Int J Lab Hematol 2011;33:146–153.
10 Zorzoli M, Rossi F: Case studies on ESA-doping as revealed by the Biological Passport. Drug Test Anal 2012;4:854–858.
11 Lamon S, Giraud S, Egli L, Smolander J, Jarsch M, Stubenrauch KG, Robinson N: A high-throughput test to detect CERA doping in blood. J Pharm Biomed Anal 2009;50:954–958.
12 Leuenberger N, Lamon S, Robinson N, Giraud S, Saugy M: How to confirm CERA doping in athletes' blood? Forensic Sci Int 2011;213:101–103.
13 Bidlingmaier M, Suhr J, Ernst A, Wu Z, Keller A, Strasburger CJ, Bergmann A: High-sensitivity chemiluminescence immunoassays for detection of growth hormone doping in sports. Clin Chem 2009;55:445–453.
14 Sottas PE, Baume N, Saudan C, Schweizer C, Kamber M, Saugy M: Bayesian detection of abnormal values in longitudinal biomarkers with an application to T/E ratio. Biostatistics 2007;8:285–296.
15 Sottas P-E, Robinson N, Saugy M: The athlete's biological passport and indirect markers of blood doping. Handb Exp Pharmacol 2010;195:305–326.
16 Schumacher YO, d'Onofrio G: Scientific expertise and the athlete biological passport: 3 years of experience. Clin Chem 2012;58:979–985.
17 Schumacher YO, Saugy M, Pottgiesser T, Robinson N: Detection of EPO doping and blood doping: the haematological module of the athlete biological passport. Drug Test Anal 2012;4:846–853.
18 Gore CJ, Parisotto R, Ashenden MJ Stray-Gundersen J, Sharpe K, Hopkins W, et al: Second-generation blood tests to detect erythropoietin abuse by athletes. Haematologica 2003;88:333–344.
19 Sottas PE, Robinson N, Giraud S, Taroni F, Kamber M, Mangin P, et al: Statistical classification of abnormal blood profiles in athletes. Int J Biostat 2006;2:3.
20 Schänzer W: Abuse of androgens and detection of illegal use; in Nieschlag E (eds): Testosterone. Berlin, Springer, 1998, pp 545–565.
21 Van Renterghem P, Van Eenoo P, Sottas PE, Saugy M, Delbeke F: Subject-based steroid profiling and the determination of novel biomarkers for DHT and DHEA misuse in sports. Drug Test Anal 2010;2:582–588.
22 Shackleton CH, Phillips A, Chang T, Li Y: Confirming testosterone administration by isotope ratio mass spectrometric analysis of urinary androstanediols. Steroids 1997;62:379–387.
23 Schulze JJ, Lundmark J, Garle M, Ekström L, Sottas P-E, Rane A: Substantial advantage of a combined Bayesian and genotyping approach in testosterone doping tests. Steroids 2009;74:365–368.
24 Sottas P-E, Saugy M, Saudan C: Endogenous steroid profiling in the athlete biological passport. Endocrinol Metab Clin North Am 2010;39:59–73.
25 Mareck U, Geyer H, Opfermann G, Thevis M, Schänzer W: Factors influencing the steroid profile in doping control analysis. J Mass Spectrom 2008;43:877–891.
26 Erotokritou-Mulligan I, Bassett EE, Kniess A, Sonksen PH, Holt RI: Validation of the growth hormone (GH)-dependent marker method of detecting GH abuse in sport through the use of independent data sets. Growth Horm IGF Res 2007;17:416–423.

27 Guha N, Erotokritou-Mulligan I, Burford C, Strobridge G, Brigg J, Drake T, Bassett EE, Cowan D, Bartlett C, Sönksen PH, Holt RI: Serum insulin-like growth factor-I and pro-collagen type III N-terminal peptide in adolescent elite athletes: implications for the detection of growth hormone abuse in sport. J Clin Endocrinol Metab 2010;95:2969–2976.

28 Erotokritou-Mulligan I, Eryl Bassett E, Cowan DA, Bartlett C, Milward P, Sartorio A, Sönksen PH, Holt RI: The use of growth hormone (GH)-dependent markers in the detection of GH abuse in sport: physiological intra-individual variation of IGF-I, type 3 pro-collagen (P-III-P) and the GH-2000 detection score. Clin Endocrinol (Oxf) 2010;72:520–526.

29 Kniess A, Ziegler E, Thieme D, Müller RK: Intra-individual variation of GH-dependent markers in athletes: comparison of population based and individual thresholds for detection of GH abuse in sports. J Pharm Biomed Anal 2013;84:201–208.

30 Cox HD, Lopes F, Woldemariam GA, Becker JO, Parkin MC, Thomas A, Butch AW, Cowan DA, Thevis M, Bowers LD, Hoofnagle AN: Interlaboratory agreement of insulin-like growth factor 1 concentrations measured by mass spectrometry. Clin Chem 2014;60:541–548.

31 Thevis M, Thomas A, Schänzer W: Detecting peptidic drugs, drug candidates and analogs in sports doping: current status and future directions. Expert Rev Proteomics 2014;11:663–673.

32 Suhre K, Shin SY, Petersen AK, Mohney RP, Meredith D, Wägele B, Altmaier E; CARDIoGRAM, Deloukas P, Erdmann J, Grundberg E, Hammond CJ, de Angelis MH, Kastenmüller G, Köttgen A, Kronenberg F, Mangino M, Meisinger C, Meitinger T, Mewes HW, Milburn MV, Prehn C, Raffler J, Ried JS, Römisch-Margl W, Samani NJ, Small KS, Wichmann HE, Zhai G, Illig T, Spector TD, Adamski J, Soranzo N, Gieger C: Human metabolic individuality in biomedical and pharmaceutical research. Nature 2011;477:54–60.

33 Rochat B, Favre A, Sottas PE: Metabotype analysis for personalized biology: a new bioanalytical territory for high-resolution MS. Bioanalysis 2013;5:1149–1152.

34 Sottas PE, Vernec A: Current implementation and future of the athlete biological passport. Bioanalysis 2012;4:1645–1652.

35 Van Renterghem P, Sottas PE, Saugy M, Van Eenoo P: Statistical discrimination of steroid profiles in doping control with support vector machines. Anal Chim Acta 2013;768:41–48.

36 Sottas PE, Kapke GF, Leroux JM: Adaptive Bayesian analysis of serum creatinine as a marker for drug-induced renal impairment in an early-phase clinical trial. Clin Chem 2012;58:1592–1596.

37 Sottas PE, Kapke GF, Leroux JM: Adaptive Bayesian approach to clinical trial renal impairment biomarker signal from urea and creatinine. Int J Biol Sci 2013;9:156–163.

Neil Robinson, PhD
Swiss Laboratory for Doping Analyses
University Center of Legal Medicine Geneva and Lausanne
Chemin des Croisettes 22
CH–1066 Epalinges (Switzerland)
E-Mail robinsonjahr@gmail.com

Next Generation "Omics" Approaches in the "Fight" against Blood Doping

Guan Wang[a, b] · Antonia Karanikolou[a] · Ioanna Verdouka[a]
Theodore Friedmann[c] · Yannis Pitsiladis[a, b]

[a]University of Brighton, Eastbourne, UK; [b]Reference Collaborating Centre of Sports Medicine for Anti-Doping Research, International Federation of Sports Medicine (FIMS), University of Rome Foro Italico, Rome, Italy; [c]Friedmann Lab, Department of Pediatrics, The University of California School of Medicine, San Diego, CA, USA

Abstract

Despite being prohibited by the World Anti-Doping Agency (WADA), blood manipulations such as the use of recombinant human erythropoietin and blood transfusions are a well-known method used by athletes to enhance performance. Direct detection of illicit blood manipulation has been partially successful due to the short detection window of the substances/methods, sample collection timing, and the use of sophisticated masking strategies. In response, WADA introduced the athlete biological passport (ABP) in 2009, which is an individualised longitudinal monitoring approach that tests primarily haematologic biomarkers of doping in order to identify atypical variability in response(s) in athletes, highlighting a potential doping violation. Although the implementation of the ABP has been an encouraging step forward in the quest for clean/drug-free sport, this detection method has some limitations. To reduce the risk of being detected by the ABP method, athletes are now resorting to microdoses of prohibited blood boosting substances to prevent abnormal fluctuations in haematologic biomarkers, thereby reducing the sensitivity of the ABP detection method. Recent studies from numerous laboratories, including our own, have confirmed the potential of transcriptomic microarrays, which can reveal distinct changes in gene expression after blood manipulations, to enhance the ABP. There is, therefore, an urgent need to intensify research efforts that involve transcriptomics and other state-of-the-art molecular methods, collectively known as "omics", e.g., proteomics (proteins) and metabolomics (metabolites), in order to identify new and even more robust molecular signatures of blood manipulation that can be used in combination with the ABP and, intriguingly, even as a stand-alone test.

© 2017 S. Karger AG, Basel

Rationale for an Omic-Based Solution with Particular Reference to Blood Doping

Blood doping is known to improve performance in elite athletes [1]. Despite being prohibited by the World Anti-Doping Agency (WADA), blood manipulations such as the administration of recombinant human erythropoietin (rhEPO) and blood transfusions are allegedly often used by athletes to enhance performance. The performance-enhancing drug rhEPO is structurally similar to endogenous erythropoietin, hence direct detection of this drug is challenging. In addition, there remains no direct detection method for autologous blood transfusions, and this also represents a significant limitation of the current anti-doping system. Historically, direct methods have been applied to detect doping agents such as analytical testing of blood and urine. Despite some success, direct approaches suffer from numerous important shortcomings such as the short detection window of substance(s), the timing of the sample collection, and the involvement of sophisticated doping [2]. This situation has led to the introduction of indirect methods aimed at detecting the physiological/biochemical changes caused by the action of doping substances and methods, and for a prolongation of their respective direct detection window. This latter approach represents the basis for the athlete biological passport (ABP) – an individualised longitudinal monitoring method introduced by WADA in 2009 that relies on identifying intra-individual abnormal variability over time for selected haematological and steroidal parameters to detect blood and exogenous steroid manipulation, respectively [3]. More precisely, the ABP approach uses bayesian networks for the evaluation of the likelihood of doping based on several putative doping-related biomarkers, which can then be used as evidence for disciplinary sanction. Bayesian networks are interpretable and flexible models representing the probabilities of causal relationships between multiple interacting variables [3, 4]. In the anti-doping field, the adaptive model estimates the probability of doping based on previous individual test history data and numerous factors known to influence the doping biomarkers. This feature allows the model to remove the variance due to intersubject differences and factors such as sex, ethnicity, altitude exposure, age, and sporting discipline [4]. Ideally, a next generation ABP may well reduce or even eliminate doping. However, in the real world, the evolution of doping practices often succeeds in evading, at least partially, some of the very best anti-doping strategies.

Rapid technological progress in whole human genome characterisation allows application of state-of-the-art molecular methods, collectively known as "omics", e.g., proteomic (proteins) and metabolomic (metabolites) technologies for research and clinical use. The omic signature concept offers new and exciting possibilities in the "fight" against doping. The premise of the next generation omic approach to detect doping is based on the presumption that drugs and other doping methods will cause profound and, therefore, detectable changes in the way in which many of the 21,000 or so genes in the human body will be uniquely expressed in response to a specific doping substance or method, therefore constituting a unique omic signature of exposure to the specific doping practice. This presumption is consistent with the general idea of biological "homeostasis" – the tendency of a living system to avoid perturbations of its established physiology and its established state of function. It is only in the past few years that this concept has begun to be tested experimentally, largely with support from WADA. The idea of a molecular-based anti-doping test has received considerable support from the WADA research funding programme with a significant proportion of the WADA research effort being devoted to the identification of an omic signature of blood doping [5, 6]. Given this focus, this chapter will address the potential of next generation omic approaches to improve drug detection, with particular reference to blood doping.

Summary of Research Findings using Omic Approaches for the Detection of Blood Doping

A genome is defined as the entire collection of genetic information encoded by a particular organism [7]. By semantic association, the words transcriptome, proteome, and metabolome refer to the entirety of all transcripts, proteins, and metabolites expressed by a genome at a specific time and collectively encompass the so-called omic cascade [8]. For example, using microarray technology, a characteristic gene expression signature of a particular stimulus can be revealed by assessing the transcription state of cells within experimental samples [9]. A gene expression response to a variety of doping substances and methods with particular reference to the detection of blood doping has been the focus of a handful of antidoping research laboratories. The general idea being that if a particular blood doping method, such as rhEPO administration, yields a specific gene expression signature, this unique attribute could lead to the development of new methods with improved discriminatory power relative to traditional detection protocols (i.e., isoelectric focusing, sarcosyl polyacrylamide gel electrophoresis, and ABP). Some initial support for this hypothesis emerged from a WADA-funded study conducted by Varlet-Marie et al. [10]. Using serial analyses of gene expression, these authors identified 95 genes whose differential expression was subsequently tested by quantitative real-time polymerase chain reaction (PCR) in 2 athletes. These athletes were treated first with high doses of rhEPO and then with microdoses; 33 marker genes for rhEPO administration were identified during the high-dose regimen and 5 remained differentially expressed with microdoses of rhEPO. A transcriptomic-based approach has also been applied with some success to other doping methods and substances used by athletes. For example, characteristic gene expression profiles have been shown in 6 subjects after autologous blood transfusion (ABT) [11]. Similarly, a WADA-funded study investigating the effects of training, altitude exposure, and sex differences on whole blood gene expression in response to ABT (3 bags of blood re-infused) using 41 candidate genes, reported changes in 16 of the 41 genes after transfusion, thus enabling ABT to be distinguished from normal variations in the athletes' gene expression subject to different training regimens (i.e., power or endurance athletes) and from altitude exposure [12]. The main limitations of this study were the small number of ABT participants ($n = 4$ with ABT vs. 47 without), the limited choice of genes, the quantitative PCR platform used for gene expression profiling, and the high volume of blood transfused [12]. The investigators used several statistical methods to evaluate the potential bias that may arise from sex, sport, age, collection time, and the discriminant performance of the selected genes [12]. Although preliminary, these results were very promising.

In line with these encouraging results, we conducted a study to identify the whole transcriptome signature of ABT using microarray analysis. Briefly, 15 healthy Caucasian males (20–35 years, body mass index ≤30) received a saline injection for the control phase, and then donated 1 bag of blood (500 mL) 14 days later, which was stored at 4°C for 36 days before reinfusion. For the ABT phase, whole blood samples were collected at baseline (4 and 1 days before blood reinfusion) and 3, 6, and 12 h, and 1, 2, 3, 6, 9, and 15 days after blood reinfusion, respectively [13]. For the control phase, whole blood samples were collected at the same time points, except for the 15-day sampling [13]. Transcriptional profiling revealed that hundreds of transcripts were altered by ABT. Compared to baseline, the main expression patterns of these genes were an up-regulation during the first 3 days after reinfusion and a down-regulation 6, 9, and 15 days after reinfusion. The range of fold changes in gene expression varied from 1.5 to 2.3 across time points. Genes which differentially expressed during the first 3 days after ABT were linked with iron homeostasis, anti-inflammatory activity, and host defence pathways, and genes expressed 6 and 9 days after blood reinfusion were related to haeme biosynthesis, the chemokine signalling pathway, and with immune responses. The down-regulation of genes linked to haeme biosynthesis could be related to alterations in erythropoiesis, as revealed in previous studies [13, 14]. In addition, reticulocyte percentage was significantly decreased 3, 6, 9, and 15 days after the blood reinfusion compared to baseline and in line with the observed gene expression changes. Although preliminary, these results are encouraging and would appear to support the detection of ABT using whole genome expression analysis. In addition to ABT, there have been numerous other attempts by multiple groups to investigate the global gene expression patterns in whole blood or lymphocytes for the detection of testosterone, anabolic steroids, recombinant human growth hormone, rhEPO, and gene doping indicating the discriminatory potential of transcriptomic markers to detect doping [5]. These results suggest that an omic-based anti-doping approach involving gene expression profiles, in the first instance, may represent a sensitive method for the detection of rhEPO and possibly other forms of blood doping.

On the basis of the promising omic results by Varlet-Marie et al. [10], significant funding from WADA was invested in our laboratories for a series of closely related studies aimed at evaluating the efficacy of an omic solution for the detection of rhEPO doping. The first study in the series was conducted at sea level in Glasgow (Scotland, UK) with Caucasian endurance trained males [15] and at moderate-altitude in Eldoret (Kenya) with Kenyan endurance runners [16] who abstained from official sporting competition for the entire duration of the study. The specific aims of the first study were:

- To determine and compare the effects of rhEPO administration on blood parameters and exercise performance in endurance-trained males living and training at or near sea level with another cohort living and training at moderate altitude in Kenya.
- To establish adequate molecular methods and molecular work flow to enable valid and optimal assessment of blood gene expression.
- To assess the effects of rhEPO on blood gene expression profiles in endurance-trained volunteers living and training at or near sea level.
- To replicate and compare the effects of rhEPO administration on blood gene expression profiles in another cohort living and training at moderate altitude in Kenya.
- To validate the gene microarray-based findings using another specific and sensitive quantitative gene expression technology.

In an attempt to achieve these ambitious goals, 39 endurance-trained males, 19 based at sea level (Glasgow) and 20 based at moderate altitude (Eldoret, 2,100–2,800 m above sea level, a.s.l.), received 50 IU $\times$ kg^{-1} body mass subcutaneous rhEPO injections for 4 weeks. Blood was obtained 2 weeks before, during, and 4 weeks after administration. Blood, urine, and saliva samples were collected at 20 time points per volunteer (i.e., 20 time points $\times$ 39 subjects), and specifically processed and stored at –80 °C for future analysis; results from this first study are beginning to emerge [15, 16]. Briefly, relative to baseline, running performance in sea level Caucasian trained men was significantly improved by approximately 6% after rhEPO administration and remained significantly enhanced by approximately 3% 4 weeks after rhEPO administration; these effects on performance coincided with an increase in maximum aerobic capacity (maximal oxygen uptake, $\dot{V}O_{2\,max}$) and total Hb$_{mass}$ [15]. Of particular interest was the finding that rhEPO administration improved $\dot{V}O_{2\,max}$ and time trial performance to a similar extent in Kenyan and Scottish runners although haematocrit and haemoglobin concentrations were higher in Kenyan than Scottish runners prior to rhEPO and similar at the end of administration [16]. In terms of the transcriptomic data, hundreds of genes were differentially expressed during rhEPO administration relative to baseline levels [17]. Notably, a few of these genes were already up-regulated after only a single rhEPO injection, while further genes were differentially expressed during rhEPO and remained differentially expressed up to 4 weeks after administration compared to baseline. Given the potential impact of these findings, and in line with the omic literature, a subset of target genes (n = 45) were further validated using another quantitative gene expression technology in both cohorts [17]. From the outcomes of our first WADA-funded rhEPO study, it is clear that significant progress was made towards successfully achieving the initial objectives. Specifically, this study successfully identified, replicated, and validated the whole blood molecular signature of rhEPO administration and as such provided good evidence to support the idea that gene biomarkers have the potential to improve the performance of current anti-doping methods such as the ABP.

According to testimonies, athletes are now resorting to microdoses of rhEPO injected intravenously to restrain abnormal fluctuations in the haematological parameters used as biomarkers of doping, thereby reducing the sensitivity of the ABP detection method and the window of detection by anti-doping methods. As such, it would appear that athletes are currently microdosing with rhEPO to minimise the risk of being caught via currently applied detection methods [18, 19]. Interestingly, in the study by Varlet-Marie et al. [10], 5 genes remained differentially expressed following both high doses and microdoses of rhEPO. While these results were generated using serial analysis of gene expression, an earlier technology, in a few subjects only, the data supported the idea that gene expression profiles may provide a sufficiently sensitive method to detect microdoses of rhEPO, especially when the whole genome is interrogated. Given the microdosing issue, WADA funded a rhEPO microdosing study to assess whether the candidate markers of rhEPO we previously identified could detect microdoses of rhEPO. In this study, 14 healthy endurance-trained subjects not involved in competition were required to participate in a randomised, double-blind, placebo-controlled crossover microdose rhEPO regimen necessitating the collection of 364 whole blood samples (i.e., 13 time points × 14 subjects × 2 trials). The aim of the rhEPO microdose regimen was to increase haemoglobin mass (Hb_{mass}) while deliberately avoiding large fluctuations in reticulocytes. Briefly, each subject received rhEPO injections (NeoRecormon; Roche, Welwyn Garden City, UK) subcutaneously twice per week for 7 weeks with the dosage ranging from 20 to 40 IU × kg^{-1} body mass. Blood samples were collected in triplicate at baseline and then once a week during rhEPO administration and for 3 weeks after rhEPO administration (i.e., 13 blood samples per subject). $\dot{V}O_{2\,max}$ and repeated sprint ability were also assessed at baseline and during the week after the last rhEPO/placebo injection. Using similar analytical methods as in our first study, 9 of the 45 previously identified genes were validated during the microdosing regimen. In a related study involving ABT, 27 of the 45 previously identified genes were found to be significantly down-regulated 6, 9, and 15 days after ABT in 7 healthy Caucasian males [20]. Taken together, these results provide further evidence to support a transcriptomic-based solution for the detection of blood doping.

Given the promising results described previously, it is necessary to evaluate the effects of major confounders on the discovered molecular signature of blood doping, such as the effects of altitude and/or exercise. Both natural or simulated altitude training is used by athletes for performance enhancement [21], although the optimal regimen and the magnitude of the ergogenic effect of natural altitude training are unclear, and there appears to be only a small/no effect of simulated altitude on performance [22]. Only the "living high – training low" altitude training method using natural altitude and developed by Levine and Stray-Gundersen [23] appears modestly effective in terms of performance benefit [22]. In addition, it remains uncertain to what extent these performance-enhancing effects of altitude are due to augmented erythropoiesis [22]. Regardless of the mechanism(s) for performance benefits of natural and simulated altitude, altitude exposure may potentially influence the haematological indices of blood doping [24, 25]. Some athletes may, therefore, claim altitude exposure as a source of variation in their individual blood variables to mask blood doping practices, such as the administration of rhEPO. There is an urgent need, therefore, to develop specific and robust testing models that can differentiate altitude training from blood doping combined (or not) with altitude exposure. Therefore, the aim of a third research project funded by WADA and currently going on in our laboratory is to compare blood gene expression profiles altered by rhEPO from altitude exposure in order to provide a set of candidate genes that can be used to differentiate rhEPO from altitude training. In our first altitude study, 20 endurance athletes (50% males) spent approximately 2 weeks at an altitude above 2,000 m a.s.l., and serial blood samples were collected prior, during, and after altitude exposure. Although preliminary, the results revealed that 13 of the 45 previously identified genes from the first study demonstrated non-significant changes in gene expression in response to altitude; nevertheless, using the same markers, the rhEPO effect on gene expression was longer lasting and greater than the altitude endurance training, favouring the application of these biomarkers, combined with current anti-doping strategies to detect blood doping. On the basis of these results, we designed and conducted a second altitude study with particular focus on longer (for approx. 4 weeks) and higher altitude exposure (approx. 2,500–3,000 m a.s.l.); whole transcriptome analysis is currently underway. It should be noted that none of the athletes participating in any of the rhEPO administration studies described in this chapter and linked with the authors were involved in competition during the study periods and for approximately 8 weeks following the completion of each study; athletes were only permitted to participate in one rhEPO study. Daily iron supplementation was given throughout the rhEPO administration.

Blood samples for anti-doping purposes are often collected at sporting or training venues after intense exercise [26]. It has previously been shown that exercise significantly influences gene expression profiles of peripheral blood mononuclear cells and white blood cells [27, 28]. It was essential, therefore, to define the effects of exercise on blood gene expression profiles and particularly on the molecular signature of blood doping. In order to provide a set of robust candidate genes that can be used for the detection of blood doping with particular focus on rhEPO in the first instance, whole blood gene expression assessment was recently conducted at baseline and during and after intense exercise following treatment with microdoses of rhEPO or placebo in the aforementioned double-blinded rhEPO trial. In particular, a modified Wingate test comprising 10 sprints of 10 s at baseline and during the week after microdoses of rhEPO was carried out in order to provide a set of robust candidate genes that can be used to detect rhEPO doping, but also to examine the effects of rhEPO on progressive anaerobic fatigue and repeated sprint ability. The ability to reproduce maximal performance in subsequent short-duration sprints separated by brief recovery periods is a key performance requirement in most team and some individual sports [29]. For example, the International Tennis Federation recently adopted the ABP programme, while there is anecdotal evidence in football that doping may be higher than perceived by sport authorities [30]. While there was no clear improvement in measures of anaerobic performance following microdoses of rhEPO, $\dot{V}O_{2\,max}$ was significantly increased by an average of 3.9%. In terms of omics, 17 of all previously validated rhEPO transcripts were differentially expressed immediately following intense exercise when compared to baseline, but this altered expression rapidly subsided within 30 min after exercise, thereby arguing against exercise/training being a significant confounder. Further replication of this important finding is currently underway in our laboratories. Specifically, a whole-blood transcriptional microarray analysis of high-intensity interval exercise is being conducted as part of an international collaboration with the Gene SMART (skeletal muscle adaptive response to training) study. The Gene SMART study aims to identify the gene variants that predict the skeletal muscle response to both a single bout and 4 weeks of high-intensity interval training [31]. The data generated will be used to inform on the precise time course of sample collection in order to ensure the validity of the blood gene expression data. A transcriptomic-based anti-doping approach is envisaged to reduce the pressure on athletes who currently need to wait 2 h after training or competition before a blood sample is taken for the ABP.

Necessary Next Steps for the Application of an Integrative Omic Solution to the Detection of Blood Doping

Based on the transcriptomic findings to date, some summarised in this chapter, it is evidently clear that once confirmed and validated the integration of the blood gene biomarkers into the ABP will further enhance the detection capacity of the ABP. The idea being to build on the current ABP approach by combining the next generation omic signatures, currently being determined in the first instance as the blood transcriptome, with the currently employed haematological parameters and in doing so attempt to create a unique ABP model with greatly improved specificity and sensitivity not amenable to manipulation: the so called "integrated omic solution." It is essential, therefore, that there is a focus on the next steps needed to bring to fruition an integrative omic solution as quickly and as cost effectively as possible. Determining the inter- and intrasubject variability in gene expression as well as factors that can affect these profiles (i.e., subject, age, sex, altitude, exercise, and analyses) is an important necessary next step to assess the feasibility of the proposed integrative omic concept. Next steps will require normal reference ranges for all confounders that can impact on blood gene expression to be generated. For example, strenuous endurance exercise can induce changes in some blood parameters not only by the well-described increase in plasma volume known as the athlete's pseudoanaemia [32] but also by exercise-induced haemolysis due to metabolic modifications, oxidative stress, and repeated foot impact [33–35]. In addition to the preliminary exercise studies summarised above, the effects of more prolonged strenuous endurance exercise (lasting over 2 h) such as cycling stage racing and marathon running on blood gene expression profiles need to be investigated. As most blood parameters differ substantially between males and females, the currently used reference ranges for the ABP were determined separately for each sex [36, 37]. A similar approach needs to be applied to omic profiles in order to evaluate sex differences. Injury-related immobility also has the potential to affect blood gene profiles, as it has been reported that immobility for a period of 4 weeks reduces Hb_{mass} by approximately 19% in a competitive international female athlete [38]. Research to date has suggested that ethnicity and residence at altitude only minimally influence the blood gene expression signature of rhEPO doping [17].

In addition to determining the biological variability in omic measures, markers, and confounders, successful implementation of an omic anti-doping solution will require the analytical variability of the finally chosen omic measures to be determined given the importance of pre-analytical and analytical factors in any anti-doping rule violation procedure. This analysis will need to be repeated for other tissue/sample types (e.g., whole blood, blood fractions, urine, saliva, and hair) in order to assess which of these matrices have anti-doping potential. For example, all WADA-funded studies conducted in our laboratories have involved the collection of numerous tissue/sample types thereby creating a unique omic biobank for future research use. It is anticipated that most future anti-doping studies utilising omics will involve more sophisticated technologies such as RNA sequencing given the capacity of these technologies to interrogate the whole transcriptome with improved dynamic range and quantification. Approaches that interrogate the entire genome, transcriptome, and metabolome have increased capacity to measure rapidly and in the near future, inexpensively, a large number of molecular signatures, which will collectively help decision making when identifying and differentiating numerous doping substances and methods by ABP experts when reviewing longitudinal profiles. Integrating these technologies will, however, introduce new challenges such as the need for more specialist technical and analytical expertise, which typically translates into more costly research. Inevitably, normal reference ranges will also need to be generated for all omic measures to be adopted before final implementation. Adopting an integrative omic anti-doping approach will require the entire road map outlined here to be undertaken and in line with other areas of modern biomedical research involving omic technologies. As such, the focus of our latest research project funded by WADA aims to evaluate a number of previously addressed factors/confounders that could influence the successful implementation of an integrative omic solution to detect blood doping, and, specifically, to develop unique omic reference data to determine the analytical variability of selected omic technologies with particular focus on gene expression in blood, and the validation of the proposed integrative omic approach to the detection of rhEPO.

Concluding Remarks

There has been more than 1 decade of significant anti-doping omic research due to the substantial investment in research, mainly by WADA and more recently by the International Olympic Committee, with the aim to develop the next generation anti-doping approach involving omics with improved discriminatory power relative to traditional detection methods. The closely interconnected studies conducted to date in a handful of research laboratories systematically evaluated an omic solution to detect blood doping with particular reference to rhEPO doping. For example, relative to baseline, hundreds of genes were differentially expressed (i.e., switched "on" and "off") during rhEPO administration. Notably, a few of these genes were switched "on" after only a single rhEPO injection, while further genes being switched "on" during rhEPO administration and remained switched "on" up to 4 weeks after the last rhEPO injection. A subset of these genes reflecting rhEPO was further validated using a complementary gene expression technology under different conditions, such as blood transfusion, altitude training, and exercise training to ensure the robustness of the technology and approach. From the outcomes generated to date, in more than a single laboratory, it is clear that significant progress has been made towards successfully developing the next generation anti-doping test involving new state-of-the-art technologies typically associated with discovery and treatment of cancer and other serious medical conditions. Despite these encouraging results, anti-doping omics has not progressed to the point that actionable findings are widely recognised and/or an omic anti-doping test implemented. The future of impactful anti-doping omics lies in large-scale collaborative and multicentre research programmes with shared biobanks. Only this "paradigm shift" in anti-doping research involving omics can "fast track" the development of the next generation anti-doping capacity. Major progress in modern biomedical research has strongly relied on international collaboration involving such omic technologies in human, animal, and cell culture studies. The future of anti-doping research must, therefore, emulate this process, with particular reference to advances in personalised medicine. For example, in cancer research, omic technologies are systematically advancing personalised medicine and making good progress despite numerous setbacks; these setbacks can also be expected in anti-doping research. International consortia could work together to design and conduct the necessary studies needed to generate the data required to construct a new ABP-like model specific to rhEPO and blood doping in the first instance – a proof of principle before tackling other substances and methods.

References

1 Malm CB, Khoo NS, Granlund I, Lindstedt E, Hult A: Autologous doping with cryopreserved red blood cells – effects on physical performance and detection by multivariate statistics. PLoS One 2016;11:e0156157.
2 Vernec AR: The athlete biological passport: an integral element of innovative strategies in antidoping. Br J Sports Med 2014;48:817–819.
3 Sottas PE, Robinson N, Saugy M: The athlete's biological passport and indirect markers of blood doping. Handb Exp Pharmacol 2010;195:305–326.
4 Sottas P-E, Robinson N, Saugy M, Niggli O: A forensic approach to the interpretation of blood doping markers. Law Prob Risk 2008;7:191–210.
5 Funded Research Projects. Montreal, WADA, https://www.wada-ama.org/en/funded-research-projects (accessed February 21, 2017).
6 Little C: WADA Sets Priorities for USD 12 Million Research Pot: Using Chemistry and Omics to Study Doping 2015. http://fasterskier.com/fsarticle/wada-sets-priorities-for-12-million-research-pot-using-chemistry-and-omics-to-study-doping/ (accessed February 21, 2017).
7 Snyder M, Gerstein M: Genomics. defining genes in the genomics era. Science 2003;300:258–260.
8 Reichel C: OMICS – strategies and methods in the fight against doping. Forensic Sci Int 2011;213:20–34.
9 Bilitewski U: DNA microarrays: an introduction to the technology. Methods Mol Biol 2009;509:1–14.
10 Varlet-Marie E, Audran M, Ashenden M, Sicart MT, Piquemal D: Modification of gene expression: help to detect doping with erythropoiesis-stimulating agents. Am J Hematol 2009;84:755–759.
11 Pottgiesser T, Schumacher YO, Funke H, Rennert K, Baumstark MW, Neunuebel K, Mosig S: Gene expression in the detection of autologous blood transfusion in sports – a pilot study. Vox Sang 2009;96:333–336.
12 Gore C, Ashenden M, Hahn A, Moerkeberg J, Damsgaard R, Belhage B: The effect of training, altitude exposure and an athlete's sex on expression of genes known to change following autologous blood transfusion. Montreal, WADA, 2015, https://www.wada-ama.org/sites/default/files/resources/files/08c05gg_gore_0.pdf (accessed February 21, 2017).
13 Leuenberger N, Bulla E, Salamin O, Nicoli R, Robinson N, Baume N, Saugy M: Hepcidin as a potential biomarker for blood doping. Drug Test Anal 2016, Epub ahead of print.
14 Damsgaard R, Munch T, Morkeberg J, Mortensen SP, Gonzalez-Alonso J: Effects of blood withdrawal and reinfusion on biomarkers of erythropoiesis in humans: implications for anti-doping strategies. Haematologica 2006;91: 1006–1008.
15 Durussel J, Daskalaki E, Anderson M, Chatterji T, Wondimu DH, Padmanabhan N, Patel RK, McClure JD, Pitsiladis YP: Haemoglobin mass and running time trial performance after recombinant human erythropoietin administration in trained men. PLoS One 2013; 8:e56151.
16 Wondimu DH, Durussel J, Mekonnen W, Anjila E, Ongaro N, Rutto M, Wilson T, Mooses M, Daskalaki E, Pitsiladis YP: Blood parameters and running performance of Kenyan and Caucasian endurance trained males after rHuEpo administration (abstract). Med Sci Sports Exerc 2013;45(suppl):1758.
17 Durussel J, Haile DW, Mooses K, Daskalaki E, Beattie W, Mooses M, Mekonen W, Ongaro N, Anjila E, Patel RK, Padmanabhan N, McBride MW, McClure JD, Pitsiladis YP: Blood transcriptional signature of recombinant human erythropoietin administration and implications for antidoping strategies. Physiol Genomics 2016;48:202–209.
18 Ashenden M, Varlet-Marie E, Lasne F, Audran M: The effects of microdose recombinant human erythropoietin regimens in athletes. Haematologica 2006; 91:1143–1144.
19 Ashenden M, Gough CE, Garnham A, Gore CJ, Sharpe K: Current markers of the athlete blood passport do not flag microdose EPO doping. Eur J Appl Physiol 2011;111:2307–2314.
20 Salamin O, Barras L, Robinson N, Baume N, Tissot JD, Pitsiladis Y, Saugy M, Leuenberger N: Impact of blood transfusion on gene expression in human reticulocytes. Am J Hematol 2016; 91:E460–E461.
21 Millet GP, Roels B, Schmitt L, Woorons X, Richalet JP: Combining hypoxic methods for peak performance. Sports Med 2010;40:1–25.
22 Bonetti DL, Hopkins WG: Sea-level exercise performance following adaptation to hypoxia: a meta-analysis. Sports Med 2009;39:107–127.
23 Levine BD, Stray-Gundersen J: "Living high – training low": effect of moderate-altitude acclimatization with low-altitude training on performance. J Appl Physiol 1997;83:102–112.
24 Ashenden MJ, Hahn AG, Martin DT, Logan P, Parisotto R, Gore CJ: A comparison of the physiological response to simulated altitude exposure and r-HuEpo administration. J Sports Sci 2001;19: 831–837.

25 Ashenden MJ, Gore CJ, Parisotto R, Sharpe K, Hopkins WG, Hahn AG: Effect of altitude on second-generation blood tests to detect erythropoietin abuse by athletes. Haematologica 2003; 88:1053–1062.
26 Rupert JL: Transcriptional profiling: a potential anti-doping strategy. Scand J Med Sci Sports 2009;19:753–763.
27 Buttner P, Mosig S, Lechtermann A, Funke H, Mooren FC: Exercise affects the gene expression profiles of human white blood cells. J Appl Physiol 2007; 102:26–36.
28 Connolly PH, Caiozzo VJ, Zaldivar F, Nemet D, Larson J, Hung SP, Heck JD, Hatfield GW, Cooper DM: Effects of exercise on gene expression in human peripheral blood mononuclear cells. J Appl Physiol 2004;97:1461–1469.
29 Girard O, Mendez-Villanueva A, Bishop D: Repeated-sprint ability – part I: factors contributing to fatigue. Sports Med 2011;41:673–694.
30 Hart S: World Anti-Doping Agency calls on the football authorities to do more to combat doping. The Telegraph, February 12, 2013.
31 Pitsiladis YP, Tanaka M, Eynon N, Bouchard C, North KN, Williams AG, Collins M, Moran CN, Britton SL, Fuku N, Ashley EA, Klissouras V, Lucia A, Ahmetov II, de Geus E, Alsayrafi M: Athlome Project Consortium: a concerted effort to discover genomic and other "omic" markers of athletic performance. Physiol Genomics 2016;48:183–190.
32 Ashenden M: Contemporary issues in the fight against blood doping in sport. Haematologica 2004;89:901–903.
33 Weight LM, Darge BL, Jacobs P: Athletes' pseudoanaemia. Eur J Appl Physiol Occup Physiol 1991;62:358–362.
34 Lombardi G, Lanteri P, Fiorella PL, Simonetto L, Impellizzeri FM, Bonifazi M, Banfi G, Locatelli M: Comparison of the hematological profile of elite road cyclists during the 2010 and 2012 GiroBio ten-day stage races and relationships with final ranking. PLoS One 2013; 8:e63092.
35 Telford RD, Sly GJ, Hahn AG, Cunningham RB, Bryant C, Smith JA: Footstrike is the major cause of hemolysis during running. J Appl Physiol 2003;94:38–42.
36 Yusof A, Leithauser RM, Roth HJ, Finkernagel H, Wilson MT, Beneke R: Exercise-induced hemolysis is caused by protein modification and most evident during the early phase of an ultraendurance race. J Appl Physiol 2007;102:582–586.
37 Sharpe K, Hopkins W, Emslie KR, Howe C, Trout GJ, Kazlauskas R, Ashenden MJ, Gore CJ, Parisotto R, Hahn AG: Development of reference ranges in elite athletes for markers of altered erythropoiesis. Haematologica 2002;87:1248–1257.
38 Schumacher YO, Ahlgrim C, Ruthardt S, Pottgiesser T: Hemoglobin mass in an elite endurance athlete before, during, and after injury-related immobility. Clin J Sport Med 2008;18:172–173.

Prof. Yannis Pitsiladis, MMedSci., PhD, FACSM
University of Brighton, Welkin House
30 Carlisle Road
Eastbourne BN20 7SN (UK)
E-Mail y.pitsiladis@brighton.ac.uk

Integration of the Forensic Dimension into Anti-Doping Strategies

François Marclay · Martial Saugy

Swiss Laboratory for Doping Analyses, University Center of Legal Medicine Geneva and Lausanne, Epalinges, and Centre Hospitalier Universitaire Vaudois and University of Lausanne, Lausanne, Switzerland

Abstract

Traditionally, research in anti-doping has been stimulated by the need for technological improvements to accommodate the expansion of the list of prohibited substances and methods. Nevertheless, in recent years, anti-doping found itself at a crossroads due to the increasing complexity and constant refinement of doping methods. As illustrated by the 2012 USADA (United States Anti-Doping Agency) versus Lance Armstrong case, a change in paradigm was necessary. The exploration of new scientific avenues to understand the mechanisms of doping and pinpoint its practice was most needed to allow designing more efficient preventive or disruptive strategies. In this context, and at the time of writing in 2017, transposing the concept of forensic intelligence to anti-doping was identified as a promising approach to address the different aspects of doping, from the individual athlete to organized doping and trafficking of substances in a proactive rather than a reactive way. Indeed, collection, structuring, and logical processing of multiple sources of information, and not strictly results of bioanalytical testing of urinary and blood samples, can bring additional value to detect and describe potential, emerging, or existing doping issues. This anti-doping intelligence can provide anti-doping authorities and relevant stakeholders with timely, accurate, and usable information for decision making to solve, reduce, and/or prevent doping-related activities. The integration of intelligence to complement other anti-doping approaches is a potentially major step forward in the development of more effective and robust anti-doping strategies.

© 2017 S. Karger AG, Basel

Introduction

Traditional Approach and Challenges of Anti-Doping

Due to the continuous evolution of the list of prohibited substances and methods, research is mostly focused on the development of bioanalytical tools to analyze doping agents in biological fluids. Therefore, technological improvements, proficiency testing programs, quality management audits, accreditation surveys, and international standards for laboratory requirements naturally constitute a priority for laboratories accredited by the World Anti-Doping Agency (WADA) [1]. David Howman, WADA's director general at the time, declared [2]:

> Testing is – and always has been – the bedrock of the fight against doping in sport; science being used against science, with the hope that "our" science – that of the anti-doping community – one day becomes too sophisticated for athletes to risk doping.

This statement implies that most of the burden of the fight against doping lies on the shoulders of accredited laboratories with hopes of solving the problem by decisive improvements in analytical methods. However, due to operational constraints, researchers are bound to feed the disciplinary process of anti-doping rather than making room for thinking outside of the box [3, 4]. Indeed, up until the past few years, the community paid only peripheral attention to understanding the whole issue using strong scientific data and alternative sources of information. As consequence to a case-by-case and justice-driven approach, anti-doping continued to lack a strategic vision to cope with the complexity of the doping phenomenon.

Actually, the use of a prohibited substance or a prohibited method by an athlete is only 1 of the 10 rule violations described in the World Anti-Doping Code [5]. Nevertheless, there is a paucity of research efforts dedicated to investigating possession, trafficking, and administration of prohibited substances to any athlete, despite evidence of doping networks and a gray/black market for prohibited substances pointing to the need for an in-depth assessment and development of specific strategies [6–9]. The 3rd version of the Code, which came into force in January 2015, widened the scientific horizon by including an intelligence aspect and stressing the necessity to implement investigative tools [5]. The Code lays emphasis on improved sharing of information between anti-doping partners and enhanced accountability of athlete support personnel.

Doping and traditional criminality share many similarities in view of their mechanisms and legal context. Forensic intelligence is particularly interesting as this concept has enhanced the understanding of criminality and helped generate better-informed security solutions. The overriding hypothesis is that implementing a proactive forensic intelligence program allied to existing testing strategies could significantly improve anti-doping outcomes.

An Illustrative Doping Investigation
In 2012, the USADA (United States Anti-Doping Agency) versus Lance Armstrong case illustrated the invaluable role of criminal investigations to detect highly professionalized organized doping. Despite the lack of direct bioanalytical evidence, the investigation was successful in obtaining sworn testimony from 26 individuals, including 15 riders and 11 teammates of Lance Armstrong. In particular, 9 of his teammates were also clients of Dr. Michel Ferrari who supervised the doping program. The evidence collected during this case covers the entire career of Lance Armstrong and was of documentary, scientific, direct, and/or circumstantial nature [10, 11]. A large amount of data, including laboratory blood test results, collected throughout his career were subjected to longitudinal assessment. The sum of these approaches allowed the use, possession, and distribution of doping agents by Lance Armstrong to be unequivocally determined.

Rationale and Hypotheses on Areas for Improvement
The Lance Armstrong case illustrates a tactical use of information to provide investigative leads and to feed the judicial process. However, the case would hardly have come into scrutiny without confessions or denunciations. Therefore, a more systematic and in-depth use of data is necessary for proactive detection and identification of suspicious activities. Taking action in a timely fashion is of utmost importance to effectively deter

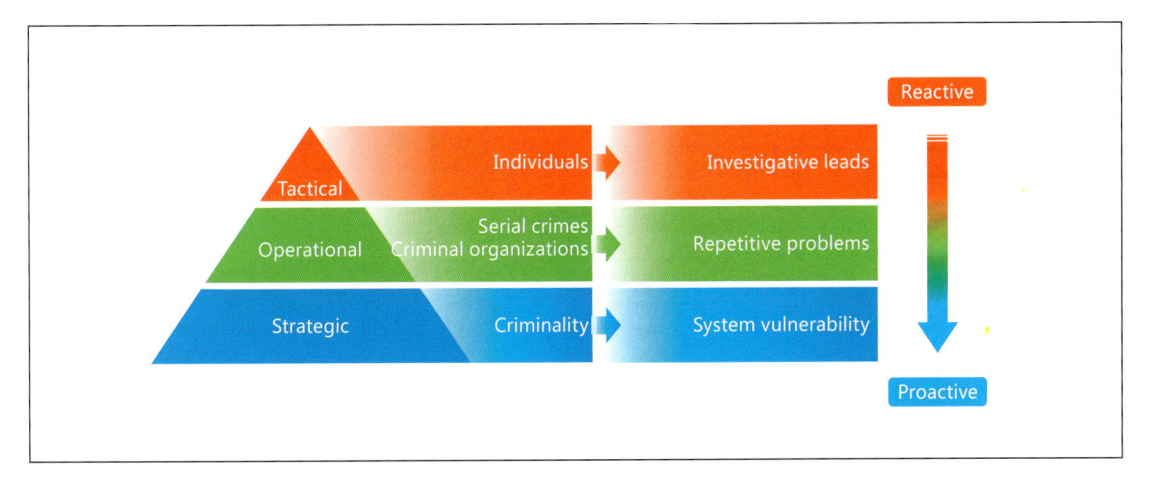

Fig. 1. Aims of each level of forensic intelligence: from the reactive micro-level of *tactical intelligence* to the crime reduction planning meso-level of *operational intelligence* and the future-oriented and proactive global level of *strategic intelligence*.

athletes from doping. The opportunity to gather broader, yet equally relevant, sources of information should be taken to better understand doping and its countless variations in order to implement effective action aimed at reducing risk, preventing substance use, legitimating observed results, or leading to punishment by courts. In this way, forensic intelligence can be used to develop more specific and efficient models to prevent and/or reduce doping in sport.

Forensic Intelligence

General Concept

In forensic science, the Locard exchange principle that "every contact leaves a trace" has been at the core of much of the field since almost a century. The trace may be defined as "an apparent sign (not always visible to the naked eye), the vestige of a presence or an action." [12]

Forensic intelligence brings a broad logical dimension to the interpretation of this mark, signal, or physical object detected and collected after litigious activity. The characteristics of these remnants are extracted and described before being integrated with information previously collated about the phenomenon. Inference structures are then constructed following logical analysis of the data to reveal a network of hypothesized links between all information. This gathering of information about the criminal phenomenon can inform decision making of tactical, operational, or strategic nature in the area of law enforcement in order to solve, reduce, or prevent crime. As such, forensic intelligence relies on 3 functional levels, namely tactical intelligence, operational intelligence, and strategic intelligence (Fig. 1).

These different levels operate on an increasing spatial and temporal dimension and interact, sharing a logical reasoning on the trace data and other numerous sources of information.

Levels of Intelligence

Tactical Intelligence

Tactical intelligence is a reactive approach supporting real-time decision making of frontline law enforcement officers and proposing investigative leads at case level. The logical analysis of traces provides accurate, timely, and usable infor-

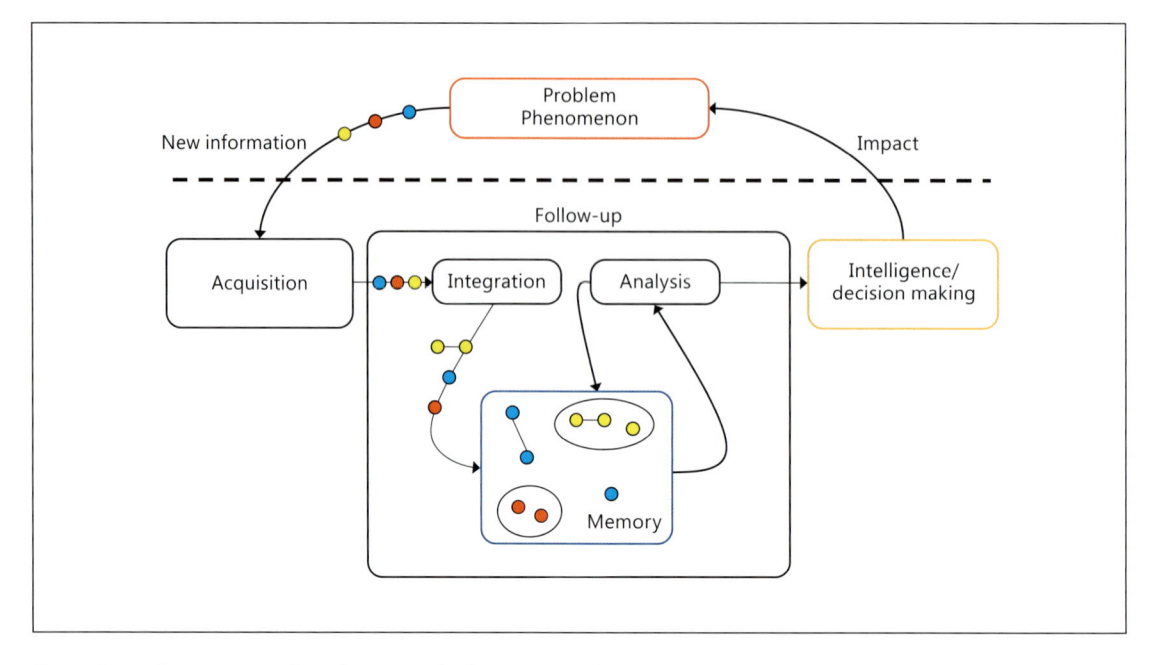

Fig. 2. Logical processing of newly acquired information and integration into a structured memory containing previously stored information [16]. The analysis is iterative and cyclic, allowing transforming raw data into timely and usable information to support decision making and impact on criminality.

mation for crime detection, for identification, localization, and arrest of potential offenders, and evidence for prosecution in court [13]. The approach is short term and case-by-case oriented, seeking to highlight the activity of an individual offender and single criminal events [14].

Operational Intelligence
Operational intelligence calls for a larger organization level to provide a comprehensive understanding of criminal trends, to ensure a follow-up, and to help in the coordination of actions [14]. The idea is to impact on repetitive problems such as serial crimes, the activities of criminal organizations, or illicit drugs trafficking with more proactive and mid-term oriented problem solving. This approach assists the targeting and deployment of law enforcement resources and the planning of actions for crime reduction or prevention [15].

With the help of exploratory, statistical, and visualization methods, extensive amounts of information are logically processed to detect geographical and/or temporal problems, to determine the type of offenders, and to identify criminal patterns. O*perational intelligence* supports intelligence-led policing with continuously refined and updated knowledge.

Strategic Intelligence
Strategic intelligence operates at a more global level of organization. Criminality is a complex phenomenon evolving over space and time due to changes in factors such as demographics, economics, and politics. *Strategic intelligence* is multivariate to better describe and understand the mechanisms behind criminality as part of a changing environment [14]. The approach is future oriented, intending to prevent the development of criminal activity by proactively identify-

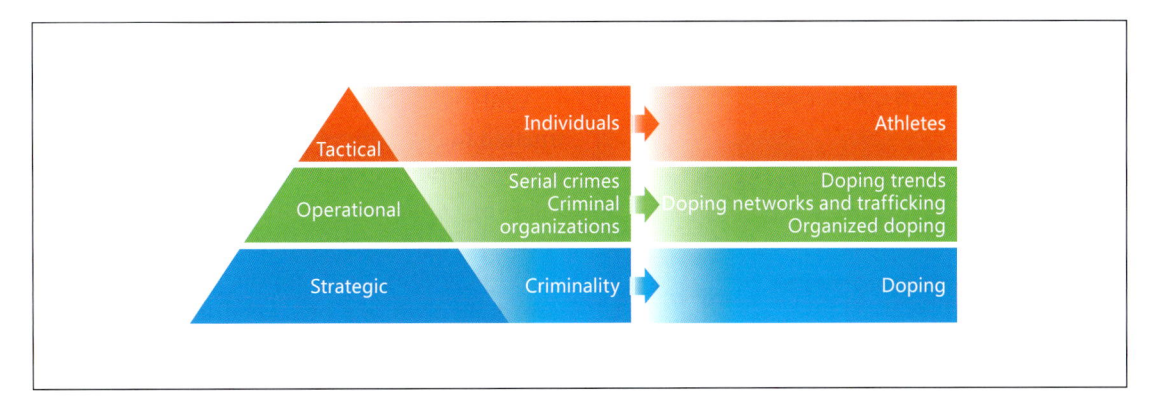

Fig. 3. Transposition of forensic intelligence into anti-doping intelligence.

ing and resolving vulnerabilities of the system. This approach seeks to impact on the whole phenomenon rather than on specific criminal activities. *Strategic intelligence* is conducive to proposing long-term problem-solving policies as well as preventive and educational interventions or programs.

Structured Memory
The operation of forensic intelligence depends on a structured memory of traces and information to gather knowledge and produce intelligence. This organized repertoire represents the knowledge we have at a certain time about the criminality under consideration, such as current criminal problems, serial crimes, and linked cases (Fig. 2).

In practice, information on a criminal phenomenon is first acquired and then integrated into a follow-up framework. Characteristics of these new data are extracted and sorted out prior to being merged with previously memorized information, allowing inference structures to reveal a network of hypothesized links. The reasoning process is entirely based on postulating and testing assumptions on the relation between items organized in the memory. The analysis is interpretative, and each new piece of information may confirm the predicted truth value of hypothesized links and/or connect sets of information originally considered as distinct. Conversely, the logical process may question or even exclude the existence of links previously assumed. Newly acquired information can be organized in a short-term memory for direct exploitation on a specific criminal case or integrated into a long-term memory to depict criminal trends or series or to identify vulnerabilities.

Perspectives for Anti-Doping
Transposition of the Concept

Forensic intelligence can be transposed into anti-doping intelligence by relying on a similar methodology and shifting the paradigm to the problem of doping in sport (Fig. 3).

At a tactical level, the focus of anti-doping intelligence would be on the athletes as individual offenders. The exploitation of traces, including bioanalytical results, documents linked to the practice of doping, and the distribution, administration, and/or consumption of doping agents, would serve to instigate investigative leads on athletes and/or individuals responsible for the doping activity. Likewise, this process would bring scientific evidence to legitimate punishment from anti-doping authorities.

At an operational level, attention would be placed on trends in the abuse of prohibited substances and doping behaviors in general, orga-

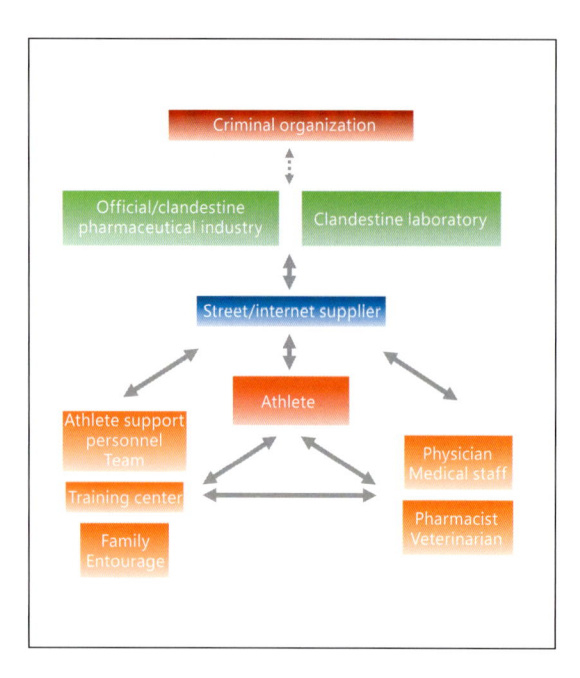

Fig. 4. Doping network and the diversity of potential links between its different intermediaries.

nized doping, and the trafficking and/or distribution of doping agents. Seriality can be defined as the recurring character of these activities. For instance, the use of hormones and/or peptides represents a form of systematic doping as the methodology involves continuous intake over long periods of time rather than a single intake. In other words, a doping program, or protocol, is followed. The exploitation of traces would serve to detect these issues, to assess their temporal and geographical dimensions, and to identify their mechanisms.

At a strategic level, the focus is on understanding the whole doping phenomenon. The reasoning would seek to determine the human, environmental, economical, or even political, factors of doping initiation among sport practitioners. The strategic dimension of intelligence seeks to prevent the phenomenon by proposing solutions to minimize, if not neutralize, the influence of predisposing and facilitating factors.

Organized Doping: Trafficking and Distribution of Doping Agents – Overview

With the 2016 WADA prohibited list being estimated to cover more than 700 substances, trafficking of doping agents is a lucrative business following complex pathways and may involve criminal organizations [17].

While doping may appear self-motivated, it always involves one or several intermediates in the supply or/and use of doping agents. These entities may include the relatives and entourage of the athlete, medical staff, athlete support personnel, teammates, chemists, biologists/pharmacists, pharmaceutical industries, and clandestine laboratories, which may even be further connected to criminal organizations, drug smugglers, and dealers (Fig. 4).

Intelligence Approach to Organized Doping

Except in a few jurisdictions, doping networks benefit from relative safety created by the lack of collaboration, and legal ground, in sharing relevant information held by organizations such as WADA, national and regional anti-doping organizations, national and international sports federations, WADA-accredited laboratories, national customs and border agencies, national police services, and INTERPOL (the International Criminal Police Organization). Logical processing of information after collection and structuring may prove useful and particularly efficient for identifying, neutralizing, disrupting, and/or preventing systematic doping or trafficking networks [13]. Forensic methodologies have been developed to fight illicit drug trafficking and the counterfeiting of pharmaceuticals [18]. With doping agents covering a large part of these categories of substances, this methodology can be transposed to anti-doping.

With online sales showing a growing popularity, strategic internet monitoring reveals useful information. Search engines and automatic alert systems on specific keywords allow listing and following online sales websites to obtain a large panorama of the market and to detect the emergence of new trends [19]. The extraction of digital data on the website coding may indicate the origin of the products and sales areas across the world, the geolocation of the retailer, and, at times, even the supplier's identity. Such an analysis may also highlight links between online sales websites and, therefore, refine the comprehension of the structure and activity of the market. The analysis of forums, blogs, social networks, and other online media also contributes to increasing the knowledge on distribution networks. These tools provide an overview of supply and demand and an estimation of consumption prevalence.

Drug profiling of seized products also generates relevant information to infer the source of production. The extraction of the physical and chemical profiles can highlight links between products to apprehend the organization of illicit drug trafficking [19, 20]. Physical profiling in the form of an optical examination of the packaging and product provides important information on the producer and its modus operandi. Chemical profiling in the form of the identification and quantification of the active compound and excipients of the seized product can highlight links between similar products or, alternatively, between different products from the same production line [21, 22].

Inference models are built upon physical examination, chemical characterization, digital data, and other circumstantial data to link product seizures, bring to light distribution networks, and identify supply sources. The models serve to evaluate the state and activity of gray and black markets to support decision making and prioritizing [23].

Similar chemical and/or physical profiles can indicate a link between separate product seizures or a priori unrelated trafficking cases [20]. *Strategic intelligence* can serve to visualize the organization of trafficking networks, from production to distribution, to identify key points and tendencies in the supply and use of illicit products. This approach can help refine the targeting of athletes or sports teams, identify doping promoters, and deploy adequate operations to dismantle core ramifications of doping networks. The overall advantage is to elicit information of a complementary nature compared to the current practice.

Establishing an intelligent system is dependent upon the will of governments and on anti-doping authorities to cooperate and legislate the sharing of sensitive data. This sharing of knowledge on doping activities between all the anti-doping stakeholders would require a principal location to gather information and reduce its fragmentation. Indeed, despite the existence of databases such as the WADA anti-doping administration and management system, others at individual national anti-doping organizations, the athlete biological passport, and the urinary steroidal passport at accredited laboratories and investigation information, a global organized forensic intelligence system is lacking. A coordination structure would help to communicate relevant and timely information among anti-doping professionals to elaborate efficient action strategies.

Highlighting Doping with Comprehensive and Indirect Approaches

Collaborative research between experts in the fields of analytical chemistry, endocrinology, genetics, pharmacology, physiology, and sports medicine is needed to adequately address and understand the specificities of each doping situation [24]. Collating analytical results, which may include atypical findings and previous adverse analytical findings, longitudinal monitoring of biomarkers, individual physiological characteristics of the athlete, epidemiological, sociological, circumstantial, and other relevant information, and products of intelligence, could all provide a fit-for-purpose logical framework. Information gathering can help refine the targeting of suspicious athletes to identify the likely cheaters. This process can also strengthen the use of nonbioanalytical data to detect and assess a rule violation and to support cases brought to court.

Accordingly, the athlete biological passport aims at the indirect detection of blood doping and takes into account natural variations over time to set personalized and adaptive confidence intervals and limits [25, 26]. Likewise, steroidomics aims at the discovery of biomarkers of doping with synthetic analogues of androgenic anabolic steroids or indirect doping with selective estrogen receptor modulators, aromatase inhibitors, or human chorionic gonadotropin. The modification of the steroid profile is processed through chemometric models taking into account the global steroid metabolism to distinguish between a natural physiological condition and steroid misuse [27]. From a *tactical intelligence* perspective, athletes are targeted based upon alerts generated when abnormal variations are detected. This increases the efficiency of doping controls and the deterrence of blood doping [28]. Likewise, within an *operational intelligence* framework, longitudinal monitoring of athletes highlights trends amongst the sports community.

Detection and Monitoring of Doping Phenomena

Anti-doping intelligence can help in the detection and description of a potential, emerging, or existing, yet unnoticed, trend in the consumption of doping agents. Information may come from numerous sources such as sociological studies on substance use, a notice of release from the pharmaceutical industry on a new medication with performance-enhancing properties, and statistics of law enforcement authorities on trafficking. Exploiting these elements and internet monitoring can serve to define testing strategies to detect substance misuse and to measure variations in prevalence between sports disciplines, genders, and across space and time [29]. *Operational* and *strategic intelligence* strategies could be adapted to the peculiarities of each doping situation. Tailor-made strategies might offer additional value as long as they remain consistent with the Code's principle of universality.

Operational intelligence can help in prioritizing areas where anti-doping resources are needed to provide a more proactive response to short-circuit potential or emerging trends or to address existing problems with innovative actions. Similarly, *strategic intelligence* can result in the inclusion of a substance or method to the list or the monitoring program, the adjustment of existing law policies, the development of preventive or educational programs, or, conversely, the decision not to legislate or to cancel a regulation as the problem.

Conclusion and Perspectives

The constant refinement and increasing complexity of doping methods require a change in paradigm in anti-doping. Traditionally, research in the field has been focusing on technological improvements required to accommodate the expansion of the list. Nevertheless, while bioanalytical methods keep improving, the problem simultaneously evolves towards more specialized doping. The 2012 USADA versus Armstrong case is a striking example of very elaborate doping where no adverse analytical finding was reported over the course of an entire and extremely successful road cycling career.

Regardless of the individual or organized character of doping, mechanisms of criminal nature for the production and distribution of prohibited substances are involved. This lucrative business sees a growing number of producers and trafficking routes, hence the difficulty to disrupt doping when solely focusing on testing. Athletes being end-products of the business, a focal point on these individuals has limited leverage and deterrent effect on doping networks. Accredited laboratories unarguably possess state-of-the-art technology. However, the efficiency of testing depends, foremost, upon the capacity of timely and accurately targeting the most likely cheaters. This crucial point remains challenging.

Therefore, efficient preventive or disruptive strategies rely on the exploration of new scientific avenues to understand and highlight doping mechanisms. In this context, anti-doping intelligence is an innovative approach to address the different aspects of doping, from the individual level up to the organized doping and trafficking level in a proactive rather than reactive way. Through structuring and logical processing of multiple sources of information, anti-doping intelligence can bring additional value to detect and describe potential, emerging, or existing doping trends. In turn, anti-doping authorities and partners of the fight can be provided with timely, accurate, and usable information for decision making to solve, reduce, and/or prevent a phenomenon. Further evaluating and putting to test the different intelligence concepts in the field is essential to build an operational system. If such a system can be coordinated by the different partners of the fight against doping, supplied and supported by these professionals, there is no doubt a major step forward could be made.

References

1 World Anti-Doping Agency: The 2016 International Standards for Laboratories. Montreal, WADA, 2015, www.wada-ama.org (accessed May 2016).
2 Howman D: Current limitations in analytical strategies. Bioanalysis 2012;4: 1535–1536.
3 Marclay F, Mangin P, Margot P, Saugy M: Perspectives for forensic intelligence in anti-doping: thinking outside of the box. Forensic Sci Int 2013;229:133–144.
4 Marclay F, Jan N, Esseiva P, Mangin P, Margot P, Saugy M: Le changement de paradigme du renseignement forensique pour la lutte contre le dopage organisé et le trafic de substances interdites. Rev Int Criminol Police Tech Sci 2013;4:451–472.
5 World Anti-Doping Agency: The World Anti-Doping Code, the Code. Montreal, WADA, 2015, www.wada-ama.org (accessed May 2016).
6 Jan N, Marclay F, Schmutz N, Smith M, Lacoste A, Castella V, Mangin P: Use of forensic investigations in anti-doping. Forensic Sci Int 2011;213:109–113.
7 Donati A, World Anti-Doping Agency (WADA): World Traffic in Doping Substances. Montreal, WADA, 2007, www.wada-ama.org (accessed May 2016).
8 Waddington I: Sport, Health and Drugs: A Critical Sociological Perspective. London, Spon Press, 2000.
9 Lentillon-Kaestner V: The development of doping use in high-level cycling: from team-organized doping to advances in the fight against doping. Scand J Med Sci Sports 2013;23:189–197.
10 United States Anti-Doping Agency: U.S. Postal Service Pro Cycling Team Investigation. Statement from USADA CEO Travis T. Tygart regarding the U.S. Postal Service Pro Cycling Team Doping Conspiracy. Colorado Springs, USADA, 2012, http://cyclinginvestigation.usada.org (accessed May 2016).
11 United States Anti-Doping Agency: U.S. Postal Service Pro Cycling Team Investigation, Reasoned Report. Colorado Springs, USADA, 2012, http://d3epuodzu3wuis.cloudfront.net/ReasonedDecision.pdf (accessed May 2016).
12 Margot P: La trace comme vecteur fondamental de la police scientifique; in Ricordel I (ed): L'expertise en police scientifique. Montrouge, Montauban, 2011.
13 Ribaux O, Walsh SJ, Margot P: The contribution of forensic science to crime analysis and investigation: forensic intelligence. Forensic Sci Int 2006;156: 171–181.
14 Ratcliffe JH: Integrated Intelligence and Crime Analysis: Enhanced Information Management for Law Enforcement Leaders. Washington, United States Department of Justice, Office of Community Oriented Policing Services (COPS), 2007, http://www.jratcliffe.net/wp-content/uploads/Ratcliffe-2007-Integrated-intelligence-and-crime-analysis.pdf (accessed May 2016).
15 Ribaux O, Girod A, Walsh SJ, Margot P, Mizrahi S, Clivaz V: Forensic intelligence and crime analysis. Law Prob Risk 2003;2:47–60.
16 Ribaux O, Genessay T, Margot P: Les processus de veille opérationnelle et science forensique pour suivre des problèmes de sécurité; in Leman-Langlois S (ed): Sphères de surveillance. Montreal, Presses de L'Université de Montréal, 2011, pp 137–158.
17 World Anti-Doping Agency: The World Anti-Doping Code, the 2016 Prohibited List. Montreal, WADA, 2015, www.wada-ama.org (accessed May 2016).
18 Dégardin K, Roggo Y, Been F, Margot P: Detection and chemical profiling of medicine counterfeits by Raman spectroscopy and chemometrics. Anal Chim Acta 2011;705:334–341.
19 Pazos D, Giannasi P, Rossy Q, Esseiva P: Combining Internet monitoring processes, packaging and isotopic analyses to determine the market structure: example of gamma butyrolactone. Forensic Sci Int 2013;230:29–36.

20 Morelato M, Beavis A, Tahtouh M, Ribaux O, Kirkbride P, Roux C: The use of forensic case data in intelligence-led policing: the example of drug profiling. Forensic Sci Int 2013;226:1–9.

21 Been F, Roggo Y, Degardin K, Esseiva P, Margot P: Profiling of counterfeit medicines by vibrational spectroscopy. Forensic Sci Int 2011;211:83–100.

22 Esseiva P, Dujourdy L, Anglada F, Taroni F, Margot P: A methodology for illicit heroin seizures comparison in a drug intelligence perspective using large databases. Forensic Sci Int 2003;132:139–152.

23 Esseiva P, Ioset S, Anglada F, Gaste L, Ribaux O, Margot P, et al: Forensic drug intelligence: an important tool in law enforcement. Forensic Sci Int 2007;167:247–254.

24 Bowers LD: Anti-dope testing in sport: the history and the science. FASEB J 2012;26:3933–3936.

25 Sottas PE, Robinson N, Saugy M: The athlete's biological passport and indirect markers of blood doping. Handb Exp Pharmacol 2010;195:305–326.

26 Robinson N, Saugy M, Vernec A, Sottas PE: The athlete biological passport: an effective tool in the fight against doping. Clin Chem 2011;57:830–832.

27 Boccard J, Badoud F, Grata E, Ouertani S, Hanafi M, Mazerolles G, et al: A steroidomic approach for biomarkers discovery in doping control. Forensic Sci Int 2011;213:85–94.

28 Robinson N, Dollé G, Garnier PY, Saugy M: 2011 IAAF World Championships in Daegu: blood tests for all athletes in the framework of the athlete biological passport. Bioanalysis 2012;4:1633–1643.

29 Pitsch W, Emrich E: The frequency of doping in elite sport: results of a replication study. Int Rev Sociol Sport 2012;47:559–580.

François Marclay, PhD
Intelligence Manager
Cycling Anti-Doping Foundation (CADF)
Chemin des Croisettes 22
CH–1860 Aigle (Switzerland)
E-Mail Francois.Marclay@cadf.ch

Next Generation Anti-Doping Approaches

How to Develop Intelligence Gathering in Efficient and Practical Anti-Doping Activities

Mathieu Holz[a] · Jack Robertson[b]

[a] European Regional Office, World Anti-Doping Agency (WADA), Lausanne, Switzerland; [b] Head Office, WADA, Montreal, QC, Canada

Abstract

Prior to the formation of the World Anti-Doping Agency (WADA), the fight against doping in sport was not unified; instead, it relied on individual approaches established by various stakeholders to make it effective. The scandal of the Festina Affair, during the Tour de France 1998, and other drug doping scandals revealed the ineffectiveness and inadequacy of such an approach. The resulting media scandal raised public authorities' awareness about the necessity to deal with doping in sport with a harmonized and a more effective approach. The International Olympic Committee interceded and convened a World Conference on Doping, bringing together all parties involved in the fight against doping. As a result, WADA was established on November 10, 1999, in Lausanne to promote and coordinate the fight against doping in sport internationally. In this regard, the World Anti-Doping Code (WADC or the Code) is the core document harmonizing anti-doping rules and regulations within sport organizations and public authorities. The Code was instrumental in introducing the concept of "nonanalytical" rule violations, which are emphasized within the revised 2015 Code. Nonanalytical rule violations allow anti-doping organizations (ADOs) to apply sanctions in cases where there is no positive doping sample, but where there may still be evidence that a doping violation has occurred. This recognition of "nonanalytical" rule violations by WADA is the concrete result of taking into account lessons learned from prior infamous doping scandals. Thus, intelligence gathering, particularly through cooperation with global law enforcement agencies, is a key tool in the fight against doping. The 2015 Code and the international standards on testing and investigations establish and implement intelligence gathering as part of ADOs' routine activities in the fight against doping in sport.   © 2017 S. Karger AG, Basel

Intelligence Gathering: A Key Tool in the Fight against Doping

In the late 1990s and early 2000s, several major scandals impacted top level sport and highlighted large scale doping practices. Those scandals, due to their importance and large media coverage, revealed to a stunned public the "dark side" of elite sports.

In July 1998, Belgium physiotherapist Willy Voët of the Festina Team and personal physiotherapist to Richard Virenque was stopped by French customs officers as he attempted to drive across the Belgian-French border. What began as a routine control stop led to one of the biggest doping scandals in cycling history. Inside the car, provided by Tour de France organizers and sporting team colors, customs officers discovered and seized 235 vials of erythropoietin (EPO) coming from 3 laboratories in Germany and Switzerland, 120 capsules of amphetamines, 82 solutions of human growth hormone, and 60 vials of testosterone, corticoids, and amphetamines. This seizure indicated large scale doping practice within the Festina team and a criminal investigation was initiated for the smuggling and illegal importation of prohibited substances. Although initially downplayed by organizers and some sport officials, the existence of widespread and systematic doping amongst Festina riders was soon recognized. The complete team was excluded from the Tour de France for unethical behavior. In November 1998, doping tests conducted on Festina riders highlighted their use of EPO and amphetamines. As a result, 2 Festina senior managers were given a 1-year suspended sentence. Richard Virenque, the Festina team leader, was discharged for eliciting other riders to take doping substances. The French criminal court also underlined and criticized various cycling authorities for their passive approach regarding doping issues [1].

A few years later, in June 2003, the US Anti-Doping Agency (USADA) received an anonymous phone call from Trevor Graham, a US sprint coach, accusing several top level US athletes of doping with a substance unknown at that time. USADA also collected information regarding the source of this substance: Bay Area Laboratory Co-Operative (BALCO) and the nickname of this steroid substance "The Clear." As evidence, USADA received from the same source a syringe containing traces of tetrahydrogestrinone (THG). Based on this intelligence, the UCLA Olympic Analytical Laboratory developed a testing process for THG; 550 athletes were subsequently tested and 20 were found positive for THG. In September 2003, a US Federal investigation led by the IRS CID (Internal Revenue Service Criminal Investigations Department), the FDA/OCI (Food and Drug Administration Office of Criminal Investigations), and USADA resulted not only in a seizure of BALCO doping substances, but also a list of user names and doping protocols. Top level US athletes were implicated from various sport leagues, including the MLB (Major League Baseball) and NFL (National Football League), various disciplines, including track and field, boxing and cycling, as well as Olympic Games' winners. This investigation led to one of the biggest doping scandals in the US history. Marion Jones and Tim Montgomery were some of the most famous US athletes linked to the BALCO scandal. The owner of BALCO and later Jones plead guilty and received jail sentences for their involvement in the BALCO affair.

In 2004, during an interview between a *Diário AS* journalist and the Spanish professional road racing cyclist Jesús María Manzano-Ruan, information was disclosed regarding the cyclist's former team Kelme. Manzano-Ruan detailed systematic and widespread doping activities inside his team under the guidance and eye of several team doctors, including Eufemiano Fuentes. In 2006, the Central Operation Unit of the Spanish Guardia Civil started the "Operation Puerto," an investigation into the alleged doping practices of Eufemiano Fuentes [2]. In May 2006, 5 men were arrested by the Guardia Civil, accused of doping practices with riders. During searches, which included Fuentes's residence, investigators found thousands of doses of anabolic steroids, more than 200 bags of blood substances (blood and blood plasma), and machines to process and transfuse blood. A list of 200 Spanish and other nationality athletes was also found, with top level athletes from various sports including cyclists. In

November 2006, the Spanish newspaper *El Mundo* obtained access to analyzed results of the bags of blood seized by the Guardia Civil. Based on the analysis of the blood bags, the journalists reported an overview of Dr. Fuentes's doping program. A few weeks before a race, riders would contact Fuentes to have blood withdrawn. The blood would then be processed, separating the red blood cells from the blood plasma. The red blood cells would then be infused back into the cyclist shortly before or during competition. Per the Code, the reintroduction of autologous blood (blood doping) is a prohibited method. The blood levels of the cyclists would be closely monitored. If hematocrit levels were too high in comparison with the athlete's classical average, blood plasma enhanced with EPO would be re-injected in order to dilute red blood cells and avoid doping detection.

Due to inadequacies in the law and other factors, those deemed culpable during Operation Puerto were not brought before a Spanish court of criminal law until 2013. At the conclusion of the trial, Dr. Fuentes and others were found guilty and were given minimal to suspended sentences. Dr. Fuentes openly stated he assisted top levels Spanish riders and athletes of other sports and discussed a willingness to identify all his former clients. However, the identities of the athletes who provided the blood bags still remain unknown. The trial judge rendered a decision that the case would not be investigated further and ordered destruction of the blood bags rather than handing them over to the Spanish Anti-Doping Agency. Appeals against this decision were filed by the Prosecution, the Spanish National Anti-Doping Organization (NADO), UCI (the International Cycling Union), and WADA. In July 2016, a decision by a Spanish judge allowed WADA to access the blood bags. WADA extracted plasma, whole blood, and condensed blood fractions and transported them to a WADA-accredited laboratory for further analysis.

On December 3, 2014, the German Television channel ARD aired a documentary "The secrets of doping: how Russia makes its winners." [3]. This documentary disclosed the existence of a sophisticated doping system within ARAF (All-Russia Athletic Federation – the governing body for the sport of athletics in the Russian Federation). The documentary revealed the involvement of athletes, coaches, and national and international sports federations, as well as the Russian Anti-Doping Agency (RUSADA) and the WADA-accredited anti-doping laboratory of Moscow.

Following these revelations, WADA took the opportunity provided by the 2015 World Anti-Doping Code (WADC) to launch investigations. In fact, Article 20.7.10 of the Code regarding the roles and responsibilities of WADA specifies: "to initiate its own investigations of anti-doping rule violations and other activities that may facilitate doping." On December 16, 2014, WADA formed an independent commission (IC) composed of Richard W. Pound, Prof. Richard H. McLaren, and Gunter Younger [4].

The IC was supported by a US-based private investigator company as well as the WADA Intelligence and Investigations Department and WADA staff. Much of the information on which IC investigators worked on were provided by whistle-blowers, and more particularly by Yulia Stepanova (800-m athlete) and her husband Vitaly Stepanov (former RUSADA employee). Thanks to their unwavering courage and convictions, IC investigators were provided with first-hand evidence (audio and video records) that gave a clear vision of the backstage.

The IC has identified failures within the International Association of Athletics Federations (IAAF) and the Federation of Russia that prevented or diminished the possibility of an effective anti-doping program. The IC report spoke of a deeply rooted culture of cheating within Russian athletics as well as corruption and bribery within the IAAF.

Based on its findings, the IC recommended that WADA:
- Declare ARAF and RUSADA to be Code non-compliant.
- Withdraw the Moscow anti-doping laboratory accreditation.
- Remove the Moscow laboratory director from his position.

The IC also recommended that IAAF suspend ARAF.

At the same time, in the framework of the Memorandum of Understanding signed in 2009 between WADA and INTERPOL (International Criminal Police Organization), the IC forwarded an intelligence report to INTERPOL [5]. French financial prosecution services initiated investigations on criminal conducts done by individuals within the IAAF. Mr. Lamine Diack, former IAAF president, was placed under formal inquiry along with his personal lawyer and advisor as both are suspected of corruption for doping cover-up. INTERPOL released a red notice on Mr. Papa Massata Diack, the son of Lamine Diack and IAAF marketing consultant [6]. The investigations are currently ongoing.

As a result of the IC investigations:
- On November 10, 2015, WADA temporarily suspended the accreditation of the Moscow anti-doping laboratory; his director, Dr. Grigory Rodchenkov, was fired by Russian authorities.
- On November 13, 2015, IAAF suspended ARAF.
- On November 18, 2015, WADA suspended RUSADA.
- On January 2016, IAAF Ethics Commissions issued life ban to Papa Massata Diack, Valentin Balaknichev (former IAAF treasurer), and Alexei Melnikov (former Russian coach); the former head of the IAAF Anti-Doping Unit received a 5-year suspension.
- On April 15, 2016, the Moscow anti-doping laboratory was revoked [7].

Fearing for his life, Dr. Rodchenkov fled to the USA with the support of a US producer and film director. In February 2016, within 2 weeks, Viatcheslav Sinev (former chairman of the Executive Board of RUSADA from 2008 to 2010) and Nikita Kamaev (the former CEO of RUSADA from 2011 to December 2015) died suddenly.

On May 12, 2016, Dr. Rodchenkov claimed in *The New York Times* that he covered up positive tests at the Winter Olympics Games in Sochi. This cover-up was done with the support of the Federal Security Service of the Russian Federation: the FSB. FSB is the Russian secret service and successor of the KGB.

On May 19, 2016, WADA appointed Prof. Richard H. McLaren as an independent person (IP) to investigate these allegations on doping during the Sochi Winter Olympics. The IP was seconded by an English-based private investigator company, WADA Intelligence and Investigations Department, and relevant scientists. Investigations were conducted by the IP within a very limited time: 57 days.

The IP investigation team led to the following key findings [8]:
- The Moscow laboratory operated, for the protection of doped Russian athletes, within a state-dictated fail-safe system, described in the report as the *disappearing positive methodology*.
- The Sochi laboratory operated a unique sample swapping methodology to enable doped Russian athletes to compete at the Games.
- The Ministry of Sport directed, controlled, and oversaw the manipulation of athlete's analytical results or sample swapping, with the active participation and assistance of the FSB, CSP (Center of Sports Preparation of National Teams of Russia), and both Moscow and Sochi laboratories.

While the IP led investigations, it appeared that what happened during Sochi as described by Dr. Rodchenkov was an exceptional situation. More particularly, a specific adaptation of a well-established doping cover-up system directed during many years by and with the support of the Russian authorities.

Following catastrophic results at the 2010 Winter Olympics in Vancouver, a new Deputy Sports Minister was appointed, Yuri Nagornykh. A "win at all costs" mentality appeared to ensure Russia a maximum of success in various sports, but more particularly the Olympic ones.

In this regard, from late 2011 to August 2015, the Moscow laboratory operated under the State directorate oversight and control of its anti-doping operational system. The objective was to enable Russian athletes to train and compete while using doping substances. As required to be part of the state system, the Moscow laboratory was an essential component of this regime. Information has emerged that purports that any Russian athlete not protected by the different mechanisms in place during the sample collection and transport process, would be protected by a fail-safe protective shield at the laboratory where the disappearing positive methodology took place. If the first analytical screen of the athlete samples revealed an adverse analytical finding, the laboratory stopped the process and referred immediately to a liaison person within the Ministry of Sport. The liaison person identified the relevant athlete and provided this code sample number to RUSADA. Once clearly identified, the athlete case was referred to the Vice Minister of Sport who decided *save* or *quarantine*. If the order was *save*, the sample was reported as negative findings. The laboratory information management system was also manipulated to reflect this negative analysis. For *quarantine*, the laboratory followed up the analytical process and reported an adverse analytical finding.

This elaborate plan was executed at the Moscow laboratory. During the Olympic Games, the Olympic Anti-Doping Laboratory hosted many international observers [9]. The disappearing positive results would obviously not work under the guise of the international observers. To resolve this issue, a sample swapping plan was developed by the Russian Ministry of Sport, the Moscow laboratory, the CSP, and FSB. Months before the Sochi Games, a pool of clean urine was prepared under the control of the CSP. The plan was for this clean urine to be tested instead of the doped athletes urine. In the dark of night, a joint operation took place involving the Sochi laboratory director and FSB. The urine samples of preselected Russian athletes, tainted with doping substances, were replaced by clean urine of the corresponding athlete. FSB officers, registered as plumbers by the accreditation service, managed to open the tamper-proof bottles containing the urine of doped athletes. This urine was exchanged with the clean urine, and Dr. Rodchenkov added table salt or diluted water in order to match the specific urine gravity as registered on the doping control form. Then the urine bottles filled with clean urine were ready for normal testing the subsequent morning.

Following these allegations, IP investigators conducted a forensic investigation of the plastic cap of the urine kit and on the urine itself. For every urine sample bottle examined, the IP investigation team and forensic expert identified scratches and marks revealing evidence of tampering (caps had been removed and reused). Furthermore, analytical analysis of the same samples by the London anti-doping laboratory revealed that they had a salt level 6 times higher than the average salt level of the human body. DNA analysis also revealed that in 3 samples the DNA did not match that of the athlete. Forensic evidence (scratches and marks, salt and DNA analysis) confirmed interview evidence provided by whistle-blowers.

Since 2015, WADA had the capacity to lead the investigations. Investigations are particularly effective when based on evidence provided by whistle-blowers. They are the only persons who could help investigators to break the "law of silence" and shed light on what really went on in terms of doping.

WADA developed a whistle-blower policy "Speak up" (https://speakup.wada-ama.org/

WebPages/Public/FrontPages/Default.aspx) to ensure that evidence provided by whistle-blowers is properly followed up, and whistle-blowers receive guidance and legal advice to protect their integrity during investigations.

Lessons Learned from Doping Scandals

Two fundamental aspects emerge from the analysis of these major scandals:
1. The necessity to cooperate with law enforcement authorities.
2. The importance of intelligence gathering.

These two aspects are interrelated, and integrating these activities with anti-doping practice would ensure a much higher likelihood of successful investigative outcomes.

Cooperation with law enforcement is essential. These scandals highlight systematic and complex doping networks with international connections. In some instances, several similarities with organized crime appear. In fact, investigators identified structured groups, defined as 2 or more people, established over time and acting accordingly to commit doping rule violations. This complexity makes proving such anti-doping rule violations (ADRVs) far beyond the ability of most anti-doping organizations (ADOs). First of all, an appropriate legal framework is a prerequisite to legally lead investigations. Unfortunately, very few countries have passed legislation providing their ADOs with the legal framework to lead investigations – even on a basic administrative level. Moreover, many of the ADOs lack the necessary human and material resources as well as any investigative experience. Currently, only a very small number of ADOs have the necessary financial and human resources, or the appropriate legal framework, to conduct investigations. Despite this, select ADOs have signed cooperation agreements or memorandums of understanding with appropriate national law enforcement agencies in order to collect intelligence or operational data they would not be able to collect by themselves. Such agreements allow the ADOs to have a deeper inside view of doping networks and a better understanding of their mechanisms.

Signed cooperation agreements allow law enforcement agencies, within defined limits, the ability to share intelligence with ADOs. This is one of the key issues for ADOs: to gather enough intelligence and evidence to bring forth one or more ADRVs as defined by the Code. Intelligence, in combination with or in the absence of analytical evidence, increasingly plays a vital role in identifying, targeting, and ultimately catching doping athletes. These data are invaluable to ADOs in their file preparation against athletes involved in doping. In addition, this intelligence provides ADOs a better understanding of the role and involvement of the athlete's entourage in ADRVs. ADOs are better able to determine how and at what stage the coach, medical staff, team management, and the manager (etc.) were possibly involved in an ADRV. Changes in the revised 2015 WADC (or the Code) allow ADOs to penalize the entourage more efficiently.

Several types of intelligence are gathered and analyzed during an investigative process and provide a clearer overview about ADRVs.

Information on Persons

The objective of intelligence gathering and/or an investigative process is to identify and target the main individuals involved in doping and to assess their level of involvement. Gathered intelligence will help identify the collusion between athletes, medical staff, managers, and coaches inside or outside the team. But this intelligence will further help identify suppliers of doping substances. Investigations conducted on former Tour de France riders revealed the performance- and image-enhancing drug (PED) suppliers could be individuals without any professional or working relationship with the involved team. This problem is more difficult to solve for investigators conducting surveillance, for example. In fact, due to the large number of persons working around the team and the open configuration of the Tour de France, it is very difficult to identify the PED supplier among all the others. Therefore, strong evidence or first-hand information from insiders is very helpful.

Information on Substances

An important objective is to identify what PED substances are most likely being utilized and the intended effects (muscle mass gain or performance enhancement) for athletes. The substance(s) could be already known (possibly combined with others), which may or may not be easily detected by testing. More challenging for ADOs are those substances not yet known. These can be unapproved medicines, a substance still under clinical trial, or worse, substances whose development was terminated for severe potential health risks, or substances not intended for human consumption. In many cases, these types of unknown substances create difficulties for investigators in bringing forth criminal charges.

Example. In early summer 2011, Belgium law enforcement seized a sample of TB 5OO (thymosin β_4), a substance for veterinary use only, purchased on the Internet, and sold by an Australian veterinary laboratory company. The purchaser was a former Belgium rider and current VIP driver for a Belgium cycling team participating in the 2011 Tour de France.

Belgium law enforcement was initially unclear as to whether they should qualify this veterinary substance as a doping substance in the framework of the prohibited list. Intelligence gathered from INTERPOL's member countries underlined the fact that TB 500 is used primarily for race animals (horses and dogs). It acts on the muscular system and has anabolic properties. The WADA Prohibited List Expert Group had previously declared TB 500 a doping substance and prohibited its use in and out of competition under category S2 Peptide Hormones, Growth Factors, Related Substances, and Mimetics. As a result of the WADA Prohibited List Committee's declaration on TB 500, Belgium law enforcement initiated a criminal investigation.

Other forms of intelligence are important for understanding doping protocols, the process, and techniques used to avoid anti-doping detection. In the same way, investigations could provide information on the methods of concealment and the means in which doping athletes or their entourage hide, transport, and smuggle their PED substances.

Information about Financial Aspects

Very often, investigations provide evidence regarding the price of the doping substances and by consequence identify the financial issues and network involved. For example, a 10-mg vial of TB 500 costs about USD 400. During the investigation of the Austrian company HumanPlasma, top level athletes paid tens of thousands of Euros for EPO doses and a blood doping protocol. This type of sophisticated product and treatment are not within the financial reach of most athletes. This is far removed from the low-cost/basic anabolic steroid products purchased on thousands of different websites. Analyzing PED price and payment structures provided investigators with a better understanding of the network set up to supply athletes with both expensive and inexpensive substances.

Cooperation Agreement between INTERPOL and WADA

In the light of these elements, cooperation with law enforcement is a clear necessity. WADA integrated this strategy early and signed a cooperation agreement with the INTERPOL General Secretariat in 2009 [10].

INTERPOL is the world's largest international police organization, with 190 member countries. INTERPOL has 4 strategic priorities:

1. To provide a secure global police communication network for connecting the National Central Bureau (NCB) with national law enforcement agencies for all 190 member countries.
2. To provide around-the-clock support to policing.
3. To provide training to build crime-fighting capacity.
4. To assist in the identification of crime trends and criminal behavior.

The INTERPOL General Secretariat is stationed in Lyon, France, but operates from 7 regional offices (Argentina, Cameroon, Côte d'Ivoire, El Salvador, Kenya, Thailand, and Zimbabwe) and 2 representative offices (at the United Nations in New York and at the European Union in Brussels).

Each INTERPOL member country maintains an NCB staffed by national law enforcement officers. The NCB is the designated contact point for the General Secretariat, regional offices, and other member countries requiring assistance with overseas investigations, and the location and apprehension of fugitives. It is also the gateway for police information sharing and cooperation between national police organizations and their foreign counterparts.

The role of an NCB is to participate in all of INTERPOL's activities, providing constant and active cooperation – compatible with the laws of their respective countries – so that INTERPOL can achieve its aims.

INTERPOL runs 15 databases regarding individuals and notice alerts, which include forensic data (i.e., fingerprints and DNA), travel and official data (i.e., stolen or lost documents, such as passports), stolen property (i.e., motor vehicles or works of art), firearms, and organized crime networks. In 2013, 1.2 billion inquiries were conducted on these databases with an average of 3,000,000 searches per day.

This agreement between WADA and INTERPOL is the outcome of 2 primary developments. During the 4th Annual Meeting of INTERPOL's NCBs, attendees underlined the need for better coordination in the fight against doping, specifically the trafficking of doping substances by organized crime groups. Furthermore, WADA recognized the importance of cooperation with INTERPOL to facilitate the exchange of information on doping. In February 2009, a cooperation agreement was signed between both organizations. As a result, within INTERPOL, a position was created for a criminal intelligence officer to coordinate anti-doping activities. Annually, WADA provides financial and technical support to this officer and their mission.

The main objectives of this cooperation agreement are:

- Establishing a framework for cooperation to facilitate the exchange of expertise along with the prevention and suppression of doping and trafficking in doping.
- Supporting enforcement of national and international anti-doping measures.
- Cooperating in the collection, storage, and exchange of information.
- Arranging information sessions and seminars to raise awareness about the trafficking of doping substances.

From a practical point of view, the WADA-positioned INTERPOL officer supports INTERPOL member countries facing complex doping investigations with international connections. This support includes, but is not limited to, the following points:

- Create a network of "points of contact" within relevant international law enforcement agencies specializing in the fight against doping.
- In conjunction with WADA's Science Department and/or WADA's expert groups, to provide technical and scientific support for criminal investigations, lead or coordinate international investigations (on request), arrange ad hoc working group meetings, and liaise with the World Customs Organization to enhance customs cooperation and enforcement-related activities.

- Facilitate the exchange of operational data among INTERPOL's member countries [11], more particularly through the "Project Energia" [12].
- Inform INTERPOL member countries and WADA about new doping substances and trends discovered during investigations.
- Support WADA's mission and related activities.

Within the framework of this multilateral cooperation, it is important to underline the "international" scope of the trafficking of doping substances. As for classical doping substances, the chemical raw material is primarily produced in Eastern Asia and sent via parcel deliveries (air, road, or sea freight) to underground laboratory locations throughout the world. There, the raw material is converted to final products (e.g., vials and pills), often with the relevant marketing (logo or brand name). Finally, the doping substances are forwarded to the final consumer for consumption or redistribution via small parcels either directly or through remailer(s) depending of the network structure. A large percentage of the consumers reside in the United States, Western Europe, and Australia. However, the consumer population base is quickly spreading to all corners over the globe.

Traffickers have the further burden of hiding illicit drug profits. Money laundering through real estate investments is quite common.

The complexity of the money laundering schemes and the size of the clandestine laboratories vary greatly. In many cases, the underground PED laboratory is a spare household room with basic equipment and void of any semblance of sterility. Product purity is a common complaint on Internet bodybuilding steroid/PED discussion forums. In contrast, law enforcement investigations uncover large and sophisticated laboratories. For example, an international, multiagency task force has unveiled one of the largest global PED manufacturing facilities located in Eastern Europe. This laboratory had a production area of 400 m^2, utilizing industrial scale equipment and employing several people. Due to lax laws within this Eastern European country, this company is allowed to openly mass manufacture PEDs for sale on the open Internet. These PED products are then smuggled via parcel delivery services to global destinations.

These diverse investigations highlight the unlimited demand of doping substances to millions of consumers worldwide. These consumers range from top level athletes to scores of anonymous users. The priority of these investigations has recently risen as law enforcement organizations have slowly but progressively come to recognize the health consequences of consuming PEDs (e.g., anabolic steroids or growth hormone). PEDs and methods are now being viewed as a societal health issue not confined to sport only.

INTERPOL has also entered the arena in the fight against doping. In 2010, in the framework of the cooperation agreement between INTERPOL and WADA, the INTERPOL General Secretariat was contacted by USADA's Chief Executive Officer (CEO) Travis Tygart. USADA and US law enforcement sought INTERPOL's assistance in arranging an operational meeting with relevant European law enforcement agencies regarding the US-led investigation against members of the US Postal (Cycling) Team, including Lance Armstrong. The Project Energia, led by an INTERPOL anti-doping unit in coordination with the School of Forensic Science at the University of Lausanne, aimed to produce a cross intelligence analysis regarding information on the supply and demand of PEDs as well as information on seized products [12].

Following this request and at the end of 2010 [13], an operational meeting was arranged and conducted at the INTERPOL headquarter in Lyon. This meeting gathered representatives from relevant US agencies (FBI, FDA/OCI, US Postal Inspection Service, and the Los Angeles Public Prosecutor's Office), the European Union

(French Gendarmerie, Swiss Customs, Italian NAS Carabinieri, Belgium Police, Spanish Guardia Civil, Spanish National Police, and Italian, Belgium, and Spanish prosecutors), representatives from the AFLD (French Anti-Doping Agency) (CEOs, the Head of the Control Department and the Head of the Science Department), and USADA's CEO Tygart. During this multilateral meeting, investigators exchanged intelligence and operational data regarding the case. The attending public prosecutors determined the types and terms of international legal assistance required via MLATs (mutual legal assistant treaties). Such meetings allow investigators to discuss case intelligence and operational data without delay pending the official and often time-consuming MLAT process. The participation of the AFLD was an opportunity for US representatives to better understand the challenges of conducting anti-doping controls at the Tour de France and more specifically on the US Postal Team and its famous leader, Lance Armstrong.

The USPS (US Postal Service) case shows the importance of intelligence gathering and the necessity to work in close cooperation with relevant law enforcement agencies with their accompanying powers in order to conduct complex and international doping investigations on top level athletes. Without this cooperation, ADOs are disadvantaged to investigate – let alone solve – complex doping cases.

While only a few NADOs are implementing a complete intelligence and investigation team (investigators and analysts), more and more NADOs are hiring former police or custom officers. They provide their experience to the NADO to lead investigations regarding ADRVs (interviews and investigations) as well as a network with the national or international law enforcement. To support these NADOs and facilitate the exchange of information, WADA set up and chaired a NADO investigator working group once or twice a year. Evidence, guidance on investigations, case debriefing, and good practices are shared.

Following the fruitful cooperation example between WADA and INTERPOL, WADA obtained a similar cooperation agreement with the World Customs Organization. Globally, numerous illicit PED parcels are seized by national customs organizations on a daily basis. In Australia and the United Kingdom, customs agencies readily share information relating to these PED seizures with their anti-doping counterparts. This information includes the type and quantities of PEDs seized, information on the senders and, most importantly, the names, addresses, and contact telephone numbers of the recipients. In some cases, the intended PED recipients were identified as top level athletes in registered testing pools. Thus, this shared intelligence has resulted in nonanalytical charges and sanctions.

The Drafting of the 2015 World Anti-Doping Code and Enhancement of the International Standards on Testing and Investigations for Implementing Intelligence Gathering in the Fight against Doping

The 2015 WADC came into effect on January 1, 2015. After 2 years of drafting, continuous consultations with stakeholders, and numerous revisions, a consensus-revised document was created. The 2015 WADC enhanced ADOs ability to fight against doping and thereby protect the clean athlete.

To ensure the proportionality and legal viability of these new measures, the WADC development was done in close collaboration with Mr. Jean Paul Costa, the former president of the European Court of Human Rights. This was especially important in that the revised Code enhanced penalties and further sought to punish nonathletes involved in doping conspiracies. The 2015 Code increases penalties against intentional sports cheaters but also affords flexibility in lessening penalties for those situations when doping was deemed not a deliberate act or involved substances with limited or no performance benefit. Additionally, the 2015 Code permits members of the athlete's entourage (e.g., medical staff, coaches, and/or managers) to be sanctioned when it is proven that they have been involved in doping or concealing the use of prohibited substances by an athlete. Intelligence gathering/sharing and investigations are often required to develop evidence of doping by an athlete or prove the knowledge and involvement of entourage personnel. The US-led investigation against the USPS Cycling Team highlighted the importance and necessity of intelligence gathering, conducting investigations, and collaborating with government police agencies in detecting and successfully proving nonanalytical doping cases.

The 2015 Code and, more particularly, the international standards on testing and investigations (ISTI) affirm this new approach in the fight against doping, as testing alone is not always sufficient to detect ADRVs. When testing falls short in revealing the use of prohibited substances and/or prohibited methods by cheaters, the analysis of analytical evidence (i.e., suspicious longitudinal testing markers) in combination with "nonanalytical" anti-doping intelligence (i.e., whereabouts failures, performance results, evidence brought forward through an investigation, and testimonies) can lead to ADRVs and subsequent sanctions. The potential of a nonanalytical approach requires ADOs to develop efficient and effective intelligence gathering and investigation functions.

The 2015 Code and the related ISTI place new burdens of responsibility on the ADOs regarding intelligence gathering and investigations. The 2015 Code requires ADOs to obtain, assess, and process anti-doping intelligence from all available sources, to be used to help deter and detect doping, via the development of an effective, intelligent, and proportionate test distribution plan and/or the planning of targeted testing, and/or by establishing the basis of an investigation into a possible ADRV(s). ISTI objectives are to establish standards for the efficient and effective gathering, assessment, and processing of intelligence regarding these purposes.

ISTI 2015 establishes standards for conducting efficient and effective investigations on:
- Atypical findings and adverse passport findings.
- Analytical or nonanalytical information or intelligence related to an ADRV.
- Athlete support personnel or any other persons involved in an ADRV.

For the greater majority of ADO staffs, the added new tasks to gather, assess, and utilize intelligence as well as conduct effective and efficient investigations will be challenging. To aid ADOs, WADA has developed basic and higher level training courses and workshops on intelligence gathering and investigations. The intended purpose is not to transform ADO staff members into investigators but rather provide them with some basic skills and tools to manage these new responsibilities.

The main objectives of the WADA basic training are to:
- Understand definitions.
- Determine the types of intelligence available to the anti-doping community.
- Efficiently collect, store, and manage information.
- Produce relevant test distribution plans.
- Create a network of "intelligence managers" amongst ADOs.

WADA has its own ad hoc anti-doping intelligence network (ADIN) through its daily work with NADOs, regional ADOs, and international sports federations. With the implementation of ISTI 2015, WADA's objective is to set up a more formalized intelligence network within NADOs and international federations. Of course, within the anti-doping community, networks of bilateral cooperation already exist wherein staffed ADO investigators collaborate on cross border investigations. As previously indicated, WADA's intelligence course and guidelines [14] will provide guidance on this type of intelligence sharing and cooperation network. WADA is aware, for a number of reasons, that all ADOs are not on the same level in terms of intelligence gathering and investigation capacities. This training aims to provide common skills for select ADO staff members. Attendance on the course, information sharing, and/or collaborative efforts will facilitate greater communication between ADOs and, therefore, enhance international cooperation.

As investigations require skilled staff, WADA promotes joint task force operation gathering from different NADOs as well as some international sports federations for a short period of time. This approach has enhanced the intelligence manager network and strengthens trust among different organizations.

Anti-Doping Administration and Management System

The Anti-Doping Administration and Management System (ADAMS) is currently the clearinghouse of all anti-doping information. ADAMS contains athlete whereabouts, biological passports, testing data, and therapeutic use exemptions. ADAMS is used by 107 international sports federations and 150 NADOs (+ regional ADOs) and 34 laboratories. Furthermore, ADAMS continues to be used by major event organizers during competition events.

In July 2016, the ADAMS data repository contained more than 380,000 athlete profiles, 16,000 therapeutic use exemptions, and more than 1,200,000 analytical results reported by WADA-accredited laboratories.

ADAMS is a fundamental tool for ADOs' day-to-day work activities. As with all aging software, ADAMS needs to be updated and improved to include a future framework of intelligence gathering and investigations. In this regard, WADA is currently developing an ADIN within the new ADAMS project. The new version of ADAMS is to be significantly more intuitive for its users and will offer a number of new helpful features.

ADIN will have different functions to support ADOs particularly regarding information gathering and sharing. ADIN will be a secure platform where ADOs will share and store information regarding anti-doping issues. Based on its legal framework, each ADO will decide to disclose fully or partially some information. Then, information could be shared directly or via cooperation agreements.

To facilitate ADO work, ADIN will integrate a search engine to facilitate data correlation and help ADOs to identify patterns and relationships. ADIN, working as a new module of ADAMS, will allow a good flow of communication in a secured environment for the benefit of information gathering and ADO activities.

Cooperation between the Anti-Doping Science and Law Enforcement Communities

In October 2014, WADA organized the "Science and Investigations Symposium" in Istanbul [15], which gathered collectively for the first time the heads of anti-doping laboratories and representatives of law enforcement, WADA's science and investigative departments, international pharmaceutical industries, the United Nations Office on Drugs and Crime, and European Monitoring Center for Emerging Doping. This symposium congregated these diverse organizations with varying responsibilities, expertise, and approaches in the fight against doping, but who have had limited or no prior exchanges. Regardless of the differing roles, the symposium showed how collaboration was mutually beneficial for countering doping, such as WADA-accredited laboratories lending their analytical expertise and testing on doping substances seized by police authorities. Chemical examination for example could provide useful information on the productions in clandestine laboratories or similarities with other criminal cases. On the other hand, law enforcement can provide useful PED trend analyses developed during the course of an investigation. One of the positive outcomes resulting from this symposium was that it developed a "forensic network" where experience and operational information are shared directly between stakeholders.

Conclusion

Over the past 20 years, several scandals requiring police-led investigations have plagued top level sports, highlighting both large scale and sophisticated doping cases. These revelations have severely damaged the general branding of sport and have forced governments to act more decisively. The creation of WADA (after the Festina scandal) was the response of the public authorities and the international sport movement to have a unified and harmonious worldwide campaign for doping-free sport.

Upon review, several lessons are drawn from these scandals. First of all, cooperation with law enforcement is a necessity for efficient anti-doping measures. The involvement of law enforcement (police and/or customs) investigators was a common and defining factor in each of these doping scandals. Through these police investigations, ADOs were often able to identify ADRVs from their law enforcement partners. Early on, WADA recognized and integrated this necessity, which prompted signing a cooperation agreement with INTERPOL in 2009. This agreement better facilitated the exchange of intelligence and enhanced international cooperation between the international sport and the law enforcement community relating to doping investigations.

The 2015 WADC gave WADA and ADOs investigative power regarding ADRVs and other activities that may facilitate doping. WADA used this ability following allegations of doping activities in the Federation of Russia. Consequently, the WADA Intelligence and Investigations Department was involved in investigations led by the IC as well as the IP. Combined with first-hand evidence provided by whistle-blowers, the investigative capacities of WADA represent a step forward in the protection of clean athletes.

References

1 Blandine Hennion: Affaire Festina: UCI et FFC retrouvent l'honneur en appel. Libération, March 6, 2002, http://www.liberation.fr/sports/2002/03/06/affaire-festina-uci-et-ffc-retrouvent-l-honneur-en-appel_395961.
2 Operación Puerto. Fuentes: "Me indigna la filtración selectiva". El País, July 5, 2006, http://elpais.com/diario/2006/07/05/deportes/1152050423_850215.html.
3 Seppelt H: The secrets of doping: how Russia makes its winners. ARD, 2014, https://www.youtube.com/watch?v=iu9B-ty9JCY.
4 Independent Commission Report 1. Montreal, WADA, 2015, https://www.wada-ama.org/en/resources/world-anti-doping-program/independent-commission-report-1.
5 INTERPOL supporting French investigation into athletics corruption. http://www.interpol.int/en/Internet/News-and-media/News/2015/N2015-185.
6 INTERPOL issues Red Notice against Papa Massata Diack at France's request. http://www.interpol.int/News-and-media/News/2016/N2016-005.
7 WADA Revokes Accreditation of Moscow Laboratory. Montreal, WADA, 2016, https://www.wada-ama.org/en/media/news/2016-04/wada-revokes-accreditation-of-moscow-laboratory.

8 McLaren Independent Investigation Report – part 1. Montreal, WADA, 2016, https://www.wada-ama.org/en/resources/doping-control-process/mclaren-independent-investigations-report-into-sochi-allegations.
9 Athlete Outreach and Independent Observer Mission at the center of WADA Sochi 2014 role. WADA to run independent observer and athlete outreach programs, monitor therapeutic use exemptions and retain right of appeal for anti-doping decisions at Winter Games. Montreal, WADA, 2014, https://www.wada-ama.org/en/media/news/2014-02/athlete-outreach-and-independent-observer-mission-at-the-center-of-wada-sochi.
10 Doping. http://www.interpol.int/fr/Crime-areas/Crimes-in-sport/Doping.
11 INTERPOL issues global alert for potentially lethal illicit diet drug. http://www.interpol.int/en/News-and-media/News/2015/N2015-050.
12 Project Energia. A criminal intelligence initiative to combat the traffic in performance-enhancing drugs. https://www.interpol.int/Crime-areas/Crimes-in-sport/Doping/Project-Energia.
13 Macur J, Schmidt MS: Lance Armstrong doping inquiry intensifies. The New York Times, November 16, 2010, http://www.nytimes.com/2010/11/17/sports/17cycling.html?_r=0.
14 Guidelines – Information Gathering and Intelligence Sharing. Montreal, WADA, 2015, https://www.wada-ama.org/en/resources/world-anti-doping-program/guidelines-information-gathering-and-intelligence-sharing.
15 Science and Investigations Symposium. Istanbul, October 28–29, 2014. https://www.wada-ama.org/sites/default/files/resources/files/wada-marclay-swiss-customs.pdf.

Mathieu Holz
World Anti-Doping Agency (WADA)
Maison du Sport International
Avenue de Rhodanie 54
CH–1007 Lausanne (Switzerland)
E-Mail mathieu.holz@wada-ama.org

Education in Anti-Doping: The Art of Self-Imposed Constraints

Sigmund Loland

The Norwegian School of Sport Sciences, Oslo, Norway

Abstract

The pillars of anti-doping are detection, deterrence, and prevention. Detection takes the form of testing for banned substances. Deterrence builds on testing and gathering evidence. Athletes who test positive are exposed to penalties. The main tool of prevention is education. Education takes many forms and can be implemented in many ways. This chapter addresses the nature and challenges of current anti-doping education. Firstly, general goals of education and their connection to sport are discussed. Secondly, three normative interpretations of sport are presented, and their implications for anti-doping education are examined. Instrumentalist interpretations and interpretations with emphasis on performance and enhancement challenge the anti-doping campaign. A human excellence interpretation is advocated in which anti-doping is considered a consistent and integral part of sport. Thirdly, future challenges for anti-doping education are reflected upon.

© 2017 S. Karger AG, Basel

Introduction

The anti-doping movement bases its work on three pillars: detection, deterrence, and prevention. Testing for banned substances, gathering evidence, and imposing penalties for doping violations serve both detection and deterrence goals. With good testing systems, no athlete using prohibited means or methods should feel secure. The main tool of prevention is education [1]. Education, however, is more difficult to define. What is its nature and goals? How can education be conducted within the anti-doping campaign?

I will answer these questions in three steps. Firstly, I will reflect upon the ideals of education and their connection to sport. Secondly, I will present three normative interpretations of sport and discuss their implications for education in anti-doping. Thirdly, I will reflect upon future challenges for anti-doping education.

My discussion is focused primarily on organized, competitive sport, as this is the main sphere for current anti-doping efforts. In the final section, I will discuss the need for more general educational efforts when it comes to the use of performance-enhancing means and methods in society.

Educational Ideals

Ideals of education lie at the core of human culture. Children are not born as blank slates but with multiple predispositions. Socialization into a culture emphasizes and encourages some of these predispositions while restricting and even sanctioning others. In cultures with totalitarian value structures, socialization and education often take the form of nonreflective practices. Definitions of value, a good life, and a good society are taken as given and not under dispute. Open, democratic societies are characterized by what sociologists refer to as reflexivity [2]; the insight that schemes of socialization and education are based on certain norms and values, and could have been different. Societies shape and construct the norms and values into which citizens are socialized. A high level of reflexivity in a society implies continuous critical discourse on socialization and education, and opens for a diversity of life forms.

In reflexive, democratic societies, a predominant ideal of education is that children have the right to an open future [3]. Children are to be brought up not by "guardians" but by "gardeners" [4] and exposed to the many possibilities of life. The goal of education is responsible, moral agents who, when a certain level of maturity is reached, can make informed choices of their own way of life.

In the development of these educational ideals, sport has played an interesting role. Ancient Greek ideals pointed to the significance of an all-round education in which bodily abilities and skills were as important as intellectual ones [5]. The Olympic Games were a cornerstone in the definition of Greek identity. The Olympic athlete was seen as an expression of human beings at their best.

The rise of modern competitive sport in 18th- and 19th-century England was intimately linked to the educational ideals of "Muscular Christianity" [6]. This ideal was integrated in Baron Pierre de Coubertin's Olympic ideology, the so-called Olympism. Being the official value system of the Olympic Movement, Olympism is an educational philosophy advocating the optimal blend of sport and culture in the all-round development of the young [7, 8].

Empirically informed studies with a social science perspective point to a less idealistic reality [9]. Sport's educational value cannot be taken for granted. On the contrary, sport is considered an ambiguous field, in particular in its competitive forms. Competition creates value tensions.

On the one hand, competition can trigger instrumental attitudes with victory as the goal that justifies most means. Sport can be cynical, aggressive, and destructive. On the other hand, competition can cultivate advanced forms of cooperation governed by rules commonly accepted by all. Sport can exert a cultivating force of friendship and community [10].

Sporting games are socioculturally constructed practices and develop according to the norms and values of the sociocultural contexts to which they belong. In what follows, I will explore three main normative interpretations of sport and their implications for education in anti-doping in more detail.

Sport as a Means: Instrumentalism

In the instrumental interpretation, sport is a struggle for profit and/or prestige of many kinds: personal, social, national, and ideological. Sport has no characteristic value of its own. Its value depends upon its efficiency in reaching external goals. Hence, sport has really no substance as an educational field. If fair play pays off, fair play is the norm. If foul play is an efficient means, foul play can be justified.

Empirically, pure instrumentalism is hard to find. Individuals and groups involved in sport have complex motivational structures, including a sense of the values of the practice. Some sport cultures, however, are marked by a predominant instrumental attitude. The commercial and political significance of sport increased dramatically in the post-Second World War period. During the same period of time, applied biotechnology developed, in particular within the military complex. Drugs were designed to stay alert, to provide energy, and to increase strength and aggression. Athletes, coaches, and medical experts found new areas of application in sport. Hoberman [11] talks of this period as a "dehumanization of sport." Dramatic events such as the 1960 Rome Olympic Games death of cyclist Knud Enemark-Jensen turned doping into a public issue. The International Olympic Committee installed a doping ban in 1967. In addition to health concerns, drug-enhanced performance is seen to violate the ideals and "spirit of sport." The 1999 establishment of the World Anti-Doping Agency (WADA) represents a qualitative step towards an independent and globally harmonized campaign against doping.

Sport cultures dominated by instrumental attitudes are not sensitive to these concerns. In totalitarian states, sport serves ideological purposes. The sport policy of the former German Democratic Republic is perhaps the clearest example. If drug use contributed to sport success and ideological prestige, so be it [12]. In sport cultures dominated by commercialism, anti-doping easily loses meaning as well. Entertainment sport is sometimes described as "the business of selling audiences to advertisers." Sport is not even part of the equation. If drug use enhances performance and contributes to commercial success, it is considered a justifiable means.

In instrumentalist sport cultures, educational efforts in anti-doping must launch revolutionary attacks on the basic value structure and aim at a cultural change. This is a hard task. Socialization and education of coaches and athletes take the form primarily of informal education. Learning occurs in daily interaction in local practice communities. Formal educational programs of limited duration have limited effect [13]. If anti-doping is not an integrated part of the basic value orientation in sport, it becomes a vulnerable and possibly an impossible task.

Sport and Human Enhancement

Contrary to the instrumentalist position, most interpretations of sport take seriously the idea that sport has characteristic norms and values that ought to be respected. One such view is that a core value of competitive sport is performance and progress. Sport is about testing and to a certain extent transcending traditional human limitations. At its best, it conveys no less than a concrete and embodied message of the possibilities of human enhancement: of what we can become.

This is not dissimilar from key ideals of de Coubertin's Olympism. He wrote on the record as holding the same function in Olympism as the law of gravity in Newton's theory of gravity: it was "the eternal axiom" [7, p. 139]. Elite athletes develop natural talent with hard training and efforts. To de Coubertin, they are admirable role models. What are the implications of the enhancement view when it comes to anti-doping?

Scholars such as Tamburrini [14] and Foddy and Savulescu [15] argue that the use of performance-enhancing drugs is closely linked to the logic of sport. In future society, enhancement regimes are to be found in many spheres of life, and the belief in sport as a "clean island" in a "polluted sea" is anachronistic and unrealistic. At its best, sport demonstrates the possibility of liberation from the deterministic laws of physiology. Competent and careful use of performance-enhancing drugs coheres with the norms and values of sport.

Human enhancement interpretations build on a value theory of sport. Within competitions, clear restrictions apply. Evaluating and comparing athletic performances depend upon common standards, rule adherence, and fair play. Outside of the competitive setting, however, athletes should be free to choose whatever performance-enhancing means and methods they prefer.

In the human enhancement scenario, there is no place for the ban on doping and testing and penalty regimes. Anti-doping rules cannot be justified. There is, however, a clear belief in education. Athletes should be educated to make informed and responsible choices. Actually, Brown [16] considers this a core educational value of sport. Anti-doping rules appear as unjustified paternalism.

Liberal enhancement positions are controversial [17]. There is general support of the ideal of athlete education. A main criticism, however, is that liberal doping policies counteract this ideal and do not take seriously the social reality of competitive sport [18]. Athletic careers start at an early age. Most teenage athletes have not yet reached the level of maturity and insight to make informed and responsible choices. Moreover, athletes are part of competitive supporting systems that rely on sporting success: leaders, coaches, and medical experts. If the system opens for drug use, there is a strong coercive effect [19]. The athlete's position becomes a vulnerable one. Anti-doping arguments with an emphasis on protection of the athlete seem well justified.

Sport and Human Excellence

A third normative interpretation of sport is of a more restrictive kind. Sport is seen as a significant arena for developing human excellence and moral virtues; justice, self-respect and respect for others, courage, and solidarity [20]. Different from the liberal enhancement interpretation, a performance is not considered admirable independent of out-of-competition means. Murray [21] refers to sport as the virtuous development of natural talent towards human excellence. What matters is the manner in which performance development takes place. What are the criteria of "virtuous"? What, more specifically, are acceptable and non-acceptable means?

In answering, Bernard Suits' [22] celebrated theory of games can be of help. Games are defined by a set of constitutive rules that make sense only within the context of the activity they define. Take soccer as an example. From the instrumentalist perspective, if the aim is to move a ball over a line between two poles, a ban on the use of hands is inefficient and simply irrational. Games, however, cannot be understood in pure instrumentalist terms. In soccer, the ban on handball has a constitutive function and defines the practice. Rules express a particular noninstrumental logic. The reason to accept a ban on certain efficient means is found by looking at the meaning and value of the activity itself. Rules open for a series of experiential values: fun, joy, mastery, excitement, tension, and uncertainty. Playing a game, Suits [22] says, is "the voluntary attempt to overcome unnecessary obstacles." The logic of games is the logic of play.

A long tradition of scholars with Johan Huizinga [23] as the most prominent has advocated the particular potential of play as a significant sphere of human development. Whether in art, music, love, professional life, or sport, individuals flourish when fully absorbed in the activity in which they take part. Play cultivates creativity, freedom, and joy. The idea has support from psychologists who talk of the significance of "peak experiences" [24] or "deep flow" [25]. Morgan [26, p. 211ff] refers to the "gratuitous logic" of sporting games: They have a power of opening for such experiences. If practiced with an emphasis on freedom and responsibility, sport engages the whole human being and stimulates development of talent in admirable ways. Sport opens for development of human excellence.

What are the implications for anti-doping education? As with the enhancement perspective, the excellence interpretation requires fair play in competition. Here, however, the idea of constraints to make an activity meaningful and valuable is further extended. Outside of competition, critical distinctions are made between admirable, acceptable, and nonacceptable out-of-competition means and methods. Some rules of thumb can be drawn [18]. As long as they do not represent significant health risks, new and efficient training methods and techniques are admirable. As long as there is equal access for all, the same can be said of innovation in sport equipment; a more elastic pole for the pole jump and the carving ski in alpine skiing enhance learning and mastery. The less athlete influence on and control over a technology, however, the more problematic it tends to become. Use of hypoxic chambers to enhance the oxygen-carrying capacity of the blood is a twilight zone [27]. Use of powerful and potentially dangerous means such as anabolic steroids is considered nonacceptable, as it tends to move the responsibility for performance from athletes towards medical expertise and external support systems.

The human excellence scenario is not without its critics, either. Hunt et al. [28] characterize the anti-doping campaign a moral crusade with an inefficient testing and penalty system. The critique should be taken seriously. On the other hand, requirements on complete efficiency are just as unreasonable in the anti-doping field as in more general drug-restrictive campaigns in society. The question is not whether doping can be eradicated, but what approach to doping can minimize its prevalence and negative consequences. In the current situation, a ban policy has the main justification of protecting athletes' status as responsible, moral agents in search of excellence.

Challenges to Education in Anti-Doping

There is a general trend in modern society towards enhancement of many kinds: cognitive enhancement, sexual enhancement, image enhancement, and physical enhancement [29]. Anti-doping is part of a more extensive cultural struggle in which instrumentalism, liberal enhancement views, and more restrictive views of human excellence represent different and to a certain extent contradictory positions. How can restrictive anti-doping education in sport succeed in this context? Upon which premises ought it be based?

Both human excellence and human enhancement proponents point at the significance of education. A first step could be a general acknowledgement of the educational ideal of free and responsible moral agents in pursuit of human excellence. Some enhancement means and methods may empower individuals, for instance by decreasing negative effects of injury and illness, or of aging. Other enhancement strategies may alienate and depower individuals. Enhancement of physical appearance easily becomes a matter of external expectations and social coercion. From a human excellence perspective, doping in sport falls on the negative side.

A second and related step is to acknowledge that human excellence is expressed differently in different social practices. In sport, excellence is expressed in developing athletic performance. From an anti-doping point of view, use of, for instance, anabolic steroids disturbs this picture. In medicine, excellence is shown in a doctor's capability of reducing or eliminating illness and pain and in a patient's recovery. Use of anabolic steroids as therapy may be an important means in this process. Different human practices have different goals that allow for different means and methods. A ban on drugs in sport does not necessarily imply negative views on the use of the same biomedical means in other spheres of life. Different means in the many and diverse settings of life can still contribute to the same overarching goal: the empowerment of individuals as free and responsible moral agents.

A third step is to design educational programs that work across a world of social and cultural diversity. The anti-doping campaign is universal. WADA has global responsibility. The ambition is to fight doping in all sports and in all national, social, and cultural systems. Individualist cultures are challenged by collectivist cultures, pro-enhancement cultures stand in opposition to more restrictive interpretations of human excellence. Are really ideals of human excellence as sketched above universally applicable?

I have indicated a way to proceed by finding common ground in the logic of play and games. Play and games are found in all cultures, and a sense for the experiential qualities of sporting games seems to be universal. No culture embraces uncritically instrumentalization of games. Most social and cultural systems have ideals of human excellence and admirable performance, and they are often expressed in direct and embodied ways in traditional play and games, and in sport. In spite of sociocultural diversity, a socioculturally sensitive and at the same time shared idea of the unacceptability of some means and methods is not unrealistic. This could be fertile terrain from where educational efforts could depart.

Concluding Comments

Sport is an ambiguous social practice. It can be an important part of flourishing lives and societies, and it can take the form of cynical exploitation and instrumental attitudes in a struggle over prestige and profit.

The anti-doping campaign is based on a value choice. It is an attempt to protect and strengthen what is considered to be "the spirit of sport"; sport as a sphere of human excellence. Challenges come from brute instrumentalism and from more liberal enhancement positions. Instrumentalism can destroy sport as we know it and leave little or no possibility for anti-doping education. Liberal enhancement interpretations challenge the detection and deterrence parts of anti-doping and leave the choice of performance-enhancing means and methods to the athlete. In the current situation, this seems sociologically naïve, as athletes are vulnerable parts in the competitive sport system.

In a human excellence interpretation, sporting games are considered to have a particular gratuitous and noninstrumental logic for strong experiential values and for the development of athletes as free and responsible moral agents. Doping reduces this possibility. Hence, anti-doping becomes an integrated part of socialization and education in sport.

Innovative biomedical means and methods can be a blessing and enhance quality of life, and they can be a curse depowering individuals, increasing social inequality, and threatening public health. To a certain extent, sport is a front zone of such tensions. Anti-doping can be a pilot test of how societies can meet these challenges.

An important educational message is that anti-doping is not primarily a policy of bans and restrictions, but, inspired by Huizinga [23] and Suits [22], a policy of self-imposed constraints to realize meaning and value in sport. These ideas are not new. The German scholar and poet Johann Wolfgang von Goethe articulates the idea eloquently with his references to mastery as "the art of constraints." Whether in art, science, music, or sport, the master excludes nonrelevant, confusing, and destructive elements and focuses on what is meaningful and valuable. The art of self-imposed constraints seems more significant than ever.

References

1. Cleret L: The role of anti-doping education in delivering WADA's mission. Int J Sport Policy Politics 2011;3:271–277.
2. Giddens A: The Consequences of Modernity. Oxford, Polity Press, 1990.
3. Feinberg J: The child's right to an open future; in Feinberg J: Freedom and Fulfillment: Philosophical Essays. Princeton, Princeton University Press, 1994, pp 76–97.
4. Bredenoord AL, de Vries MC, van Delden H: The right to an open future concerning genetic information. Am J Bioeth 2014;3:21–23.
5. Reid H: Sport and moral education in Plato's republic. J Philos Sport 2007;2:160–175.
6. Mangan JA: Athleticism in the Victorian and Edwardian Public School: The Emergence and Consolidation of an Educational Ideology. London, Cass, 2000.
7. de Coubertin P: Olympic Memoirs. Lausanne, International Olympic Committee, 1979.
8. Loland S: Coubertin's Olympism from the perspective of the history of ideas. Olympika 1995;IV:49–78.
9. Coakley J: Sport in Society: Issues and Controversies, ed 11. New York, McGraw-Hill, 2014.
10. Hyland DA: Competition and friendship. J Philos Sport 1978;5:27–37.
11. Hoberman J: Mortal Engines. The Science of Performance and the Dehumanizing of Sport. New York, Blackburn, 2001.
12. Spitzer G: Sport and the systematic infliction of pain. A case study of state-sponsored mandatory doping in East Germany; in Loland S, Skirstad B, Waddington I: Pain and Injury in Sport. Social and Ethical Analysis. London, Routledge, 2006, pp 109–126.
13. Backhouse SH, Patterson L, McKenna J: Achieving the Olympic ideal: preventing doping in sport. Perform Enhanc Health 2012;1:83–85.
14. Tamburrini CM: What's wrong with doping? in Tännsjö T, Tamburrini C (eds): Values in Sport: Elitism, Nationalism, Gender Equality and the Scientific Manufacture of Winners. London, Routledge, 2000, pp 200–216.
15. Foddy B, Savulescu J: Ethics and performance enhancement in sport: drugs and gene doping; in Ashcroft RE, Draper H, McMillan JR (eds): Principles of Health Care Ethics. London, Wiley, 2007, pp 511–519.
16. Brown M: Practices and prudence. J Philos Sport 1990;17:71–84.
17. Sandel M: The Case against Perfection. Ethics in the Age of Genetic Engineering. Cambridge, Belknap, 2007.
18. Loland S: The ethics of performance-enhancing technology in sport. J Philos Sport 2009;36:152–161.
19. Murray TH: The coercive power of drugs in sport. Hastings Cent Rep 1983;13:24–30.
20. McNamee MJ: Sport, Vices and Virtues. Morality Plays. London, Routledge, 2008.
21. Murray TH: In search for the ethics of sport: genetic hierarchies, handicappers general, and embodied excellence; in Murray TH, Maschke KJ, Wasunna AA (eds): Performance-Enhancing Technologies in Sport. Ethical, Conceptual and Scientific Issues. Baltimore, The Johns Hopkins University Press, 2009, pp 225–238.
22. Suits B: The Grasshopper. Games, Life, and Utopia. Toronto, Toronto University Press, 1978.
23. Huizinga J: Homo Ludens. A Study of the Play Element in Culture. Boston, Beacon Press, 1955.
24. Maslow AH: Religions, Values, and Peak Experiences. London, Penguin, 1964.
25. Csikszentmihalyi M: Beyond Boredom and Anxiety: The Experience of Play in Work and Games. San Francisco, Jossey-Bass, 1975.
26. Morgan WJ: Leftist Theories of Sport: A Critique and Reconstruction. Urbana, University of Illinois Press, 1994.
27. Loland S, Murray TH: The ethics of the use of technologically constructed high-altitude environments to enhance performances in sport. Scand J Med Sci Sports 2007;17:193–195.
28. Hunt TM, Dimeo P, Jedlicka SR: The historical roots of today's problems: a critical appraisal of the international anti-doping movement. Perform Enhanc Health 2012;1:55–60.
29. Murray TH: Enhancement; in Steinbock B (ed): The Oxford Handbook of Bioethics. Oxford, Oxford University Press, 2007, pp 491–515.

Sigmund Loland
The Norwegian School of Sport Sciences
PO Box 4014, Ullevål Stadion
NO–0806 Oslo (Norway)
E-Mail Sigmund.loland@nih.no

Social and Ethical Dimensions of Anti-Doping

Can We Better Integrate the Role of Anti-Doping in Sports and Society? A Psychological Approach to Contemporary Value-Based Prevention

Andrea Petróczi[a,b] · Paul Norman[b] · Sebastian Brueckner[a,c]

[a]Faculty of Science, Engineering, and Computing, School of Life Sciences, Kingston University London, Kingston upon Thames, and [b]Department of Psychology, University of Sheffield, Sheffield, UK; [c]Olympic Training Center Rhineland-Palatinate/Saarland, Saarbrücken, Germany

Abstract

In sport, a wide array of substances with established or putative performance-enhancing properties is used. Most substances are fully acceptable, whilst a defined set, revised annually, is prohibited; thus, using any of these prohibited substances is declared as cheating. In the increasingly tolerant culture of pharmacological and technical human enhancements, the traditional normative approach to anti-doping, which involves telling athletes what they cannot do to improve their athletic ability and performance, diverges from the otherwise positive values attached to human improvement and enhancement in society. Today, doping is the epitome of conflicting normative expectations about the goal (performance enhancement) and the means by which the goal is achieved (use of drugs). Owing to this moral-functional duality, addressing motivations for doping avoidance at the community level is necessary, but not sufficient, for effective doping prevention. Relevant and meaningful anti-doping must also recognise and respect the values of those affected, and consolidate them with the values underpinning structural, community level anti-doping. Effective anti-doping efforts are pragmatic, positive, preventive, and proactive. They acknowledge the progressive nature of how a "performance mindset" forms in parallel with the career transition to elite level, encompasses all levels and abilities, and directly addresses the reasons behind doping use with tangible solutions. For genuine integration into sport and society, anti-doping should consistently engage athletes and other stakeholders in developing positive preventive strategies to ensure that anti-doping education not only focuses on the intrinsic values associated with the spirit of sport but also recognises the values attached to performance enhancement, addresses the pressures athletes are under, and meets their needs for practical solutions to avoid doping. Organisations involved in anti-doping should avoid the image of "controlling" but, instead, work in partnerships with all stakeholders to involve and ensure integration of the targeted individuals in global community-based preventive interventions.

© 2017 S. Karger AG, Basel

Introduction

Athletes entering high-level sport competition are required to abide by the rules as set by the relevant governing bodies, which include a precise list of prohibited performance-enhancing practices and methods, commonly referred to as "doping." From a regulatory point of view, efforts for keeping doping out of sport are harmonised at the global level by the periodically revised World Anti-Doping Code (the Code) [1]. Activities related to the implementation of the Code (i.e., code compliance monitoring and testing as well as anti-doping outreach activities, research, and education) are overseen by the World Anti-Doping Agency (WADA). Athletes identified by their national sport organisation comprise the National or International Registered Testing Pool (N/IRTP) and are subject to the Code. Whilst anti-doping intervention via education primarily aims at athletes in the N/IRTP, preventive anti-doping efforts should also target young athletes well before they may enter the N/IRTP. Building a persuasive anti-doping culture must embrace all levels and abilities. To aid the development of effective anti-doping strategies that are ecologically valid and endorsed by the athletic community, it is paramount to have a better understanding of the factors that influence athletes' decisions about doping.

Doping is a complex phenomenon [2], which is partly reflected in the simultaneous need for performance enhancement and – justified on the values of the amateur sport – the desire to control the methods by which enhancement can be achieved [3]. In today's professionalised and commoditised sport, rules of the amateur sport such as fair play and level playing field are readily replaced by rational investments into gaining a competitive edge [3, 4]. Such investment routinely includes developing and using state-of-the-art equipment, specialised apparel, training methods, nutrition, physiotherapy, medical and psychological support, and pharmacological boosts – with only some being prohibited [5]. Thus, there exists a precisely defined set of substances and methods that are deemed to be unacceptable by the anti-doping authorities and, therefore, prohibited. Consequently, the behaviour (i.e., performance enhancement) per se is not condemned, only if it involves prohibited substances or methods. Assisted performance enhancement with permissible means (e.g., nutritional or herbal supplements, superfoods, training methods, and technological advancements) is not only tolerated but actively supported and often encouraged throughout the athletic career development [6]. This paradoxical situation creates an inherent ambiguity between the expectation for high-performing athletes and the anti-doping rules, which prohibit the use of a defined set of drugs and methods.

Doping is also a social and institutional construct [7–9] that generates tensions between values underpinning competitive sport and doping control, rendering the bioethical arguments – based on naturalness or negative health effects – unconvincing [10]. At the level where sport becomes a commodity – which is produced, sold, or used for political agendas by governments and organisations with vested interest in sport – the idealistic values of amateur sport are no longer core-governing principles of the activity but an appealing attribute of the product. One key function of anti-doping is to ensure that a "drug-free and clean" status remains a credible attribute of high-performing elite sport. Critical observers argue that doping control, which originally was born out of concerns for athletes' health, has incrementally turned into a moral crusade for preserving the noble values of "gentleman sport" for the high-performing and competitive world, which not only creates a dissoluble tension but also has a detrimental effect on the meaning of modern sport [11, 12]. After almost half a century since the first attempt for formalised doping control, doping today is more commonly seen as unethical conduct – cheating and shortcuts – than health-compromising behaviour, despite the fact that doping cannot guarantee winning or replace training and hard work.

From a strictly functional point of view, doping – through pharmacological advancements – can expand the somewhat fixed capacities of human performance [13] and thus contribute to *going faster, higher and stronger*. The history of doping clearly indicates that doping does not contravene universal moral codes but, rather, violates the agreed rules of today's sport competition which are in place to protect the intrinsic values of sport. Doping is cheating but cheating is the function of the rules. It is the set of anti-doping rules, not universal morality, that classifies some methods of assisted performance enhancement as cheating and the clandestine nature of this specific rule breaking makes doping deceitful and dishonest. Doping is also a contextualised behaviour which only lasts as long as the need or perceived need is present during the active athletic career [14], and it is often triggered by athletic-related life events such as injury or other threats to an elite athlete status [15–18]. Today's high-performing athletes are no longer amateur sports(wo)men but professionals, who continuously make investments into increasing their sport performance via hard work, training, and lifestyle that can last for decades [19]. It is not only the athletes' livelihoods, but also those of their entourage, that depend on good performance. Therefore, economic pressures of elite sport are also potential pressure points where doping use is more enticing than it would be otherwise [18, 19].

A major challenge facing anti-doping is that doping is defined in an ideological and institutional context [7], whereas traditional anti-doping education targets athletes and members of their entourage on individual terms. Restriction on how performance can be enhanced inherently limits individual fulfilment of universal values such as self-enhancement and self-direction [20], but the institutional, top-down, law-and-order approach to doping control through prohibition, detection, and punishment leaves very little room for a more rational and nuanced approach to be negotiated [9]. Furthermore, a gap between how clean sport is codified and how it is seen by the athletes themselves creates a wide zone of "permissible means of performance enhancement" which is not yet fully considered in anti-doping education.

The cumulative evidence from decades of health protection and harm reduction initiatives in the public health domain suggests that effective preventive interventions should identify the key contextual or environmental factors that influence, in some cases indirectly, the undesirable behavioural choices. Interventions that target the underlying causes (collectively referred to as *structural interventions*) are more likely to be successful and more cost effective than stand-alone individual-focused programme, and by capturing the broad target population, structural interventions remove the need to identify and target only those who are considered at risk for the unwanted behaviour. However, the success of structural interventions depends on how closely the well-intended initiatives fit with the opportunities and constraints of the microsocial environment of the target population, and what kind of support is available to facilitate their integration. Community-based interventions[1] seek consensus and conciliation between structural and individual values. Their attractiveness is underpinned by (1) the recognition of the needs of those affected, (2) the commitment to identify mutually acceptable solutions between the regulators and those subjected to the respective regulations, seeking balance between the individual and collective needs, and (3) the focus on both

---

[1] Note that community-based interventions are also referred to as "value-based interventions" although being "value based" is interpreted differently in public health than in anti-doping. We hope that with this chapter we are able to reconcile the different terminologies and provide a more encompassing definition for value-based anti-doping, which is congruent with the broader scope of structural interventions addressing critical health and social issues.

proximal and distal factors that exert influence on empowering individuals to make the right decisions.

In this chapter, we advocate a forward-looking anti-doping approach that provides a more pragmatic and functional view of doping, accepting that performance enhancement is at the core of competitive sport. This approach assumes that (1) the goal behind doping behaviour is performance enhancement – as opposed to cheating and/or gaining unfair advantage; (2) the behaviour of utilising pharmacological and technological advances to enhance athletic ability and performance per se is not condemned or prohibited; only certain means are; (3) motives and reasons for doping and anti-doping can be conflicting; (4) the influential driving forces behind doping are the beliefs about the reasons for doping use; (5) indirect influences via changing social cognitive factors (e.g., attitudes or norm perceptions) are necessary for building sustainable anti-doping culture but not sufficient to induce behavioural changes at the individual level without offering direct, practically relevant means for building or maintaining resilience to doping; and (6) processes such as moral disengagement, normalisation, and rationalisation are not driving forces for doping but coping strategies for reducing cognitive dissonance caused by having inconsistent values, thoughts, beliefs, or attitudes. We propose that effective anti-doping should recognise these contextual contingencies, be preventive, target knowledge gaps (to prevent inadvertent doping) and social cognitive factors (to promote motivations for clean sport and competition), adopt a positive approach that directly addresses athletes' beliefs about reasons for doping, and offer practical and acceptable solutions. In doing so, we focus on how the performance enhancement mindset forms [6] and raise awareness about the potential psychological risks associated with promoting and using permitted means (supplements) for performance-enhancing reasons. This is particularly important in situations where young athletes are involved because – along the transition in their sport to elite status – their "performance enhancement mindset" is still forming.

Definitions of Doping

The various definitions of doping demonstrate the conflict between moral and competitive values, which has affected the way society sees doping, as well as how anti-doping has been organized. From the societal point of view, sport is generally seen as a healthy, uplifting and character-building activity, in which using performance-enhancing substances defeats the purpose of sport and thus is morally wrong [10]. In competitive sport, these noble but archaic values of gentleman sport are in conflict with the driving forces behind high-performance sport [13, 20] as well as with the universal values of self-enhancement and self-direction [21]. From a behavioural point of view, doping can equally be seen as a motivated, effortful and goal-oriented behaviour [6, 22] that is justified on the grounds of functionality and triggered by athletic-related life events; as a deviant behaviour in terms of substance use [23], or as rule breaking and moral disengagement [24]. In contrast to all, the official definition of doping [1] does not (1) distinguish between the desired goals, (2) require intention, or (3) limit doping offences to a substance or method being artificial.

The precise definition of doping is important. Firstly, it gravely affects social science research. Surveys without a precise definition rely on personal definitions of doping and thus may not only vary widely but also differ from the official definition that is likely to be explicitly or implicitly adopted by the researchers [25]. Secondly, the definition matters for designing anti-doping interventions as definitions are inherently centred on key factor(s) which are assumed to underlie doping behaviour (e.g., gaining unfair advantage, moral disengagement, using artificial means, or increasing performance). Thus, definitions determine the behavioural components to be targeted in anti-doping efforts.

Doping Control and Deterrence

The nature of doping makes policing difficult and leads to an imperfect but costly monitoring system that has been challenged on many accounts, including the fairness principle [26], medical ethics [27, 28], and ethical, employment and privacy law issues arising from the need for constant surveillance [29–31]. Ongoing debates around doping in sport focus on the fit for purpose [32–36], justification [37, 38], effectiveness, and associated costs as deterrents [11, 39, 40]. Paradoxically, the ever-increasing severity and intensity of externally imposed sanctions intended to serve as an effective deterrent could inadvertently trigger doping use through signalling that doping is spreading in sport, hence the harsh sanctions are merited [41]. Evidence indicates that human decisions involve a combination of self-interest and internalized social norms [42]. Socio-economic models [43] suggest that the decision whether doping should be used not only depends on the outcome of the cost-benefit analysis but also on the microculture of the given sport. Athletes are more likely to refrain from doping if fellow athletes condemn such behaviour, and doping substances are absent from their repertoire. The main problem with the norm-based approach to doping is the presence of contradicting norms. Whilst aspiring athletes adopt professional norms in order to progress in the sporting career, professional athletes must subscribe to the universally accepted norms of the amateur sport, such as fair play or equal chances, with the emphasis on participation, not winning [19].

Value-based education represents a positive approach to prevention as it engages all stakeholders (athletes, coaches, and other key members of the athlete entourage) in developing and promoting the intrinsic values of the spirit of sport. A plethora of education resources and education campaigns – provided by WADA – aim to promote a global clean-sport culture. However, whilst promoting the intrinsic values to foster positive attitudes toward clean sport, it is necessary to encourage athletes to be responsible agents for their own actions. In order to be effective, value-based education must incorporate intrinsic values associated with athletic achievement, striving to go higher, stronger, and faster. In addition to the values of the spirit of sport, value-based education targeting the broad spectrum of the sporting community must acknowledge that the universal values – which are simple, broad, and readily agreed on by most at the abstract level [21] – become fragmented in everyday applications and actual situations at the individual level, and address the individual athletes' needs in a constructive, permissible, and positive way.

Motivations for Doping and Anti-Doping at the Individual Level

To date, doping control and anti-doping intervention have been characterised by targeting athletes as individual agents. Anti-doping education must encapsulate all kinds of doping offenses, regardless of the reasons and intention. However, from a psychological perspective, a differentiation must be made between accidental and deliberate doping. Accidental doping assumes no intention to use doping substances and that doping occurs because of lack of knowledge, blissful ignorance, or carelessness. The limited research available on avoiding inadvertent doping builds on theories of self-determination, planned behaviour, and self-regulation [44–46]. In contrast, deliberate doping is controlled and goal oriented. The search for the key determinants of such behaviour has predominantly drawn on social cognitive models. Although statistically significant relationships between psychosocial variables (e.g., attitudes, beliefs, norms) and self-reported doping behaviour/

intentions have been documented in the literature, causal relationships cannot be established from the cross-sectional study designs. Furthermore, a meta-analysis by Ntoumanis et al. [47] demonstrated that the relationships between doping intention and attitudes, subjective norms, and perceived behavioural control are weak. In practical terms, these findings suggest that intervention-induced changes to social cognitive factors such as subjective norms or attitudes, even if successfully made, would not necessarily translate into desirable behavioural outcomes. In contrast, the importance of the social environment has been highlighted through evidence of a strong link between doping behaviour and knowing a friend who has used doping or the widespread use of permissible supplements.

Perceived norms represent people's beliefs about what behaviour is common, generally accepted and/or expected. Research has highlighted the importance of athletes' beliefs about how widespread doping is. Self-confessed doping users have been consistently found to report a higher estimation of doping prevalence, although it remains unclear whether the perceived high doping prevalence precedes doping behaviour or is a post hoc justification for doping [48–50].

The Pragmatic View of Doping

Competitive sport does not exist in a vacuum but is inevitably affected by economic, sociological, and cultural changes in society. Pharmacologically assisted human enhancement is an emerging phenomenon that characterises the later part of the 20th century. It is not limited to doping in sport, but manifests in functional drug use to enhance human experience in the general population, including non-medical use of cognitive enhancers, fat burners, and diet pills, cosmetic surgery, and the use of doping substances (growth hormone and steroids) for cosmetic reasons. Using aids to improve the human body is no longer seen as deviant but as a normal part of human development to enhance functions and enrich experiences [51–53]. Fundamental questions for anti-doping are (1) what sets doping apart from the rest in the vast array of available chemical and technological assistance to human performance, body appearance, and experiences, and (2) it is better to focus on the "means" (doping substance and methods) or on the driving forces behind the doping behaviour. It is far too simplistic, and not supported by evidence, to argue that those who engage in doping practices consider "winning is everything." Instead, the literature suggests that motivations tied to initiating or maintaining doping use are extremely diverse [47, 54] and often tied to performance and not competition.

There are 2 advantages in considering doping as a normalised functional (as opposed to a deviant) behaviour: (1) it is in line with the contemporary approach to drug use, and (2) it can offer a practically relevant theoretical framework to anti-doping. The concept of "normalisation" in social drug research refers to an emerging consumption style that is characterised by patterns of sensible or controlled drug consumption which is rationalised and, at times, framed as a safe option [55, 56]. In sport, bodybuilders may rationalise illicit anabolic steroid use as a goal-oriented activity that is perceived to be "under control" [57, 58]. Emerging evidence for normalisation of doping by elite athletes is characterised by reference to elite sport as a profession and rationalised as a "job demand" [19, 59, 60]. Furthermore, athletes report perceived expectations from teammates or coaches "to do whatever it takes" to increase performance and see doping as a potent method to do so [61].

Bridging the gap between amateur and elite sports, the incremental model of doping behaviour asserts that doping is a learned behaviour, which stems from prolonged involvement in assisted performance enhancement [6]. Throughout their athletic career development, athletes are accustomed to using ergogenic aids to enhance their athletic performance, either directly or indirectly by aiding the recovery process between training sessions. During this time, it is reasonable to assume that athletes also form their beliefs about reasons for using some sort of assistance for performance enhancement, which then contributes to their general attitudes toward assisted performance enhancement that may influence future behavioural choices about performance-enhancing practices. Whether or not these practices involve prohibited means primarily depends on the athletes' beliefs about the reasons for, and expectations of, doping, and is influenced by individual values about sport and performance enhancement. The behavioural reasoning theory [62] distinguishes between *anticipated reasons* (justify planned behaviour in the future), *concurrent reasons* (explain current behaviour), and *post hoc reasons* (explain past behaviour). These reasons are also an integral part of the athlete's performance enhancement mindset. Owing to the legal and personal ramifications of doping, reliable evidence for reasons reported in the literature is limited to first-person post hoc justifications [59, 60], hypothetical scenarios [17], and third-person projected reasons (i.e., why athletes in general may use doping) [63]. Ongoing investigations suggest that the demarcation between different types of supplement users is primarily based on whether supplements are used for health maintenance or for performance-enhancing reasons [64].

The Importance of the "Performance Enhancement Mindset" for Doping Prevention

The "performance enhancement mindset" refers to an established "way of thinking"; that is, a mental disposition or a set of thoughts and beliefs that shape one's attitudes, beliefs, and assumptions held about the need for pharmacological assistance for performance excellence. This "performance enhancement mindset" is a powerful concept in anti-doping because it is thought to exert influence on how athletes and members of the athlete entourage interpret and respond to events, circumstances, and situations when it comes to performance excellence and enhancement.

Approaching the "athlete mindset" from a mental representation angle, a study contrasting doping simultaneously to nutritional supplements and illegal drugs revealed a telling picture about how athletes might think about doping [65]. Specifically, the study showed that doping, despite being prohibited in competition and often referred to as "illegal," was more closely aligned with supplements (representing performance enhancement and functionality) than it was with illegal drugs (representing regulated status). Such a "mental representation of doping" suggests that the key characteristic of performance-enhancing substances is more aligned with functionality than legality [6]. A review of reaction time-based attitude measures (1) showed that the mental representation of doping is a function of the behavioural path that the athlete follows and (2) provided evidence that the functional aspect of doping influences both explicit and implicit retrieval of representations of doping [66]. Notably, and most importantly for anti-doping, the functional aspect is not limited to prohibited substances but rather starts with the use of dietary supplements for performance-enhancing reasons. This characteristic of assisted performance enhancement practices that develops over time is the key tenet of the incremental model of doping behaviour [6].

Past research on mindsets in relation to sport performance has been dominated by investigations into how different mindsets contribute to elite sport performance achieving excellence in athletes and coaches [67–70]. Dweck's [71] model of fixed versus growth mindsets highlights not only societal but specifically the influence that young athletes' parents and coaches exert on an individual's belief system. The means by which athletes approach their goals – categorized as a fixed or growth mindset – are characterized not only by individual talent or abilities but also by their self-regulation skills [72]. Ryan and Deci's [73] self-determination theory – which has been extensively applied to doping behaviour [74–79] – serves as a broader framework providing theoretical underpinnings for Dweck's [71] and Kuhl et al.'s [72] work on performance mindsets. The juxtaposition of the performance enhancement mindset to Dweck's [71] fixed and growth mindset categorisation advances anti-doping by highlighting the importance of taking a holistic view of the athlete's performance enhancement mindset throughout the athlete career transition stages. The cognitive connection between permitted supplementation and prohibited doping draws attention to the potential danger of inadvertently promoting doping for advanced career stages by promoting permissible means early on or as a substitute to doping. In an era where nutritional supplements are aggressively marketed and often endorsed by elite athletes, attention must be given to the influence of habitual use of these supplements for performance enhancement on doping behaviour. Because the decision about doping or avoiding doping is made in a social and environmental context, the roles that society, the media, and the athlete entourage play in this process warrant further attention for devising holistic approaches to anti-doping.

Preventing Doping

Athletes may refrain from using doping for normative reasons (i.e., they feel that they are under obligation to comply with the anti-doping rules and stay clean), or because they have a compelling rational reason (e.g., concern for health, personal moral beliefs, or lack of need or access). The problem with the normative anti-doping approach is that the expectation about the behaviour (what the athlete *ought* to do – or not do – about doping) inherently introduces a conflict between the promoted value system for clean sport, where performance enhancement via artificial means is to be avoided, and between the intrinsic motivation and normative expectation for maximising one's athletic ability and performance. In anti-doping, it is usually taken for granted that the clear values of the normative approach (i.e., use of doping is bad and refraining from doping is good) are automatically considered in doping decisional situations. This approach has characterised the anti-doping movement for decades and has negated the fact that the individual decision-making situation about doping is constantly influenced by both internal and external factors, including beliefs about the reasons for doping.

Backhouse et al. [80] noted that the necessary ingredients of an effective preventive anti-doping education are yet to be "(i) discovered, (ii) applied and (iii) evaluated" (p. 85). Historically, anti-doping education has been characterised by didactic information transfer linked to the Anti-Doping Code compliance and health consequences. Undoubtedly, knowledge is necessary for making informed choices, and anti-doping organisations are under obligation to provide information necessary for avoiding both inadvertent doping and deliberate action. However, a sufficient level of anti-doping knowledge only prevents accidental doping (which itself is important) but does not deter motivated and rationalized doping use.

Motivation for using doping, like many other behavioural choices, stems from weighing negative and positive outcomes, including the chance of being detected and the consequences, and such motivation leads to behavioural intention and, in favourable situational contexts, to execution. Although Woolf and Mazanov [81] rightly point out that the decision about doping is not always rational, it can be viewed as a goal-oriented choice [6] that is underpinned by justifiable reasons [62]. Reasons for doping that are in line with athletes' motivation will have greater cognitive consistency and stability. In order to be effective, anti-doping interventions and preventive efforts must address doping and anti-doping from the athlete's perspective. Targeting ethical and moral aspects of doping is unlikely to serve as a strong enough deterrent because moral disengagement [24], along with normalisation and rationalisation [55, 56], are not causes of doping but coping strategies for partially resolving the conflict between attitudes towards performance enhancement as the goal and behaviour. For devising anti-doping interventions, it is important to note that cognitions related to "not doing something" are not the reverse of cognitions about "doing something." [82] Work on reasons for doping and doping avoidance has clearly shown that the predictors of anti-doping motivation are not the simple opposites of predictors of doping motivation, and vice versa [17, 83]. Furthermore, active involvement in anti-doping through building clean sport culture relies on a complimentary – but different – set of values than doping avoidance, and doping avoidance cannot be underpinned by negating the motives for doping. Thus, anti-doping strategies must be clear about the specific end goal to which measures of effectiveness should be carefully aligned.

Integration of Reason-Based Behavioural Changes into Value-Based Anti-Doping Intervention

An anti-doping intervention with high degree of legitimacy must aim for structural changes by simultaneously incorporating the stakeholders' needs and considering how alternatives for meeting these needs fit with the opportunities and constraints, as well as values held by the stakeholders. The structural change concept represents a holistic approach which recognises the shortcomings in solely targeting behaviour at the individual level and addresses this by incorporating factors both within and outside the individual's control, offering choices for achieving the desired behaviour and actively creating opportunities for positive decision making. However, structural interventions that are embodied in top-down policies without considering the needs of those affected limit individual choice and undermine responsibility. Sweat and O'Reilly [84] argue that the best outcomes from structural interventions occur when the voices of those most affected are incorporated into the design, appropriate attention is given to structural changes, and core values underpinning the interventions are clearly defined and codified. A seamless integration of anti-doping prevention and intervention in today's society and modern sport era calls for a broader interpretation of value-based education. In line with the way in which value-based interventions (also called community-based interventions) are defined in public health [84], value-based anti-doping should comprise strategies and interventions that promote and strengthen a clean sport culture via embedding core values of sport and human integrity. However, the performance-related values of athletes must also be considered and their specific needs addressed with tangible solutions and feasible behavioural choices to avoid doping. An anti-doping intervention is likely to yield the best outcomes when targeting structural changes at the global level and empowering athletes, through increased self-efficacy, to make the right choice and avoid doping. As self-enhancement, self-direction, and achievement are universally valued qualities, emphasising respect for oneself as well as respect for one's own health and body along with values of sport, fair play, and the Olympic motto[2] and Olympic creed[3], is likely to offer a good avenue for effective anti-doping intervention.

A value-based intervention will seek consensus and conciliation between structural and individual values. For example, there is a need to cre-

---

[2] Citius, altius, fortius (faster, higher, stronger).
[3] "The most important thing in the Olympic Games is not to win but to take part, just as the most important thing in life is not the triumph but the struggle. The essential thing is not to have conquered but to have fought well."

ate an anti-doping culture with strong shared values and to empower athletes with knowledge, skills, and alternatives to deal with pressure and vulnerable situations in order to make the right behavioural choices and avoid doping. A value-based intervention based on these core principles is expected to lead to improved legitimacy of anti-doping policies and practices, and result in better voluntary compliance and support. On a practical level, value-based anti-doping considers those affected and targeted for behavioural changes (i.e., athletes) as partners in the process. This approach breaks away from finding character flaws in those who dope and, rather, seeks understanding of the proximal and distal factors that could, alone or in synergy, lead to vulnerability to doping. In value-based anti-doping education, athletes are actively involved in finding solutions and are empowered to resist doping. Such an approach can be further enhanced by evident respect for athletes as responsible agents for their own actions and active reinforcement of the positive values each individual holds about him/herself. Athlete education to prevent doping is enhanced if it is (1) *pragmatic*, (2) *positive*, (3) *preventive*, (4) *proactive*, and (5) developed and delivered in *partnerships* with athletes. Figure 1 captures both the structural and the individual levels of value-based anti-doping. While promoting the positive values of sport and effective value-based anti-doping simultaneously:

- *Works on Establishing and Maintaining Legitimacy by Being Relevant, Pragmatic, and Athlete Centred.* Positive and collaborative outreach initiatives and educational strategies offer an excellent opportunity for changing the perception of anti-doping in the athletic community and build legitimacy for the anti-doping rules, regulations, and enforcement. Instead of portraying anti-doping authorities in policing roles, they can be seen as entities working in partnership with all stakeholders and, more importantly, with athletes for doping-free sport.

- *Increases Anti-Doping Literacy for Code Compliance and for Building Resilience.* Increased anti-doping literacy not only prevents inadvertent doping but also equips athletes and their entourage with accurate and up-to-date scientific knowledge. This, in turn, enables athletes to make informed decisions about doping and helps them to take responsibility and be in charge of their performance enhancement and sport career progression.

- *Works in Partnership with Athletes and Their Entourage to Build Anti-Doping Culture.* Following the principles of shared decision making that is central to health care [85], anti-doping interventions should also be developed involving all stakeholders – but most importantly athletes – from intervention mapping and process evaluation to refinement and implementation. This community-based, co-participatory framework [84, 85] would support the generation of context-sensitive behavioural strategies that are practically meaningful and acceptable to athletes as well as being feasible, sustainable, and effective.

- *Builds a Prevailing Anti-Doping Culture.* Anti-doping is justified on protecting athletes' health, rights to compete in a doping-free sport, and the positive values of sport. In search for an alternative monitoring system, researchers have turned to self-regulation and/or peer-monitoring systems. Socio-economic models suggest that the decision whether doping should be used not only depends on the outcome of the cost-benefit analysis but also on the microculture of the given sport [43]. Athletes are more likely to refrain from doping if fellow athletes condemn such behaviour, and doping substances are absent from their repertoire. However, anti-doping should also make effort to minimise the contradiction present in social norms surrounding performance enhancement versus the promoted notions of fair play.

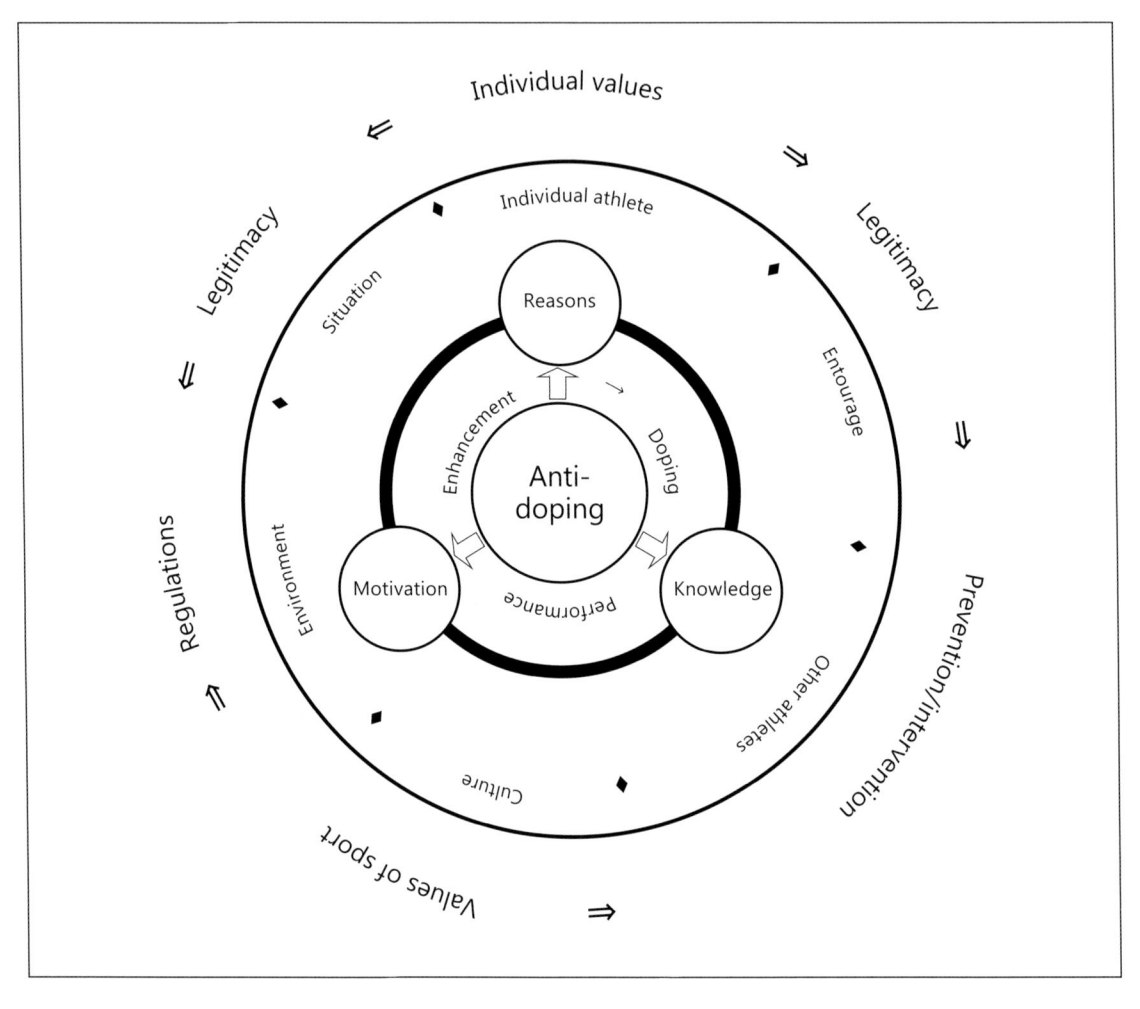

Fig. 1. The key components of anti-doping in environmental/situational context and their implications for anti-doping prevention and intervention.

- *Prevents Doping from the Onset by Managing Outcome Expectations and Mould Behavioural Strategies for Performance Goal Pursuit.* Considering doping primarily as a performance goal-driven and learned behaviour that develops over time [22], anti-doping intervention must start well before athletes reach the level of performance and competition to qualify for being included in the N/IRTP. One way to achieve that is by managing outcome expectations from doping [22] and offering help with acceptable alternatives for performance goal pursuits [6, 86].
- *Is Positive, Direct, and Targeted by Addressing Causes, Not Symptoms, and Be Practical and Specific to Sport/Athlete Groups.* Addressing inadvertent and purposive doping requires different anti-doping strategies. Inadvertent doping can be addressed by increasing anti-doping literacy for Code compliance. Interventions for deliberate doping should be based on a goal-oriented behavioural model and ad-

dress the transition phases throughout the athletic career, particularly the transition from mastery to performance goals [6]. Acknowledging valid pressure points for doping and offering practical help may also increase the perceived legitimacy of the anti-doping efforts.

- *Considers the National/Ethnic Cultural Context.* Anti-doping is the only drug prevention effort that is harmonised at the global level. The importance of matching cultural frames to messages targeting human behaviour has been long recognised in international trade and advertisements, but largely absent from anti-doping research. The established relationship between individuals and cultures and culturally relevant mindsets [87] should be taken into account in communicating anti-doping messages.
- *Selects the Appropriate Mode of Delivery.* In addition to the content, the framing of anti-doping messages should also receive attention. The efficacy of persuasive messages is influenced by congruency between message framing and the individual's motivations and motivational tendencies [88]. In contrast to the traditional didactic approach, problem-based experiential learning represents a new and pragmatic method for anti-doping education. Carefully constructed scenarios (case studies and/or problem vignettes) offer opportunities for honest discussion, practice for problem solving and facilitate active learning. A better integration of scenario-based, interactive learning into anti-doping is recommended.

The Start of a New Era: Value-Based Anti-Doping Education

In response to the changing environment and demand characteristics for current and effective anti-doping, WADA has recently adopted a pragmatic, positive approach to anti-doping with the view to foster anti-doping behaviours and create a strong anti-doping culture. In the fight against doping, value-based anti-doping education represents a new development which focuses on prevention and complements the conventional drug testing and sanctioning model. The core concept of this value-based anti-doping education lies in creating a strong anti-doping culture at the community level as the foundation for a sustainable clean sport culture through promoting the *spirit of Sport*. Referencing these universal positive values, this comprehensive community-based approach – which encourages athletes to be responsible decision makers and to improve performance in a clean way – offers a multitude of education resources including an (1) interactive eLearning tool for athletes called the Athlete Learning Program about Health and Anti-Doping (ALPHA), which promotes moral reasoning and changes attitudes by providing positive solutions to stay clean; (2) CoachTrue and the Coach's Tool Kit to assist coaches, an e-textbook for universities aiming to raise social awareness about doping in sport; and (3) a research package for anti-doping organisations (ADOs) to help them evaluate the effectiveness of their education programs as well as measure a host of environmental and individual factors that may influence doping behaviours.

The inherent challenge in preventing doping through fostering a global clean sport culture across all stakeholders, levels, and age groups is how to translate global community level value-based prevention into specific strategies and activities implemented at the individual level. In addition, addressing motivations for doping avoidance at the community level is necessary, but not sufficient, for effective doping prevention. Cultivating the intrinsic values of sport (spirit of sport) leads to positive attitudes toward clean sport, and ultimately athletes and stakeholders become more engaged in their own roles and responsibilities, and thus motivated to keep sport drug free. However, evidence from the relevant doping literature indicates that universally accepted positive values attached to the *spirit of sport* become fragmented

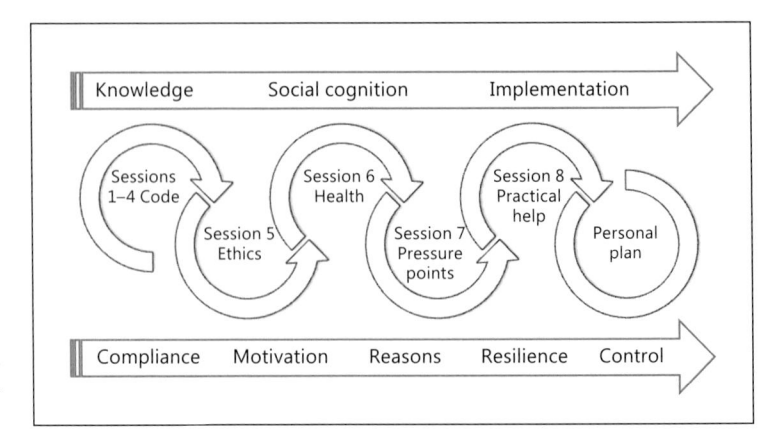

Fig. 2. Elements of the Athlete Learning Program about Health and Anti-Doping (ALPHA), mapped onto cognitive factors and practical outcomes.

when applied in actual decisional situations [61, 89]. Therefore, in addition to engendering positive intentions to avoid doping, it is also necessary to equip athletes with simple and pragmatic solutions to help them make desirable decisions in situations where the intrinsic sport values are in conflict with values attached to enhancement, improvement, and self-fulfilment. In addition, contemporary anti-doping also calls for a positive approach by which anti-doping research concentrates on what drives clean athletes to remain so, as opposed to exploring what drives some athletes to dope [90].

ALPHA: A Preventive Intervention That Works at Multiple Levels

Building on the cumulated knowledge through social science research, in 2014 WADA launched an interactive educational tool named "ALPHA" (Fig. 2). The program consists of 8 sessions and features several novel elements, including video testimonials from elite athletes, extensive resources and points of references for many aspects of athletes' lives. The unique aspects of the programme are that, for the first time, athletes' needs for performance enhancement are recognised and the programme requires athletes to be actively involved in the education process. The first 6 sessions of ALPHA follow the traditional approach to anti-doping and address the World Anti-Doping Code requirement for athletes to be educated on the following: doping control, whereabouts, therapeutic use exemptions, and result management processes, and medical and ethical reasons not to dope. Information provided in sessions 1–4 is vital to avoid inadvertent doping via establishing accurate knowledge and raising awareness of the risks associated with negligence. Medical and ethical reasons for avoiding doping justify doping control measures, and anti-doping interventions are covered in sessions 5 and 6. Building on the medical and moral foundation, athletes are encouraged to contribute to a clean sport culture that is not conducive to doping. Being equipped with values and knowledge, athletes are expected to act as responsible agents to refrain from doping as well as to avoid inadvertent doping. However, whilst it is desirable that athletes should refrain from doping, the reasons and motivation for doping are still present and thus should be addressed if the doping-free status is to be achieved or maintained. To achieve self-motivated and sustained behavioural changes via educational intervention, it is important to address athletes' reasons for doping. The reasons why athletes dope must be identified and then discounted or counteracted. Telling athletes what not to do (i.e., to avoid doping) creates a vacuum which has to be filled with advocating positive and desirable behaviour choices. The general fact is that "doping increases performance" and can only be counteracted by offering other – acceptable – alternatives for increasing performance. Athletes' reasons for doping are, therefore, addressed in session 7. Having engendered positive intentions to avoid doping, it is also necessary for athletes to have clear plans for how to deal with specific pressure points for doping, such as injury, threats to an elite athlete status, and economic pressures [15, 16, 18, 89]. In session 8, athletes are encouraged to make specific "if-then" plans (i.e., implementation intentions) [91] for these high-risk situations. For example: "*If* I feel fatigued, *then* I will make sure I get enough rest to let my body to recover (instead of using doping to keep me going)." Such planning exercises equip athletes with skills to resist pressure points to use doping and promote active involvement in avoiding doping.

With the 2 new sessions of ALPHA (7 and 8), which are rooted in a functional view of doping [6] and offer practical help on how to stay clean and how to resist the pressure to dope, ALPHA represents a holistic value-based approach and offers pragmatic and positive alternatives to the traditional normative approach to the prevention of doping. Instead of only telling athletes what they cannot do (which can come across as negative and daunting), ALPHA also takes athletes' needs to perform and succeed into consideration, acknowledges the pressure points that may serves as reasons for doping in decisional situations, and helps them to understand that a number of options and actions are available to them without doping. In summary, ALPHA addresses the 3 fundamental aspects of anti-doping depicted in Figure 1: (1) knowledge facilitates Code compliance and prevents inadvertent doping; (2) ethical and health reasons are intended to form negative attitudes towards doping (and thus affects general motives) which – through impacting on a large number of individuals – help to build a sustainable anti-doping culture within sport; and (3) the recognition of reasons for doping allows anti-doping to counteract these beliefs, offer practical help, and encourage athletes to develop plans to avoid doping in a positive and proactive way that is practically meaningful for the athletes. The inclusion of a self-affirmation exercise, which reinforces positive individual characteristics through reflection on past acts of kindness toward others [92], aims to create openness to anti-doping information and evoke motivation for active involvement in making positive behavioural choices about doping. ALPHA's new approach – which is in line with the guiding principles of the value-based intervention in public health settings – also contributes to legitimacy and helps create acceptance among athletes and their entourage by "making the athletes partners rather than objects in the process." [93]

Evaluation

Assessing the effectiveness of community-wide value-based anti-doping is challenging. The effectiveness of initiatives that directly target individuals, where the main outcome of interest is behavioural change, is typically measured directly by the achieved change in the target behaviour. Although behavioural change is also the ultimate aim behind value-based anti-doping education, the behaviour of interest (doping avoidance) is several layers removed from the intervention target (intrinsic values of sport). Even if reliable data can be gathered on behaviour – a significant challenge itself – it may not be possible to directly link changes to a specific intervention. Community-based anti-doping interventions should ideally incorporate measures beyond doping behaviour and attitudes. Having a close match between the targeted and assessed factors is critically important for demonstrating effectiveness of any specific intervention activity. For example, the effectives of modules 1–4 in ALPHA should be assessed with changes in knowledge (at individual level) and reduction in inadvertent doping rates (at community level); modules 5 and 6 should be assessed through changes in attitudes and increased positive perception of legitimacy, whereas modules 7 and 8 seek to strengthen individuals' self-efficacy to avoid doping. Making inferences from observed changes in factors not directly targeted for the effectiveness of specific anti-doping interventions is conceptually questionable because a cause-effect relationship in field settings cannot be demonstrated. Community-based structural interventions are best evaluated via changes in structures and context, possibly through changes in perceived legitimacy of anti-doping among stakeholders and the general public.

Conclusion and Perspectives

In order to fully engage athletes and key stakeholders in the process, value-based education must be interpreted in a broad sense. In addition to promoting the intrinsic values of the spirit of sport, individual athletes' performance-related values and needs must be acknowledged and addressed in a constructive, permissible, and positive way. These interventions must be theory based, underpinned by empirical evidence, targeted, relevant, and acceptable to athletes. Anti-doping organisations should avoid the image of 'policing' and reinforce the legitimacy of their actions via building partnerships with all stakeholders and consistently engaging athletes in the process in order to stay tuned into the pressures athletes are under and their needs for practical solutions for avoiding doping. Clean athletes should play a larger role in developing anti-doping education. Their views clearly suggest that clean sport culture cannot be cultivated around the demarcation between prohibited versus permitted substances, but rather it should be underpinned by the notion of not using any substances for performance enhancement. Finally, the key attributes of effective anti-doping should manifest in all ages, athletic levels, and abilities.

References

1 World Anti-Doping Code. Montreal, WADA, 2015, https://wada-main-prod.s3.amazonaws.com/resources/files/wada-2015-world-anti-doping-code.pdf.
2 Petróczi A, Strauss B: Understanding the psychology behind performance-enhancement by doping. Psychol Sport Exerc 2015;16:137–139.
3 Heikkala J: Modernity, morality, and the logic of competing. Int Rev Sociol Sport 1993;28:355–370.
4 Volkwein KA: Ethics and top-level sport – a paradox? Int Rev Sociol Sport 1995;30:311–320.
5 Loland S: Technology in sport: three ideal-typical views and their implications. Eur J Sport Sci 2002;2:1–11.
6 Petróczi A: The doping mindset – part i: implications of the functional use theory on mental representations of doping. Perform Enhanc Health 2013;2:153–163.
7 Dimeo P: A history of Drug Use in Sport 1876–1976. Beyond Good and Evil. New York, Routledge, 2007.
8 Møller V: The Ethics of Doping and Anti-Doping: Redeeming the Soul of Sport? New York, Routledge, 2009.
9 Møller V: The Doping Devil. International Network of Humanistic Doping Research. Aarhus, Books on Demand, 2008.
10 Gleaves J: Exploring new avenues to the doping debate in sports: a test-relevant approach. Fair Play 2013;1:39–63.
11 Hunt TM, Dimeo P, Jedlicka SR: The historical roots of today's problems: a critical appraisal of the international anti-doping movement. Perform Enhanc Health 2012;1:55–60.
12 Møller V, Dimeo P: Anti-doping – the end of sport. Int J Sport Policy Politics 2014;6:259–272.
13 Beamish R, Ritchie I: From fixed capacities to performance enhancement: the paradigm shift in the science of "training" and the use of performance-enhancing substances. Sport History 2005; 25:412–433.
14 Hauw D: Toward a situated and dynamic understanding of doping behaviors; in Tolleneer J, Sterckx S, Bonte P (eds): Athletic Enhancement, Human Nature and Ethics. Dordrecht, Springer, 2013, pp 219–235.
15 Mazanov J, Huybers T, Connor J: Qualitative evidence of a primary intervention point for elite athlete doping. J Sci Med Sport 2011;14:106–110.
16 Smith ACT, Stewart B, Oliver-Bennetts S, McDonald S, Ingerson L, Anderson A, Dickson G, Emery P, Graetz F: Contextual influences and athlete attitudes to drugs in sport. Sport Manag Rev 2010; 13:181–197.
17 Overbye M, Knudsen ML, Pfister G: To dope or not to dope: elite athletes' perceptions of doping deterrents and incentives. Perform Enhanc Health 2013;2: 119–134.
18 Bloodworth A, McNamee M: Clean Olympians? Doping and anti-doping: the views of talented young British athletes. Int J Drug Policy 2010;21:276–282.

19 Christiansen AV: "We are not sportsmen, we are professionals": professionalism, doping and deviance in elite sport. Int J Sport Manag Mark 2010;7: 91–103.
20 Beamish R, Ritchie I: From chivalrous "brothers-in-arms" to the eligible athlete. Changed principles and the IOC's banned substance list. Int Rev Sociol Sport 2004;39:355–371.
21 Schwartz SH: Are there universal aspects in the structure and contents of human values? J Soc Issues 1994;50: 19–45.
22 Petróczi A, Aidman E: Psychological drivers in doping: the life-cycle model of performance enhancement. Subst Abuse Treat Prev Policy 2008;3:7.
23 Lüschen G: Doping in sport: The social structure of deviant subculture. Sports Sci Rev 1993;2:92–106.
24 Boardley ID, Kavussanu M: Moral disengagement in sport. Int Rev Sport Exerc Psychol 2011;4:93–108.
25 Lentillon-Kaestner V, Ohl F: Can we measure accurately the prevalence of doping? Scand J Med Sci Sports 2011; 21:e132–e142.
26 Loland S, Hoppeler H: Justifying anti-doping: the fair opportunity principle and the biology of performance enhancement. Eur J Sport Sci 2012;12: 347–353.
27 Hilderbrand R: The world anti-doping program and the primary care physician. Pediatr Clin North Am 2007;54: 701–711.
28 McNamee M, Phillips N: Confidentiality, disclosure and doping in sports medicine. Br J Sports Med 2011;45:174–177.
29 Hanstad DV, Loland S: Elite athletes' duty to provide information on their whereabouts: justifiable anti-doping work or an indefensible surveillance regime? Eur J Sport Sci 2009;9:3–10.
30 Park JK: Governing doped bodies: the World Anti-Doping Agency and the global culture of surveillance. Cult Stud Crit Methodol 2005;5:174–188.
31 Møller V: One step too far – about WADA's whereabouts rule. Int J Sport Policy Polit 2011;3:177–190.
32 Finocoeur B, Frenger M, Pitsch W: Does one play with the athletes' health in the name of ethics? Perform Enhanc Health 2013;2:182–193.
33 Kayser B, Mauron A, Miah A: Current anti-doping policy: a critical appraisal. BMC Med Ethics 2007;8:2.
34 Kayser B, Smith ACT: Globalisation of anti-doping: the reverse side of the medal. Br Med J 2008;33:85–87.
35 Lippi G, Banfi G, Franchini M: The international anti-doping system: why it might not work. Clin Chim Acta 2009; 408:141–142.
36 Smith AC, Stewart B: Drug policy in sport: hidden assumptions and inherent contradictions. Drug Alcohol Rev 2008; 27:123–129.
37 Lippi G, Franchini M, Guidi GC: Doping in competition or doping in sport? Br Med Bull 2008;86:95–107.
38 Tamburini C: Are doping sanctions justified? A moral realistic view. Sport Soc 2006;9:199–211.
39 Kayser B, Broers, B: The Olympics and harm reduction. Harm Reduct J 2012;9: 33.
40 Pitsch W: "The science of doping" revisited: fallacies of the current anti-doping regime. Eur J Sport Sci 2009;9:87–95.
41 Van der Weele J: The signaling power of sanctions in social dilemmas. J Law Econ Organ 2012;28:103–126.
42 Anderson E: Beyond Homo economicus: new developments in theories of social norms. Philos Public Aff 2000;29:170–200.
43 Strulik H: Riding high – success in sports and the rise of doping cultures. Scand J Econ 2012;114:539–574.
44 Chan DKC, Donovan RJ, Lentillon-Kaestner V, Hardcastle SJ, Dimmock JA, Keatley D, Hagger MS: Young athletes' awareness and monitoring of anti-doping daily life: does motivation matter? Scand J Med Sci Sports 2015;25:e655–e663.
45 Chan DKC, Dimmock JA, Donovan RJ, Hardcastle S, Lentillon-Kaestner V, Hagger MS: Self-determined motivation in sport predicts anti-doping motivation and intention. J Sci Med Sport 2015;18: 315–322.
46 Chan DKC, Ntoumanis N, Gucciardi DF, Donovan RJ, Dimmock JA, Hardcastle SJ, Hagger MS: What if it really was an accident? The psychology of unintentional doping. Br J Sports Med 2016;50: 898–899.
47 Ntoumanis N, Ng JY, Barkoukis V, Backhouse S: Personal and psychosocial predictors of doping use in physical activity settings: a meta-analysis. Sports Med 2014;44:1603–1624.
48 Uvacsek M, Nepusz T, Naughton DP, Mazanov J, Ránky MZ, Petróczi A: Self-admitted behavior and perceived use of performance-enhancing vs psychoactive drugs among competitive athletes. Scand J Med Sci Sports 2011;21:224–234.
49 Moston S, Engelberg T, Skinner J: Self-fulfilling prophecy and the future of doping. Psychol Sport Exerc 2015;16: 201–207.
50 Petróczi A: Indirect measures in doping behavior research; in Barkoukis V, Lazuras L, Tsorbatzoudis H (eds): The Psychology of Doping in Sport. New York, Routledge, 2015, pp 93–110.
51 Hogle LF: Enhancement technologies and the body. Annu Rev Anthropol 2005;34:695–716.
52 Menuz V, Hurlimann T, Godard B: Is human enhancement also a personal matter? Sci Eng Ethics 2013;19:161–177.
53 McVeigh J, Evans-Brown M, Bellis MA: Human enhancement drugs and the pursuit of perfection. Adicciones 2012; 24:185–190.
54 Johnson MB: A systemic social-cognitive perspective on doping. Psychol Sport Exerc 2012;13:317–323.
55 Blackman S: Youth subcultures, normalisation and drug prohibition: the politics of contemporary crisis and change? Br Polit 2010;5:337–366.
56 Müller CP, Schuman G: Drugs as instruments: a new framework for non-addictive psychoactive drug use. Behav Brain Sci 2011;34:293–347.
57 Hoff D: Doping, risk and abuse: an interview study of elite athletes with a history of steroid use. Perform Enhanc Health 2012;1:61–65.
58 Monaghan LF: Vocabularies of motive for illicit steroid use among bodybuilders. Soc Sci Med 2002;55:695–708.
59 Lentillon-Kaestner V, Carstairs C: Doping use among young elite cyclists: a qualitative psychosociological approach. Scand J Med Sci Sports 2010;20:336–345.
60 Ohl F, Fincoeur B, Lentillon-Kaestner V, Defrance J, Brissonneau C: The socialization of young cyclists and the culture of doping. Int Rev Sociol Sport 2015;50: 865–882.
61 Pappa E, Kennedy E: "It was my thought… he made it a reality": normalization and responsibility in athletes' accounts of performance enhancing drug use. Int Rev Sociol Sport 2012;48: 277–294.

62 Westaby JD: Behavioural reasoning theory: identifying new linkages underlying intentions and behaviour. Organ Behav Hum Decis Process 2005;98:97–120.
63 Huybers T, Mazanov J: What would Kim do: a choice study of projected athlete doping considerations. J Sport Manag 2012;26:322–334.
64 The Safe You Project: Strengthening the Anti-Doping Fight in Fitness and Exercise in Youth. www.safeyou.eu.
65 Petróczi A, Mazanov J, Naughton DP: Inside athletes' minds: preliminary results from a pilot study on mental representation of doping and potential implications for anti-doping. Subst Abuse Treat Prev Policy 2011;6:1.
66 Petróczi A: The doping mindset – part ii: potentials and pitfalls in capturing athletes' doping attitudes with response-time methodology. Perform Enhanc Health 2013;2:164–181.
67 Balent B, Bosnar K: An attempt to improve operational definition of mindset in sport concept. 7th International Scientific Conference on Kinesiology, 2014, p 490.
68 Chase MA: Should coaches believe in innate ability? The importance of leadership mindset. Quest 2010;62:296–307.
69 Potgieter RD, Steyn BJM: Goal orientation, self-theories and reactions to success and failures in competitive sport. Afr J Phys Health Educ Recreat Dance 2010;16:4.
70 Sheard M: Mental Toughness: The Mindset Behind Sporting Achievement. London, Routledge, 2012.
71 Dweck CS: Mindset: The New Psychology of Success. New York, Random House, 2006.
72 Kuhl J, Kazen M, Koole SL: Putting self-regulation theory into practice: a user's manual. Appl Psychol Int Rev 2006;55:408–418.
73 Ryan RM, Deci EL: Self-determination theory and the facilitation of intrinsic motivation, social development, and well-being. Am Psychol 2000;55:68–78.
74 Barkoukis V, Lazuras L, Tsorbatzoudis H, Rodafinos A: Motivational and social cognitive predictors of doping intentions in elite sports: an integrated approach. Scand J Med Sci Sports 2013;23:e330–e340.
75 Chan DKC, Dimmock JA, Donovan RJ, Hardcastle SJ, Lentillon-Kaestner V, Hagger MS: Self-determined motivation in sport predicts anti-doping motivation and intention: a perspective from the trans-contextual model. J Sci Med Sport 2015;18:315–322.
76 Chan DK, Donovan RJ, Lentillon-Kaestner V, Hardcastle SJ, Dimmock JA, Keatley DA, Hagger MS: Young athletes' awareness and monitoring of anti-doping in daily life: does motivation matter? Scand J Med Sci Sports 2015;25:e655–e663.
77 Chan DK, Lentillon-Kaestner V, Dimmock JA, Donovan RJ, Keatley DA, Hardcastle SJ, Hagger MS: Self-control, self-regulation, and doping in sport: a test of the strength-energy model. J Sport Exerc Psychol 2015;37:199–206.
78 Hogle LF: Enhancement technologies and the body. Annu Rev Anthropol 2005;34:695–716.
79 Lazuras L, Barkoukis V, Tsorbatzoudis H: Toward an integrative model of doping use: an empirical study with adolescent athletes. J Sport Exerc Psychol 2015;37:37–50.
80 Backhouse SH, Patterson L, McKenna J: Achieving the Olympic ideal: preventing doping in sport. Perform Enhanc Health 2012;1:83–85.
81 Woolf J, Mazanov J: How athletes conceptualise doping, winning, and consequences: insights from using the cognitive interviewing technique with the Goldman dilemma. Qual Res Sport Exerc Health 2017;9:303–320.
82 Richetin J, Conner M, Perugini M: Not doing is not the opposite of doping: implications for attitudinal models of behaviour prediction. Pers Soc Psychol Bull 2011;37:40–54.
83 Engelberg T, Moston S, Skinner J: The final frontier of anti-doping: a study of athletes who have committed doping violations. Sport Manag Rev 2015;18:268–279.
84 Sweat M, O'Reilly K: Ideological barriers to structural change. Toward the model of values-based interventions; in Sommer M, Parker RG (eds): Structural Approaches in Public Health. London, Routledge, 2013, pp 83–95.
85 Coulter A, Collins A: Making Shared Decision-Making a Reality. No Decision About Me, without Me. London, The King's Fund, 2011.
86 James R, Naughton DP, Petróczi A: Promoting functional foods as acceptable alternatives to doping: potential for information-based social marketing approach. J Int Soc Sports Nutr 2010;7:37.
87 Oyserman D: Culture as situated cognition: cultural mindsets, cultural fluency, and meaning making. Eur Rev Soc Psychol 2011;22:164–214.
88 Sherman DK, Mann T, Updegraff JA: Approach/avoidance motivation, message framing, and health behavior: understanding the congruency effect. Motiv Emot 2006;30:164–168.
89 Kirby K, Moran A, Guerin S: A qualitative analysis of the experiences of elite athletes who have admitted to doping for performance enhancement. Int J Sport Policy Polit 2011;3:205–224.
90 Englar-Carlson M, Gleaves J, Macedo E, Lee H: What about the clean athletes? The need for positive psychology in anti-doping research. Perform Enhanc Health 2016;4:116-122.
91 Gollwitzer PM: Goal achievement: the role of intentions. Eur Rev Soc Psychol 1993;4:141–185.
92 Reed MB, Aspinwall LG: Self-affirmation reduces biased processing of health-risk information. Motiv Emot 1998;22:99–132.
93 Hardie M, Henne K, Mazanov J: Justice in sport. Deakin Research Communication 2013. http://www.deakin.edu.au/research/stories/2013/05/13/justice-in-sport.

Andrea Petróczi
Faculty of Science, Engineering, and Computing
School of Life Sciences, Kingston University London
Penrhyn Road
Kingston upon Thames KT1 2EE (UK)
E-Mail A.Petroczi@kingston.ac.uk

Sport, Society, and Anti-Doping Policy: An Ethical Overview

Andrew J. Bloodworth[a] · Mike McNamee[b]

[a]Department of Sport and Exercise Science, College of Engineering, and [b]College of Engineering, Swansea University, Swansea, UK

Abstract

The purpose of this chapter is to provide an overview of the philosophical and ethical underpinnings of anti-doping policy. The nature of sport and its gratuitous logic is explored. The doping rules in sport, such as the Prohibited List, are ways of drawing a line to facilitate a certain sort of competition. Sports can be understood as a means of testing the natural physical abilities of the athlete, combined with the hard work they put into improving their performance. A test promoted by the anti-doping laws. Permitting certain forms of performance enhancement would threaten the special nature of such a test. Doping can be seen as a threat to the integrity of sport, not just because of the rule breaking doping currently entails. The chapter explores the ethical issues that arise with such forms of enhancement, such as fairness, harms to health, and indeed a refusal to accept human limitations. Finally, the criteria upon which a substance or method may be prohibited by the World Anti-Doping Agency (WADA) is addressed. The 3-part criteria, concerning (1) enhancement, (2) health, and (3) the spirit of sport are described, and literature that takes a critical line is addressed. Particular reference is made to the public health agenda explicit within anti-doping policy.

© 2017 S. Karger AG, Basel

Introduction

Most individuals, irrespective of class, ethnicity, gender, or wealth, have been introduced to sports, both in the form of plays and organized competition, as part of their formal or informal upbringing. Billions of spectators watch sport every year as a spectacle of human excellence. It is unquestionably a social good. That is not to say, however, that sports do not bring in their wake other social problems such as inequality, greed, corruption, racism, and so on. Being a human practice, sports are vulnerable to human excess and distortion. The particular ethical problem that sports are perhaps most often associated with is the issue of doping. More generally, this problem or set of problems can be viewed as part of a broader ethical debate about human enhancement [1]. Is the goal of unlimited athletic perfection in itself desirable? What methods in pursuit of such a goal are desirable or even permissible? These are questions that challenge journalists and educators as much as philosophers and scientists working in sports.

The purpose of this chapter is to provide an overview to the philosophical and ethical underpinnings of anti-doping policy. To do this, it is necessary to begin with an understanding of the nature of sports themselves and their gratuitous logic. From there, we proceed to describe how doping can be understood as a threat to the integrity of sport understood from the perspective we set out. We then consider the criteria upon which a substance or method may be prohibited by the World Anti-Doping Agency (WADA) and explore the relationship between anti-doping efforts and the broader public health agenda.

Sports and Their Gratuitous Logic

Often people who have played or even coached sports all their lives have never taken the time to consider the logic of sporting activities themselves. "What is the nature and purpose of a given sport?" is a question seldom asked outside of university courses in the philosophy of sport. Yet, it is a crucial question if we are to consider the role of doping and anti-doping in sports, and how anti-doping efforts are intended to preserve the integrity of sport. To what do such efforts aim?

Sports have what is called by philosophers a "gratuitous logic" [2, 3]. In contrast to everyday life, when participating in sports (as opposed to mere play) we create and accept difficult challenges simply in order to overcome them. The challenges are defined and the ways in which they may be achieved are formalized in rules or laws that govern the activity. These rules always prohibit what seems to be the most efficient way of achieving the goal of any given sport. Indeed, playing sport requires a willingness to undertake a task using inefficient means [3]. One might summarize this by saying that in sports we try to be as efficient as possible in an inefficient system. Thus, the quickest way to score a goal in football, or a try in rugby, is outlawed by the rules of the game.

The rules of the sport also define the nature of the activity and stipulate the sorts of challenges that the competitors must face, the goal of the activity, and how it may or may not be achieved. Philosophers have split the rules up in to 2 categories: constitutive and regulative rules. The former constitute the activity, and the latter tell us how we may or may not compete. They also tend to talk about sports as purposive activities: enterprises that make distinctions between the ideas of "means" and "ends." The ends of sport are the logical goal of the activity, as opposed to the psychological or personal goals of any particular athlete. So athletes try to run faster than their opposition, score more points or goals, and so on. Equally, in playing tennis with my daughter, I may wish to focus on her self-confidence and allow her to win to experience a motivation-enhancing experience. The goals we have for a sport may or may not be logically connected to the sports. They are simply *our* goals. Nevertheless, the ends or goal of any given sport may only be achieved using certain methods or means: so one cannot use wheels or springs (or a motorbike for that matter) when sprinting; one may not grab the helmet of an opposing football player; or strike an opponent in hockey, and so on. In essence, sports are rule-governed activities. The rules tell us what we are trying to achieve, and how we may go about it.

In summary then, competitors in a sport aim at maximum efficiency in a system made inefficient by the very rules themselves. Getting better at reaching your goal via these inefficient means is the very point of sport. A football team aims to improve its capacity to score goals, while preventing the opposition doing so. Thus improvement, or indeed enhancement, is one of the central aims of sport. We aim to get better at the sports we partake in.

Doping, Anti-Doping, and Sports

In keeping with these lines of thought, we can understand doping policy in relation to the idea of inefficient means to achieve sporting goals. We noted above how there are constitutive and regulative rules for sports. There is also another, generally agreed, category: auxiliary rules. These do not define the activity, or say how to compete, but rather define how we may prepare for sports, or what we may or may not do prior to the competition.

The anti-doping rules, evident in the World Anti-Doping Code (WADC or the Code) (updated in 2015) [4] make certain forms and ways of enhancing our sporting capabilities contrary to the definition of sports themselves. WADA publishes a List of Prohibited Substances and Methods [5] defining the substances and methods prohibited in sports each year. The Prohibited List itself forms part of the rules of the sport, prescribing the ways in which athletes may legitimately improve their ability to achieve the sporting goal (e.g., scoring a goal or completing a race).

A lot of people when hearing the word "doping" have a substance such as erythropoietin, human growth hormone, or an anabolic steroid in their mind. There is not, however, merely one violation known as doping, but rather 10 described in the Code [4]. These are called anti-doping rule violations (ADRVs). Thus misleading the doping control officers as to your whereabouts, for example, may lead to an ADRV. Tampering with the sample given to a doping control officer, say by manipulating one's urine or blood sample, is another. It is important to understand their variety since any of the 10 may be the basis of a ban on athletes.[1] Not one ADRV is considered in itself more serious than any other.

While there are a range of ways in which an athlete might break anti-doping rules, the use of prohibited substances or methods with a view to enhance performance often receives the most media attention. The obvious objection to utilizing banned methods and substances is that it is cheating. To cheat is to use deceptive methods in order to gain an advantage that might otherwise be unmerited. Doping is against the rules of just about every sport.

Imagine, though, that public attitudes changed, and it was widely agreed that athletes were not prohibited from doping? What if the rules were to change? Well, of course, doping practices would no longer be thought of as cheating. What potential benefits would accrue? It has been argued that permitting doping would reduce the costs associated with anti-doping initiatives and that this policy would be better aligned with the current spirit of elite sport [6]. Any so-called open doping policy would not seek to ban the use of performance-enhancing substances, but would rather just seek to ensure such substances are being used safely [7]. Some proponents of this line have suggested a testing program that seeks merely to ensure that the athlete's use of such substances did not compromise their health to such an extent that participation would be unwise or dangerous. Response to such arguments [8] has suggested that even in an open doping environment, athletes would still seek to hide the methods they were using, in the hope of maintaining a competitive performance advantage. Holm [8], moreover, assumes that this is part of the strategy of any competitive activity.

Notwithstanding such objections, however, it is clear that if the sports rules were changed, and we were to do away with any Prohibited List of substances and methods, what we consider to be doping now would no longer qualify as cheating. It might be asked whether the current doping rules stipulate a sort of activity that is in some way better, more admirable, than competition in

---

1 For a full list of the anti-doping rule violations see Section 2 of the WADC [4]. These violations include but are not limited to the use or attempted use of prohibited substances and/or methods; failing to submit a sample for testing; being unavailable for drug testing; tampering; and possession of a prohibited substance or method.

which such methods (doping) were permitted. It is to these deeper questions we now turn. What are the philosophical and ethical foundations of current anti-doping policies?

What We Admire in Sports and How Anti-Doping Policy Might Preserve It

Currently, the decision as to whether a substance or method is placed upon the Prohibited List depends on whether it meets at least 2 of the 3 criteria stated in the WADC [4]. There are, as we noted above, a wide range of ADRVs, e.g., the use of a particular substance to act as a masking agent for a banned substance. This may be relevant for anti-doping authorities to consider, irrespective of whether the masking agent was performance enhancing or not.

The criteria used to consider whether a substance or a method should be included on the Prohibited List may be summarized as follows:
- Enhances or has the potential to enhance performance.
- Risks athlete health or has the potential to do so.
- Violates the spirit of sport as characterized by WADC.

The Code lists the kinds of considerations that the spirit of sport entails. The WADA state that the spirit of sport "is the essence of Olympism, the pursuit of human excellence through the dedicated perfection of each person's natural talents" [4, p. 14]. WADA refers to ethics, fair play, and honesty; health; excellence in performance; character and education; fun and joy; teamwork; dedication and commitment; respect for rules and laws; respect for self and other participants; courage; and community and solidarity. Note, the Code does not offer a definition but rather collates a series of principles and values, and this fact has engendered some controversy for those who say this omission creates a latitude for policy decisions that is useful [9] or useless [10] to policy makers. It has been suggested [9] that characterizing the spirit of sport as part of anti-doping policy recognizes the basis of our admiration for athletes and what is generally considered as ethically good in sports. In contrast, some critics have suggested that such a list does not reflect the values of *elite* sport that currently exist [6].

In considering revisions to the 2009 WADA code, it was widely suggested by some of WADA's stakeholders that performance enhancement – being the main purpose of doping – ought to be the sole necessary criterion for consideration on the Prohibited List. In such a scenario, a substance or method could not be banned if it did not enhance performance or have the potential to do so. Having acknowledged this possibility in early stages of the revision process for the 2015 Code, this move was eventually not retained in the final version of the WADC. Thus, a substance can be banned for a range of reasons. A substance or method might be banned if it constitutes an unhealthy form of enhancing performance. Equally, it might be prohibited if it were a means of enhancing performance that – while not necessarily unhealthy – violated the spirit of sport, as set in the Code. Finally, if an enhancing substance or method met both of the other criteria, that it both damaged health and was contrary to the spirit of sport, it too could be prohibited.

WADA's agenda extends beyond performance enhancement. A substance or method might be banned if it satisfies the health and spirit of sport criteria. This leaves room for a substance or method being banned that does not enhance performance. Waddington [11], making particular reference to the inclusion of cannabis on the Prohibited List, argues that this essentially amounts to an illegitimate extension of WADA's remit into public health issues, rather than a sports-oriented focus on performance enhancement. Others, however, might cite the importance of sports, and indeed sports people, as a source of moral education. In these terms, we might see some utility in preventing much admired athletes from engaging in recreational substance use.

The criteria utilized by WADA raise a number of interesting questions. As noted above, the spirit of sport criterion has been challenged as difficult to operationalize and vague [10]. Others, however, have contended that the spirit of sport offers an idealized version of sport, the sort of sport we ought to aspire to [9]. Retaining the spirit of sport in these terms helps to protect some unique values of sport, and the sorts of sports performances that we ought to admire. While there may be an inherent vagueness to a policy that utilizes concepts such as the spirit of sport, it is important to note that WADA's Prohibited List is not vague. WADA stipulates that their Prohibited List is final, cannot be disputed on the grounds that a substance or method for example is not performance enhancing, or does not damage the spirit of sport. Therefore, the Prohibited List [5] comprises a fairly lengthy sport rule.

With any rule, however, and particularly complex rules such as those for anti-doping, problems and issues arise. The very idea of a noncontestable system of rules for anti-doping is a nonstarter. Moreover, the application of any (e.g., anti-doping) rule can be challenged by the Court of Arbitration for Sport, if both parties agree to take their dispute there. Within any complex system of rules that cover a wide range of activities and international scope, there are problems of application and interpretation.

The effective communication of the Prohibited List is key, as is the responsibility of the athlete and their support personnel to remain abreast of any amendments to the List. This is particularly important when we consider WADA's strict liability policy. Regardless of the athlete's intention, or indeed even if they are not at fault, an athlete can still be found to have committed an anti-doping rule violation. While WADA has a therapeutic use exemption process in place whereby athletes who require a prohibited substance for legitimate medical reasons can access this treatment given certain criteria are met, this process can offer an additional layer of bureaucratic complexity.

The current Prohibited List might also be challenged on consistency of application. Some have suggested that altitude chambers or hypoxic tents, currently permitted, ultimately amount to a form of enhancement that is contrary to the spirit of sport [12]. Similar moves can be made in the context of caffeine (currently permitted but monitored by WADA), with suggestions that the use of high levels of such stimulants amounts to an unhealthy form of enhancement. In developing sports rules, however, these difficult borderline cases always arise. Indeed it might help to see them as akin to the lengthy debates that accompany the offside rule (and its application) in soccer or the integration of athletes with prosthesis in the Olympic Games. While we might strive for the most consistent and rigorous sports policy possible, if we accept the need for anti-doping rules, controversy and complexity is bound to follow.

How the Rules Attempt to Preserve an Inefficient or Gratuitous Logic of Sport

Having considered the foundation of the current anti-doping policy under the WADC, we will now reflect in greater detail on the policy itself. Is there good reason to ban doping rather than just permit such methods of enhancement? Exploring this question draws not only on sporting examples but also on broader societal practices. WADC's first criterion concerns performance enhancement. This, of course, is a central tenet of competitive sports participation, training, and indeed sports science. So, why such concern with the ethical issues that arise from enhancing processes?

In the main, the use of prohibited substances and methods in this context entails the use of medical (or, more generally, biotechnological) means to enhance sports performance. What we find here is athletes and their support personnel (whether coaches, pharmacologists, sports engineers, or sports scientists) utilizing means originally devised for therapeutic purposes, the treatment of illness and disease, and the restoration of function, for sporting advantage. It might be argued that this essentially amounts to an improper use of otherwise legitimate means. Health optimization, or enhancement, or enhanced well-being, have not been viewed traditionally as a legitimate goal of medicine, and thus ethical questions ought to be raised about using such means in this fashion [13]. This is an interesting starting point but raises further questions about why we might object on ethical grounds to such practices.

Nevertheless, beyond sporting landscapes, many people seem comfortable with the use of medical means for nonmedical ends or purposes. Consider the performance of a musician, so nervous without pharmacological intervention that they are unable to get up on stage. Neither the performance nor the performer are condemned in the manner that athletic performances that are pharmacologically enhanced are. Likewise, a very tired office worker may utilize stimulants on WADC's Prohibited List in order to get through a tough but important day. The ethical issues that arise here have not had the sort of attention that has been generated in a sporting context. There are 2 ways of responding to these sorts of challenges. One way is to argue that sports are somehow unique or special tests, where these sorts of enhancement are especially significant and detrimental to such a test. A second way of approaching such challenges is to suggest that these forms of enhancement are indeed ethically problematic, whether inside or outside of sport.

The first challenge requires an expansion of our earlier definition of sport. If we can get clear on what sort of challenges sports represent, then we may be in a position to explore more critically whether doping threatens the very basis of such a test. Douglas [14] argues that sport is a test unlike that faced by the musician or the office worker. Sport should test our natural physical abilities, and something that directly works to enhance these abilities jeopardizes the very essence that sport is designed to test. In focus group interviews with young athletes, researchers found a similar concern with the notion of "natural performance" [15], that is one where athletic merit was the determining criterion. It is also interesting that the notion of "natural performance" is referred to at the beginning of the spirit of sport section of the WADC. The term "natural" would need further explanation in order to be operationalized effectively within anti-doping policy [16]. There are a range of ways in which sporting performance is currently aided in a fashion that some might suggest is unnatural (wearing spikes in athletics, modified costumes in swimming, or high technology helmets in cycling for instance). That such examples exist, however, need not mean that we need to do away with the term altogether.

A different approach to the ethics of human enhancement would entail consideration of more general objections to such methods or means. Some legitimate objections to the use of enhancement methods might be made on the grounds of safety and fairness. Taking a substance to enhance certain capacities, be they moral, physical, or mental enhancement, can provoke concerns about side effects. Likewise, if such methods were to become widely available there may be concern about how a good might be distributed equally, so as not to compound existing inequalities.

There are, however, deeper objections to the use of such enhancement methods. These deeper objections might help to offer a stronger foundation to anti-doping initiatives. Here, we will take just one approach, intended to advocate against the drive to enhance. Michael J. Sandel's [17] *The Case against Perfection* offers a lucid account of the ethical issues that human enhancement raises, aside from the potential concerns over safety and fairness. For Sandel, the main ethical problem with such efforts is the disposition these efforts reflect. This problematic disposition appears to continually attempt to master our human nature and refuses to accept the unbidden or giftedness of our human nature.

The athlete, for Sandel, ought to work within their own limitations, instead of trying to manipulate their nature in order to enhance their chance of success. Sandel also suggests that certain values would be under threat if we accept the legitimacy of these methods of enhancement. In his subsequent analysis, Sandel claims that enhancing would be to the detriment of the virtue humility. Such a virtue encourages us to work with our limitations, and acknowledge them, rather than refuse to accept that there are aspects of ourselves that cannot be changed. Sandel also expresses concern that enhancing will encourage us to see ourselves as increasingly responsible for our success, and indeed for our failures. If we accept the legitimacy of human enhancement we might be critical of those who decide not to enhance, who "play naked" to use a sporting metaphor, referring to those who would decide to play without using performance-enhancing substances.

There are of course some challenges to Sandel's line of argument. Sandel seems to be saying that the good life consists in a life that works within the limits of our human nature. Others [7] have argued that doping is reflective of an admirable aspect of our human nature; the desire to improve and challenge ourselves. We should also note that for Sandel's line of argument to be upheld, a firm distinction between therapy and enhancement must be maintained. Sandel is not arguing against medical intervention when a sports person is injured or suffers from illness or disease, but against the use of medical means to enhance capabilities beyond normality, both inside and outside of the sporting context.

The Idea of Non-Doped Performance as Healthier than Doped Performance in Keeping with the Spirit of Sport

The second of the 3-part WADC criteria justifying banning substances or methods concern damaging of the athlete's health, or with substances and methods that are potentially damaging to health. We might take such anti-doping efforts here to be strongly paternalistic. What does this mean?

In western moral and political life and philosophy, adults are normally taken to be the captains of their own ship, so to speak. We prize our autonomy. We value the right to live our lives as we see fit, so long as we do not interfere with the life and liberty of others. Of course, we widely accept that the very young, or sometimes the old or infirm, may not be competent to choose autonomously what is in their best interests. But these represent exceptions to a general rule for respecting autonomy. To intervene over incompetent choices that might be risky or damaging for the individual making those choices is labeled "soft paternalism," where as to interfere with the choices of competent adults to prevent them harm or to do them good is called "hard paternalism" [18]. The latter is much more difficult to justify. Why accept such strong interventions in our athletic lives?

WADA's rules set clear limits (at least in the case of adult sport) on the sorts of risks competitors are permitted to take. It's not just left up to the athlete to decide whether to enhance in a risky or unhealthy way, methods that meet these criteria are not permitted. One way in which to justify such a policy would be to say that its focus is not merely paternalistic. It concerns the good not only of the athlete who would potentially dope, but of the athlete who wants to remain clean and ought not to be placed under coercive pressures. Equally, given the important role-modelling function attributed to sport, we might wish to preserve a picture of sports – at least those governed in part by anti-doping rules – that they are not excessive in the risks demanded for success.

As we have noted, in liberal societies we tend to leave people alone who might be harming themselves, providing they do not harm others and are capable of formulating rational and autonomous choices. Even this liberal approach has its limits; however, alcohol and tobacco is permitted in the UK for example to those over 18 years of age, but heroin is not. Further restraints on liberty for our own good (a legal obligation to wear seatbelts for example) suggest that at least in this respect, anti-doping policy intended to protect the health of athletes is not in contradiction with broader public policy.

While the focus thus far has been on considering ways in which the enhancement and health criteria might be combined in order to ban a substance or method, it is not a requirement of current policy that a substance or method enhances in order for it to be banned. A substance or method might be banned on the basis that it is damaging or potentially damaging to health, and violates the spirit of sport as characterized by WADA. Aside from any potential performance-enhancing effects, the combination of spirit of sport and health criteria allows WADA to address recreational substance use under the doping banner. Objections suggest that WADA's focus ought to be limited to sporting and thus enhancing matters [11]. WADA's efforts in this respect might be supported by citing for example the influence athletes have on young people, and the relationship we would at least like to see between sport and health more generally.

The Code characterization of the spirit of sport includes such values as fun and joy. Such a characterization does not seem to reflect the work that *elite* sport has become. Autobiographies from athletes such as Tyler Hamilton, admitting doping practices, also report a number of other practices, including exploitation of the therapeutic use exemption processes, the obsessive focus on training statistics, and almost reduction of the body to a machine [19]. None of this seems to fit with the Code's characterization. Elite sport in many cases seems to reflect a "win at all costs" ethos; hence, the willingness of some athletes to take risks with their health in order to improve their performance. This lack of fit with existing practices need not necessarily pose a problem for this characterization. While this ethos may not be shared unanimously, or seem particularly prominent in certain elite sport competitions, it is best to consider the characterization as an ideal rather than a description of current norms. Including this idealized conception of sport encourages us to reflect upon the sort of performances we ought to admire. The *spirit of sport* criterion reminds us to consider whether the use of certain substances and methods is reconcilable with this sporting ideal.

Conclusion

Sporting rules dictate that the achievement of the goal of any sporting activity must only be achieved with the use of stipulated means. These means enshrine a gratuitous logic that enforces inefficiency on the athletes and their support systems, who nevertheless aim to be as efficient as they can be. Certain substances and methods are prohibited, as they reflect means that challenge the sort of test that sport is designed to be. Deciding what falls under consideration, and what does not, is an ongoing and complex exercise of, or compromise between, scientific and philosophical considerations. Comparisons with societal practices more generally, and an apparently more liberal attitude toward enhancement practices, do not necessarily suggest we should permit doping in sport. Rather, they force us to reflect on the values that sport represents at its best and the very bases for our admiration of athletes. These, it seems, are protected by supporting anti-doping policy that prohibits attempts at excessively instrumental attitudes to success in sports at the expense of broader ethical and social goals and goods.

References

1 Parens E: Is better always good? The Enhancement Project. Hastings Cent Rep 1998;28:s1–s17.
2 Morgan WJ: Leftist Theories of Sport: A Critique and Reconstruction. Urbana & Chicago, University of Illinois Press, 1994.
3 Suits B: The Grasshopper: Games, Life and Utopia. Toronto, Toronto University Press, 1978/ Peterborough, Broadview Press, 2005.
4 World Anti-Doping Agency: World Anti-Doping Code 2015. Montreal, WADA, 2015, https://www.wada-ama.org/en/resources/the-code/world-anti-doping-code (accessed January 12, 2017).
5 World Anti-Doping Agency: Prohibited List. Montreal, WADA, 2016, https://www.wada-ama.org/en/what-we-do/prohibited-list (accessed January 12, 2017).
6 Møller V: The Ethics of Doping and Anti-Doping: Redeeming the Soul of Sport? New York, Routledge, 2010.
7 Savulescu J, Foddy B, Clayton M: Why we should allow performance enhancing drugs in sport. Br J Sports Med 2004;38:666–670.
8 Holm S: Doping under medical control – conceptually possible but impossible in the world of professional sports? Sport Ethics Philos 2007;1:135–145.
9 McNamee MJ: The spirit of sport and the medicalisation of anti-doping: empirical and normative ethics. Asian Bioethics Rev 2012;4:374–392.
10 Kornbeck J: The naked spirit of sport: a framework for revisiting the system of bans and justifications in the World Anti-Doping Code. Sport Ethics Philos 2013;7:313–330.
11 Waddington I, Christiansen AV, Gleaves J, Hoberman J, Moller V: Recreational drug use and sport: time for a WADA rethink? Perform Enhanc Health 2013;2:41–47.
12 Loland S, Caplan A: Ethics of technologically constructed hypoxic environments in sport. Scand J Med Sci Sports 2008;18(suppl 1):70–75.
13 Edwards SD, McNamee MJ: Why sports medicine is not medicine. Health Care Anal 2006;14:103–109.
14 Douglas TM: Enhancement in Sport, and Enhancement outside Sport. Stud Ethics Law Technol 2007;1:ukpmcpa-2293.
15 Bloodworth A, McNamee MJ: Clean Olympians? Doping and anti-doping: the views of talented young British athletes. Int J Drug Policy 2010;21:276–282.
16 McNamee MJ: Sports, Virtues and Vices. London, Routledge, 2008.
17 Sandel MJ: The Case against Perfection. Cambridge, Harvard University Press, 2009.
18 Feinberg J: Harm to Self. Oxford, Oxford University Press, 1986.
19 Hamilton T, Coyle D: The Secret Race: Inside the Hidden World of the Tour De France. London, Bantam Press, 2013.

Dr. Andrew Bloodworth
Department of Sport and Exercise Science
College of Engineering
Swansea University
Bay Campus
Fabian Way
Swansea SA1 8EN (UK)
E-Mail A.J.Bloodworth@swansea.ac.uk

A Moral Foundation for Anti-Doping: How Far Have We Progressed? Where Are the Limits?

Thomas H. Murray

Brewster, MA, USA

Abstract

Clarity about the ethical justification of anti-doping is essential. In its absence, critics multiply and confusion abounds. Three broad reasons are typically offered in anti-doping's defense: to protect athletes' health; to promote fairness; and to preserve meaning and values in sport – what the World Anti-Doping Agency (WADA) Code refers to as the *spirit of sport*. Protecting health is itself an important value, but many sports encourage athletes to take significant risks. The case against doping is buttressed by concern for athletes' health, but it cannot be the sole foundation. Promoting fairness is vital in all sports as the metaphor of the *level playing field* attests. But playing fields can be leveled by providing performance-enhancing drugs to all competitors. When doping is prohibited, fairness is aided by effective anti-doping. But the fundamental justification for anti-doping is found in the meanings and values we pursue in and through sport.

© 2017 S. Karger AG, Basel

Thomas H. Murray is president emeritus of The Hastings Center, Garrison, NY, USA, and was formerly the director of the Center for Biomedical Ethics in the School of Medicine at Case Western Reserve University in Cleveland, OH, USA.

Introduction

Why is it wrong to dope in competitive sport? Public opinion in survey after survey consistently shows strong disapproval of doping in sport [1]. Polls of athletes show, if anything, even stronger condemnation of doping [2, 3]. Not everyone agrees, however. A small but persistent chorus of dissident voices insist that anti-doping organizations, including the World Anti-Doping Agency (WADA), are misguided [4, 5]. Sometimes the critics acknowledge that doping in sport is morally problematic but insist that the lines drawn between permitted and prohibited means of enhancing performance are vague or indefensible, or that the apparatus of doping control – testing, whereabouts reporting, laboratory work, adjudication, and sanctions – is overly intrusive or not worth the effort. In short, they claim that however bad doping may be, the current cure, in the form of anti-doping programs, is worse than the disease. Certain critics insist that there is nothing wrong in the first place with using any and all performance enhancement technologies in sport or anywhere else in our lives [6, 7]. They may assert that the goal of sport is maximum performance by any means, or that using technology to extend our powers is just what humans do – a creative act of sorts. Tamburrini [8], for example, proclaims "…doping is not only compatible with, but also incarnates, the true spirit of modern competitive elite sports" [p. 200]. Other scholars disagree [9, 10].

Anti-doping critics are not going away. At times, they do a service to sport by calling attention to aspects of anti-doping that could be improved. Most of all, the critics compel us to make certain that the ethical case against doping in sport is robust. It is reassuring to have strong support among athletes and the public, but majorities, even large majorities, can be wrong. In the decades since anti-doping became prevalent in sport, weak arguments have been exposed and stronger ones developed. But the struggle to articulate and refine the case for preserving a world in which athletes can compete successfully without resorting to doping must continue. To begin, let us examine two candidate criteria that are commonly offered in defense of anti-doping: health and fairness.

Is Health the Answer?

In 1998, Juan Antonio Samaranch, then Chair of the International Olympic Committee (IOC), said "Doping [now] is everything that, firstly, is harmful to an athlete's health and, secondly, artificially augments his performance. If it's just the second case, for me that's not doping. If it's the first case, it is." With that pronouncement the then head of the IOC proclaimed a threat to athletes' health to be the central feature of what made any technology that enhanced performance an instance of doping. Though he did not explicitly say so, it seems reasonable to assume that in his view an important rationale – perhaps *the* most important or even sole rationale – for anti-doping is protecting athletes' health. Unfortunately, as a moral principle, protecting the health of athletes, though undeniably important, may not be up to the task of distinguishing clearly those enhancing technologies that should be banned from those that should be permitted or even celebrated. In philosopher-speak, its impact on athletes' health may be neither necessary nor sufficient to determine whether a technology that enhances performance should be prohibited.

Take the case of ski racing. New ski materials and designs along with new waxes, poles, and boots allow ski racers to go faster. Speedier descents down snowy slopes also mean that when racers crash they do so with greater velocity and force, increasing the possibility that whatever injuries they suffer will be severe. Yet, we cheer on skiers to go as fast as they can despite the risks. The same can be said for many other sports in which athletes are encouraged to push against the limits even at the risk of injury. Little wonder that athletes smell hypocrisy when sports officials declare that they should avoid performance-enhancing drugs because they might hurt themselves.

The mere fact that some technology that enhances performance also increases the risk to athletes' health is not a sufficient reason to ban that technology as the history of ski racing shows. Of course, some changes in equipment have the effect, as well as the intent, of reducing the likelihood of injury. The javelin, really a sort of spear, was redesigned in recent years to make it more nose-heavy resulting in a shorter flight and enhanced ability to stick in the ground rather than skid. The record with the old javelin was 104.8 m – nearly 344 ft, almost the length of a football field including end zones. The change made the distance thrown easier to measure. It also eased concerns about spearing people at the other end of the stadium.

Protecting the health and safety of athletes as well as spectators and officials is an important value in sport. But it is not the only value, and it does not always trump the other good things we pursue in sport.

Suppose sport did make health the sole criterion for deciding what was permitted and prohibited. It is likely that some (perhaps quite a lot of) standard equipment would be rejected on the grounds that it may increase risks to athletes' health. We would also face difficult judgments about the standard of proof needed. Societies struggle over how much evidence is sufficient to show that a particular thing is harmful, from exposures to chemicals in our air, food, or water to hydraulic fracturing in the extraction of oil and gas. The United States spent decades debating whether cigarette smoking caused cancer and other diseases despite an overwhelming accumulation of evidence clearly establishing the connection. It is easy to imagine that those who sell and those who use particular performance-enhancing drugs will deny their risks and play down the cogency of whatever evidence shows otherwise. Even today, there are skeptics who argue that there is inadequate proof that anabolic steroids are harmful, though there are well-qualified experts who conclude that steroids are indeed dangerous [11]. Similar skepticism abounds on erythropoietin (EPO) [12]. How is sport to decide among the various opinions?

From athletes' reports and other sources, we also have reason to worry that a drug that can be used safely in the management of a disease may have very different consequences in sport. Athletes are known to have used drugs in higher dosages and in a myriad of combinations with other drugs, far from the circumstances studied by scientists trying to establish safe dosages. Studying the impact of drugs on athletes faces 2 additional challenges. First, if the drug is banned from sport, athletes have strong motivations not to be honest if they use it. Critics cite this as a reason to lift prohibitions on drugs such as the anabolic steroids and EPO so that their impact on athletes' health could be more readily ascertained. A fair point, but this assumes that athletes will be forthcoming about how they are using the drug being studied and – a very big *and* – what other drugs they may be taking to enhance performance. Athletes have 2 reasons to be secretive: they do not want to be disqualified from competing, and they will not want to disclose whatever "secret formula" they're using lest they lose an advantage over their competitors. This last phenomenon – the never-ending quest for competitive advantage, and the fear that others have found one – turns out to be crucial for understanding the dynamics of performance-enhancing technologies in sport.

It is interesting and a bit ironic to note that Samaranch's advice to focus on health as the primary criterion is echoed by some of the fiercest critics of anti-doping. For example, in a 2008 article in the prestigious *BMJ*, 2 scholars proposed "making legal the use of drugs associated with low harm and testing health rather than testing for drugs … This view holds that if health is safeguarded it does not matter how performance is supplemented." [13, 14] Other advocates agree that "safe" drugs should be permitted in sport; one essay goes so far as to praise anabolic steroids for being "extremely safe and effective at reducing recuperation time" from injuries [15, p. 308]. The authors of the 2008 piece propose also a "harm reduction" strategy analogous to those used to reduce crime and the spread of disease for drugs such as heroin. The analogy turns out to have serious flaws, which are best exposed when the conversation turns to the second common defense of anti-doping, fairness.

Fairness and the Relentless Search for Advantage

As far as I know, people who use heroin and other narcotics are trying to get high – but they are not competing with one another to see who can get the highest. The way to win a high jump or pole vault event is, of course, precisely to get higher than anyone else. A drug addict needs only enough of his or her preferred substance to get to that individual's desired state, no more. What matters in athletic competitions is who can go fastest, highest, or farthest. If one drug, or some combination of drugs, provides an advantage, then as long as some athletes are using them, other competitors must do the same or else give up what could well be a decisive edge. In some sports, such as cycling road races, the advantage provided by a drug such as EPO, which stimulates production of oxygen-carrying red blood cells and thereby increases stamina, the difference can be as much as 5–10% [16]. You can be more talented and dedicated in your training, yet lose to the cyclist who uses EPO when you decline to do the same.

This phenomenon first became apparent to me when I spoke with elite athletes and coaches in the early 1980s. I asked why athletes used anabolic steroids or amphetamines – the performance-enhancing drugs of choice at that time. The answers were consistent and unequivocal: no athlete wants to surrender a decisive advantage to his or her competitors. That fear of losing to someone of lesser talent and commitment drove then, and drives today, some athletes to resort to banned performance-enhancing drugs and other technologies. I described this as the "coercive power" of drugs in sport [17, 18]. Coercion is typically understood to require force or threat of harm. Most athletes faced with the temptation to dope are not strictly speaking coerced. But the threat of losing their life's dream, of having what they worked for so hard and so long snatched from them because other people cheated is surely a powerful thing. Young athletes sacrifice much in order to devote themselves to their sport. Achieving their goals of an Olympic medal or a career in professional sport can be so important to them that it may be as powerful a threat to their hopes and dreams as coercion conventionally understood [19].

In sports where a banned performance-enhancing drug can be the difference between winning and finishing at the back of the pack or peleton, athletes confront three bad choices and only one good one. Of the bad alternatives, the first is to compete without doping in the knowledge that you may lose to someone who dopes. Some athletes make this choice; a very few do it and win despite the edge they have surrendered [20, 21]. A second choice is simply to cease competing, at least at this level. Many bicycle racers have now come forward to acknowledge making this choice when EPO and other drugs pervaded their sport [22]. The third option is to try to "level the playing field" by using whatever drugs your competitors use [23–25]. The fourth option is possible only where there is effective anti-doping: to compete without doping in the reasonable confidence that your fellow competitors are likewise not cheating.

It is worth noting that options three and four both attempt to "level" the playing field. Four accomplishes this by diminishing or eliminating the impact of doping on sport. Option three – using the same drugs as your competitors – illuminates the problem with relying on the principle of fairness alone to defend anti-doping. It may seem perverse but if all athletes cheat in precisely the same way, the playing field in a way has been made level. Anti-doping critics make this point frequently. It would not be unfair, they note, if all athletes were allowed to dope in comparable measure. On the other hand, as long as doping is prohibited, athletes who dope are acting unfairly to those athletes who respect the rule against doping.

The power of fairness as a moral foundation for anti-doping depends on having solid reasons for banning particular performance-enhancing technologies in the first place. If there are good reasons to ban, then fairness requires us to rigorously enforce that policy. Protecting health is certainly a good reason to prohibit certain technologies in sport where health is in fact threatened. But as stated previously, protecting health cannot be the entire story. By itself it cannot explain all that we care about in sport. For the rest of the story we have to look at meanings and values in sport.

Meanings and Values in Sport

WADA's guiding document is the WADA Code. The 2015 edition of the Code has this to say about its fundamental rationale:

Anti-doping programs seek to preserve what is intrinsically valuable about sport. This intrinsic value is often referred to as "the spirit of sport." It is the essence of Olympism, the pursuit of human excellence through the dedicated perfection of each person's natural talents. It is how we play true. The spirit of sport is the celebration of the human spirit, body and mind, and is reflected in values we find in and through sport, including:
- Ethics, fair play, and honesty
- Health
- Excellence in performance
- Character and education
- Fun and joy
- Teamwork
- Dedication and commitment
- Respect for rules and laws
- Respect for self and other participants
- Courage
- Community and solidarity

Doping is fundamentally contrary to the spirit of sport.

People quibble over the list of values enumerated in the WADA Code. The revised text now makes clear that these are only some of the values we seek in and through sport, not a comprehensive account. Critics often seize on the notion of "the spirit of sport," which on the one hand seems rather mystical and unspecific. On the other hand, however, that "spirit" is now in part spelled out as "the pursuit of human excellence through the dedicated perfection of each person's natural talents." I invite each reader to improve on this formulation or, alternatively, to show how this way of thinking about meanings and values in sport is defective. (As the source of this particular description of the spirit of sport, I am not inclined to attack it.)

Critics of anti-doping have recently come to embrace in part this account of the spirit of sport but continue to find reasons to reject efforts to ban many performance-enhancing drugs and other technologies. Here is a prominent and illuminating example:

The rules of any sport aim to define some activity which will bring out the display of certain skills or strengths, and allow the players to compete meaningfully in the expression of those skills. But the rules are essentially arbitrary. Why then do we have rules prohibiting beneficial substances? [15, p. 309]

These authors acknowledge that sport should promote meaningful competitions that exhibit certain skills; so far, this is consistent with the WADA Code. They also understand that rules are crucial in determining which skills are valued within each sport. But, they claim, these rules are "essentially arbitrary," notably when those rules ban what they describe as "beneficial substances." It is worth taking a closer look at the concept of "beneficial" and at what rules tell us about meanings and values in sport [26].

A professional golfer could find it very beneficial to use clubs that have rectangular grooves carved in their faces. These designs provide golfers much better control of balls that they hit out of the tall grass found in the rough that typically flanks the fairway of each hole. For that matter, there are specially designed golf balls that fly straight even if the golfer hits them in a way that would result in a hook or slice with other balls. Unfortunately, that professional golfer would be disqualified because those clubs and balls are banned from competition [27]. Aside from sheer perversity, why would the sport of golf ban such "beneficial" technologies? Why would any sport want to make performance more difficult?

The sport of swimming banned over a hundred bathing suits, but not until many world records had been shattered by swimmers wearing them [28]. Why would anyone want swimmers to go slower? [29].

A compact electric motor could help bicycle racers climb a long steep hill, but that is absolutely forbidden. (A gas-powered motorcycle would be even faster of course.) Why does the sport of cycling deny such "beneficial" technologies to competitors?

When it comes to sport the concept of "beneficial" means something other than merely whatever allows competitors to go faster, higher, or farther [30]. Otherwise those golf clubs and balls, slippery swimsuits, and motorized bikes would have been embraced, even celebrated – perhaps right alongside anabolic steroids, stimulants, EPO, growth hormone, and the many other substances athletes have used to enhance performance. So when Savulescu and Foddy [15] question why sport's "arbitrary" rules ban such "beneficial" technologies they fail to grasp something essential about sport – that sports regularly reject some technologies that enhance performance. Clearly, sport is about something more than simply maximum performance by whatever means possible.

Savulescu and Foddy also conflate two senses of "arbitrary." The accusation that something is arbitrary is not a compliment. It connotes autocratic, unjustified whim. But there is another sense of the term that is morally neutral. Take an example from the sport Americans call soccer and the rest of the world calls football.

In adult football, the goal is 24 ft wide by 10 ft high. I once suggested to a mostly European audience of scholars that football would have many more goals scored if only we doubled the width of the net to 48 ft. They were horrified at the thought. But surely, the current width of 24 ft is arbitrary – as is the size of the field, the number of players permitted on each side, and the rules prohibiting everyone but the goalie from contacting the ball with hands or arms. All of these rules are arbitrary in the sense that they were made by people who could have chosen different rules. Changing certain rules would alter the very nature of the sport; for example, allowing all players to catch the ball with their hands. But other changes would be more subtle, and the benign nature of their "arbitrariness" revealed. Suppose the goal was 23 ft 11 inch wide? Or 24 ft 1 inch? Football would look just as it does today. Occasionally, a ball would deflect the opposite way from it would now, but that would likely be a rare occurrence. The strategy of play would not be affected, nor would the creative tension between the goalie and the opposing team. It would remain difficult to kick the ball past a skilled goalkeeper, who would still be able to prevent many scores.

A width of 24 feet is arbitrary in the sense that it could have been otherwise, at least a bit, without fundamentally altering the nature of the game. It works well enough to allow the display of talents that make for exciting and fascinating football. Beneath this supposedly arbitrary rule is a deep and widely shared conception of what football is meant to be; in particular, the talents it displays and celebrates. Indeed, when any particular sport considers whether to change or retain a rule, to welcome or ban some technology, it does its job well when it grounds its decision in the values and meanings of that sport [31]. So it goes when golf bans certain clubs and balls, swimming bans buoyant, impermeable swimsuits, and cycling prohibits motors [32].

A vital choice that cuts across most sports, including all Olympic sports, is how to think about the role of natural talents versus pharmacologic enhancement. There is no question that athletes' performance can be boosted when some drug or combination of drugs alters their anatomy or physiology to suit the demands of their sport. Athletes who compete in the shot-put, discus, and hammer throw benefit from increased muscle, which anabolic steroids can help to build. Bike racers benefit from increased endurance; EPO is exceptionally good at doing just that. Some Olympic sports records set a decade or more ago, with the aid of performance-enhancing drugs, have not been broken. If the "spirit of sport" were maximum performance by whatever means necessary, then doping would be just another means of striving for that spirit.

If we followed the recommendations of various critics of anti-doping we could find sport welcoming a startling array of technologies from genetic manipulations to surgical alterations to a host of drugs and other ways of modifying human bodies, perceptions, and behaviors. What we cannot evade is the obligation to ask what we value in sport. Maximum performance abetted by any and all technologies is one possible answer. The anti-doping movement in sport offers an alternative: "the pursuit of human excellence through the dedicated perfection of each person's natural talents. It is how we play true. The spirit of sport is the celebration of the human spirit, body and mind…" This is an idealistic vision of sport to be sure. But it underlies, I believe, much of what draws people to the Olympic Games, to elite sports in general, and to the numberless local competitions that millions upon millions of people engage in every year [33]. Sustaining such a vision in practice against the forces of commercialism, unbridled ambition, fear, and greed is challenging. Neither can anti-doping become complacent or rely on its good intentions [34]. Anti-doping must strive unrelentingly for excellence just as the athletes it serves. Nevertheless, for everyone who plays, and everyone who watches appreciatively, the essential question for the future is what values and meanings do we seek in and through sport [35]. Our dedication to asking and answering this question should be no less than the dedication of each athlete in her or his quest for excellence.

References

1 Moston S, Skinner J, Engelberg T: Perceived incidence of drug use in Australian sport: a survey of public opinion. Sport Soc 2012;15:64–77.
2 Breivik G, Hanstad DV, Loland S: Attitudes towards use of performance-enhancing substances and body modification techniques. A comparison between elite athletes and the general population. Sport Soc 2009;12:737–754.
3 Stamm H, Lamprecht M, Kamber M, Marti B, Mahler N: The public perception of doping in sport in Switzerland, 1995–2004. J Sports Sci 2008;26:235–242.
4 Kayser B, Mauron A, Miah A: Current anti-doping policy: a critical appraisal. BMC Med Ethics 2007;8:2.
5 Ritchie I, Jackson G: Politics and "shock": reactionary anti-doping policy objectives in Canadian and international sport. Int J Sport Policy Polit 2013, pp 1–18.
6 Miah A: Enhanced athletes? It's only natural. Washington Post, August 3, 2008, pp 14–17.
7 Bostrom N: Letter from utopia. Stud Ethics Law Technol 2008;2:1–7.
8 Tamburrini C: Are doping sanctions justified? A moral relativistic view. Sport Soc 2006;9:199–211.
9 McNamee MJ, Edwards SD: Transhumanism, medical technology and slippery slopes. J Med Ethics 2006;32:513–518.
10 Sparrow R: A not-so-new eugenics. Hastings Cent Rep 2011;41:32–42.
11 Hoffman JR, Ratamess NA: Medical issues associated with anabolic steroid use: are they exaggerated? J Sports Sci Med 2006;5:182–193.
12 López B: The invention of a "drug of mass destruction": deconstructing the EPO myth. Sport Hist 2011;31:84–109.
13 Kayser B, Smith ACT: Globalisation of anti-doping: the reverse side of the medal. BMJ 2008;337:85–87.
14 Kayser B, Mauron A, Miah A: Viewpoint: legalisation of performance-enhancing drugs. Lancet 2005; 366(suppl):S21.
15 Savulescu J, Foddy B: Le Tour and failure of zero tolerance: time to relax doping controls; in Savulescu J, ter Meulen R, Kahane G (eds): Enhancing Human Capacities. Oxford, Blackwell, 2011.
16 Thomsen JJ, Rentsch RL, Robach P, Calbet JA, Boushel R, Rasmussen P, Juel C, Lundby C: Prolonged administration of recombinant human erythropoietin increases submaximal performance more than maximal aerobic capacity. Eur J Appl Physiol 2007;101:481–486.
17 Murray TH: The coercive power of drugs in sports. Hastings Cent Rep 1983; 13:24–30.
18 Johnson J, Butryn T, Masucci MA: A focus group analysis of the US and Canadian female triathletes' knowledge of doping. Sport Soc 2013;16:654–671.
19 Thompson T, Vinton N, O'Keeffe M, Red C: Victims of Lance Armstrong's strong-arm tactics feel relief and vindication in the wake of U.S. Anti-Doping Agency report. New York Daily News, October 26, 2012, pp 1–9, http://www.nydailynews.com/sports/more-sports/zone-lance-armstrong-bully-downfall-article-1.1188512.
20 Kimmage P: Rough Ride. London, Yellow Jersey Press, 2007.

21 McGee B: How dopers stole the best years of my career. The Sidney Morning Herald, October 27, 2012, pp 10–13, http://www.smh.com.au/sport/cycling/how-dopers-stole-the-best-years-of-my-career-20121026-28aif.html.

22 Kelly B: One Cyclist's Experience. Athletes Stories: In Their Own Words. Anti-Doping Research Institute, http://www.antidopingresearch.org/athletes-stories-in-their-own-words-2/.

23 Kirby K, Moran A, Guerin S: A qualitative analysis of the experiences of elite athletes who have admitted to doping for performance enhancement. Int J Sport Policy Polit 2011;3:205–224.

24 Leipheimer L: Affidavit of Levi Leipheimar. 2012, http://d3epuodzu3wuis.cloudfront.net/Leipheimer,+Levi,+Affidavit.pdf.

25 Lentillon-Kaestner V, Hagger MS, Hardcastle S: Health and doping in elite-level cycling. Scand J Med Sci Sports 2012;22:596–606.

26 Murray TH: Enhancement; in Steinbock B (ed): The Oxford Handbook of Bioethics. Oxford, Oxford University Press, 2009, pp 491–515.

27 USGA: Questions & Answers: Implementation of New Rules regarding Grooves. USGA Good Game 2009, http://cdn.cybergolf.com/images/1244/Grooves-Rule-Explanation.pdf.

28 ESPN: Swimmers bid farewell to high-tech bodysuits. Associated Press, May 24, 2010, http://sports.espn.go.com/espn/wire?section=swimming&id=5216167.

29 O'Connor LM, Vozenilek JA: Is it the athlete or the equipment? An analysis of the top swim performances from 1990 to 2010. J Strength Cond Res 2011;25:3239–3241.

30 Loland S: Technology in sport: three ideal-typical views and their implications. Eur J Sport Sci 2002;2:1–11.

31 Loland S, Hoppeler H: Justifying anti-doping: the fair opportunity principle and the biology of performance enhancement. Eur J Sport Sci 2012;12:347–353.

32 Loland S, McNamee M: Fair play and the ethos of sports: an eclectic theoretical framework. J Philos Sport 2000;27:63–80.

33 Murray T, Murray P: Rawls, sports, and liberal legitimacy; in Kaebnick GE (ed): The Ideal of Nature: Debates about Biotechnology and the Environment. Baltimore, The Johns Hopkins University Press, 2011, pp 179–199.

34 Overbye M, Wagner U: Experiences, attitudes and trust: an inquiry into elite athletes' perception of the whereabouts reporting system. Int J Sport Policy Polit 2013;6:407–428.

35 Murray TH: In search of an ethics for sport: genetic hierarchies, handicappers general, and embodied excellence; in Murray TH, Maschke KJ, Wasunna AA (eds): Performance-Enhancing Technologies in Sports: Ethical, Conceptual, and Scientific Issues. Baltimore, Johns Hopkins University Press, 2009, pp 225–238.

Thomas H. Murray, PhD
173 Crocker Lane
Brewster, MA 02631 (USA)
E-Mail thmurray46@gmail.com

Conclusion and Perspectives

David Howman

Wellington, New Zealand

Introduction

In the prior chapters of this book, leading experts across multiple disciplines have addressed specific aspects of anti-doping – regulatory and legal issues; anti-doping science; next generation anti-doping approaches; and social and ethical dimensions.

The fact that such a diverse set of expertise is required to thoroughly address the current state of anti-doping, and to identify the future opportunities and challenges facing the anti-doping community, speaks to the multiple fronts the global anti-doping community must cover to protect the clean athlete.

It is easy to forget that up until 1999 the anti-doping landscape looked very different than it does today. There was no single answer tackling doping in sport and there was no World Anti-Doping Agency (WADA).

David Howman was director general of the World Anti-Doping Agency from 2003 to 2016.

The anti-doping industry – and it is truly now a fully fledged industry – and WADA emerged from two serious crises that engulfed sport in 1998:
- First came the Festina controversy at that year's Tour de France. During the race, a large number of prohibited medical substances were found during a police raid. Several cyclists and entourage members were arrested.
- The second crisis, known as the Salt Lake City scandal, involved problems with the International Olympic Committee (IOC) and resulted in the suspension of several IOC members.

The cherished values of sport were being threatened. Doping, above all else, was identified to be the most serious threat to sport's future.

WADA: An Antidote to Doping in Sport?

WADA was formed in 1999 at the First World Conference on Doping in Sport. Representing the sport movement, the IOC invited governments of the world to Lausanne, Switzerland, with the aim of establishing an international, independent agency to combat doping in sport.

WADA started operating later that year as a unique 50/50 partnership between the sport movement and governments, with the IOC contributing half of WADA's annual budget, and national governments contributing the other half. This 50/50 split is also reflected in the composition of WADA's 38-member Foundation Board and 12-member Executive Committee.

WADA's key activities include scientific research, education, development of anti-doping capacities, and monitoring of the World Anti-Doping Code (the Code), the document that harmonizes anti-doping policies in all sports and all countries, and one of the most significant achievements in the fight against doping in sport to date [1].

Drafted in Copenhagen in 2003, the initial Code and International Standards – the *first* set of *globally consistent* anti-doping rules – were in effect in time for the Athens 2004 Olympic and Paralympic Games.

The government commitment to recognizing the Code came in the form of a UNESCO treaty: the UNESCO International Convention against Doping in Sport, which was written in record time in 2005, ratified by 30 countries, and came into force in 2006.

The Code and Standards have since been reviewed and revised twice – in 2007 (the 2009 Code) and in 2013 (the 2015 Code). There are more than 660 Code signatories, while 183 of a possible 195 countries (a 98% commitment) have ratified UNESCO's International Convention against Doping in Sport.

Values and Integrity: Twin Pillars of the Anti-Doping Movement

Despite today's "win-at-all-costs" culture continuing to threaten sport, the public and vast majority of athletes value the importance of fair play as they always have. Yet, the fact remains that within this "win-at-all-costs" culture there is a huge amount of temptation and pressure encouraging athletes to take shortcuts, enticing them with more money, with entourage members persuading the athlete to break the rules to benefit from any ill-gained success.

The public, however, continues to be disgusted by cheating. One might even say that in light of recent doping scandals, there are signs of doping fatigue. While people have not lost trust in the anti-doping movement, they have become more cynical about cheating. The anti-doping community has the responsibility to lead by example, to retain public and athlete confidence through a robust anti-doping system led by strong values and a unified, global voice for clean sport.

Ethics in sport help us distinguish what is right from what is wrong. Respect for the rules of sport and fair play, for sport opponents and officials, for honesty and ethical behavior – these values are about doing what is *right*.

Integrity aligns outward actions with inner values. A person with integrity refuses to compromise on matters of principle (e.g., honesty and fairness), even when the alternative (cheating) might seem "easier," "quicker," or "simpler."

A sport that displays integrity can often be recognized as honest and genuine in its dealings, championing good sportsmanship, and providing safe, fair, and inclusive environments for all involved. "Playing by the rules" is nonnegotiable. A sport that acts with integrity earns community confidence, trust, and support. The resulting faith and loyalty contribute to a healthy sport culture and to a business value that cannot be underestimated.

Integrity in sport can lead to:
- Increased participation – through member loyalty and attraction of new members.
- Financial viability – through membership, attraction of sponsors, and funding grants.
- On-field success – through attraction of players who want to be associated with a healthy, successful brand.

Activities and behaviors that define sport as lacking integrity include: creating an unfair advantage or manipulating results through performance-enhancing drugs, match fixing, or tanking.

Anti-social behaviors demonstrated by parents, spectators, coaches, and players also pose a significant integrity issue for sport. Such behaviors may include bullying, harassment, discrimination, and child abuse.

The integrity of a sport will be judged by its participants, spectators, sponsors, the general public, and, more often than not, the media. The survival of a sport, therefore, relies on ensuring that "the sport is the same on the outside as it is on the inside," and remains true to its values, principles, and rules.

As a young athlete in New Zealand, I was brought up on the value of fair play. At 10 years of age, I was captain of my school rugby team. I remember having to give the post-match speech. I turned to my grandmother for advice – herself, someone who held values in high esteem – and she told me how it should be done and reminded me what was important. First, show respect to your opponents and thank them for a good game. Second, show respect to the officials by thanking the referee on a job well done. And third, show appreciation of the many volunteers who make sport possible by thanking the hosts for their hospitality.

Following my 13th and final year as director general of WADA, up to the present, values remain of huge importance to me. But, it does not matter if you are director general of WADA, an athlete, or a sports fan – values remain vital if clean, honest sport is to continue to prosper. Our job in the anti-doping community is to ensure that these values are maintained, and the integrity of sport is protected, that fair play lives on, and that "play true" is our mantra.

Replacing a "War on Doping" with Protection of the Clean Athlete

For years, anti-doping has been thought of in negative terms: a war on doping; a battle between cat and mouse; and good guys versus bad guys. Yet today, it is more apparent that what we are doing in anti-doping in sport is not fighting a war on these fronts, rather we are protecting the clean athlete. This philosophical shift better captures what we in the anti-doping community stand for – ensuring clean athletes have the opportunity to compete on a level playing field. Clean athletes are the overwhelming majority, after all.

Today, under the improved rules of the revised Code, we protect the clean athlete like never before. We have longer, 4-year sanctions for intentional doping cheats; more effective testing that encourages organizations to test the *right* athlete for the *right* substance at the *right* time; and rules that better recognize that doping is less a solitary decision but more often results from the entourage encouraging the athlete to make bad decisions.

We are always increasing and improving research, both in science and also in social science, so we are able to better understand *why* an athlete dopes. To date, WADA has invested approximately USD 70 million in research, thanks to support from the IOC, governments, and other stakeholders.

WADA now has investigative power under the new Code. We cannot be the police to conduct search or seizure, but we can work with police and share information, ask people questions, form views, and build a case. More importantly, other anti-doping organizations can do the same.

We have an enhanced compliance program so that high-quality anti-doping programs are in place in every part of the world. We lead outreach and education initiatives that promote value-based education so that the athletes of tomorrow are prevented from doping. And let us not forget other crucial tools that are used to combat doping such as the athlete biological passport.

The potential is there for anti-doping to make greater progress than ever before, but for that to happen, we also require good practice from our anti-doping partners worldwide.

We also require the athletes to hold up their end of the bargain. As such, our expectations of athletes are that they make use of the system available to them. If athletes are aware of doping behavior, they can provide information to any one of the whistle-blower lines provided by WADA and its partners. Athletes have a responsibility to avoid association with banned support personnel, as is required through the new "Prohibited Association" article in the Code. And athletes also have responsibilities to complete their whereabouts reports efficiently. All these aspects are important if the system is to work in the athletes' best interests. Anti-doping organizations have a responsibility to uphold quality practice, but athletes must play their part in ensuring quality, too.

It is gratifying to see just how far we have come. The original struggle was to create a document that harmonized sanctions across every country and every sport. At the time, some stakeholders were reluctant to agree to a *2-year* sanction for a serious doping offence. Under today's Code, the sanction for serious offenders has *doubled*. This did not happen by accident. Public opinion shifted because of a constant debate that WADA has driven.

WADA has forged partnerships with INTERPOL and the World Customs Organization, the International Federation of Pharmaceutical Manufacturers & Associations, the Biotechnology Innovation Organization, and the Innovative Medicines Initiative; written models of best practice; provided education models for schools and universities; appealed many cases to the Court of Arbitration for Sport; and, much, much more.

When you consider the size of the challenge WADA faces; the limited budget (USD 30 million per year) at our disposal; and the difficulties inherent with uniting disparate bodies and countries and attempting to enhance anti-doping practice, it should not be doubted that WADA has achieved much in its short life.

Advances in Anti-Doping

Unquestionably, detection has improved in the last decade, but we cannot underestimate the extent to which people will take risks to achieve financial gain and personal glory. The reality is that, to protect clean athletes, we have reached the stage where science *alone* will not eradicate cheating or very often even detect it.

The reality is that the scientific expertise of those who choose to dope – many of whom are assisted by an entourage with increasing scientific and medical expertise designed solely to cheat and avoid detection – is often able to keep ahead of the science of the anti-doping community or at least the practical application of science in the accredited laboratories when analyzing collected samples, which of course the laboratories neither collected nor selected for collection.

The clever cheating athlete, on the other hand, is becoming better at cheating, more sophisticated, and *funded* more extensively. Look at the money to be made in sport today: most reasonably good footballers in the Premier League earn more than WADA's annual budget – 1 player! That clever cheating athlete might now feel quite confident in the view that he or she will avoid detection under the historical approach.

What has become more telling is that the mode of evidence collection need not simply nor solely be through sample collection and analysis of blood and urine. Already we have moved far from being reliant only on such processes – perhaps to the discomfort and concern of many – but to successfully gathering information and sharing intelligence as powerful evidence against those who have cheated with impunity.

Nonanalytical cases are mounting, from the days of BALCO (the Bay Area Laboratory Co-

Operative) and Tim Montgomery, to regular cases around the world in which authorities exchange data on a growing basis and gather evidence to proceed with these cases.

One only has to remind people that Lance Armstrong and Marion Jones competed for many years, were tested many times, and were never found to have an adverse analytical finding, and yet cheated throughout.

In her 2004 autobiography, *Life in the Fast Lane*, Jones [2] specifically wrote that she had not taken drugs and sued those who suggested she cheated. It was the investigative process – during which Jones lied to federal agents about her drug use – that led to the eventual charge of perjury to which she confessed, receiving a 6-month prison sentence in 2008.

Armstrong went on for many years bullying and threatening anyone who dared to challenge him. In fact, if he had not returned to competition in 2009, following his retirement in 2005, he might have got away with it all.

Investigations now form an integral part of any effective and efficient anti-doping program. There are of course ways and means of obtaining evidence through such inquiries.

Criminal Underworld and Black Market Pharmaceuticals

It has been estimated that at least 25% of the world's pharmaceutical products emanate from the black market and that 50% or more of the drugs sold on the Internet are counterfeit. They are nonsanitary and potentially dangerous to health. Some of the products are readily available through the Internet; some are "stolen" during research and development stages of the regulated industry.

The incentive to engage in drug trafficking has existed for several years and remains high. In many parts of the world, this activity is legal, and the financial returns are vast. For example, an initial investment of USD 100 can yield a return of between USD 1,000 and 10,000.

All governments might appropriately recognize this intrusion; it is a criminal matter if laws are in place, and the police will act if there are compelling penalties.

The illicit substances are sourced from raw materials obtained on the Internet and put together in unregulated, nonsanitized "kitchen laboratories." They do not just go to elite athletes or their entourage. They go to high school students who want to "look good," to security agents, to armed forces, and to ordinary people in gymnasia. As a matter of public health, this should be of concern to governmental authorities.

The criminal underworld makes money out of this activity, but it is also engaged heavily in other aspects challenging the integrity of sport. WADA is well aware that the same people who engage in the distribution and trafficking of prohibited substances are involved in bribery, corruption, money laundering, illegal betting, and fraud.

Clearly, WADA does not have the mandate, jurisdiction, or expertise to engage these underworld figures, but WADA is able to share information with the relevant authorities such as INTERPOL and others.

Our good and growing arrangements and agreements with the regulated pharmaceutical industry ensure that evidence of the black market supply is provided to the industry and to regulators. Partnerships with the pharmaceutical and biotechnology industries also allow WADA to receive information on compounds that have the potential for abuse in sport during their research and development stages, giving WADA the opportunity to develop detection methods at a much earlier stage.

In sport, there continues to be the "dopey" doper who is regularly caught through standard testing protocols, with a large number still risking in-competition testing. This doper effectively catches himself. On the other hand, there is the "sophisticated" doper who continues to get away with cheating.

Some might say the sophistication has expanded since the advent of WADA. Some might say that it has advanced even further through the introduction of the biological passport. Whatever the genesis, increasing sophistication is undoubted.

From microdosing to manipulation, the clever doper, aided, abetted, and considerably financed by clever entourage members continues to evade detection through the analytical process. And we continue to be haunted by the impunity with which, for example, many have treated human growth hormones and other prohibited substances.

WADA is under no illusion that it faces a huge struggle to keep pace with the techniques of the sophisticated dopers, but this must continue to be the aim – indeed, we need to get in front. If that means thinking more like the bad guys, then so we shall – and we shall encourage our researchers to do the same. To counter cheats, you have to change the whole way of looking at things.

There are significant costs involved – legal costs, testing costs, research costs, transport of samples costs, and others – that do not need any further clarification or explanation. Regrettably, cost can be used as an excuse by those responsible for anti-doping programs *not* to undertake the best possible approach.

To put cost into perspective, the sport industry brings in at least USD 800 billion a year. How can spending USD 400–500 million to protect the integrity of such a business be considered a significant amount of money in comparison? In fact, one could easily mount an argument that sport is not spending *enough* to defeat the biggest scourge it currently confronts.

The challenge also requires a funding level that is more commensurate with the size of the problem. What *should* be spent to protect the integrity of sport?

The Trickle-Down Effect of Doping

Why are athletes being tempted to dope? And, why is it becoming an issue for society in general? Is it just because substances are so much more readily available than they were, say, 10 years ago, or is it due to a quantum shift in moral attitudes?

WADA suspects it is a combination of both, but there is no doubt that attitudes towards doping have changed. Values generally across our societies have changed, and there are studies to prove that "cheating" in its many forms is not only commonplace but also considered acceptable in many countries, just so long as you do not get caught.

Cheating pervades all levels of the social spectrum. We have major scandals involving politicians that are fiddling with their expense forms and stories of tax evasion. A poignant example from the world of academia is the controversy surrounding dozens of students attending a Harvard undergraduate class admitting to plagiarism in an open book examination. As a Harvard dean aptly remarked, "Without integrity, there can be no genuine achievement."

WADA continues to deliver anti-doping messages and information through its education and outreach programs and spurs on its partners worldwide to replicate the WADA model, but we also need there to be a greater recognition that doping is wrong – on all levels.

It is not just at the elite level of sport that doping exists – we are now experiencing a significant "trickle-down" effect.

There are examples of high school athletes choosing to dope in order to try and win professional contracts – a particular problem with schoolboy rugby in South Africa, for example.

We hear of veteran recreational cyclists and runners taking prohibited substances, both to cheat their way to contention and to prolong their careers. Indeed, there was even the recent case of a national sports federation board member testing positive after competing in an amateur event.

Should there be a greater sense of outrage? Otherwise the trickle-down effect we are now witnessing from the elite to amateur and youth level could become a torrent.

Athletes

WADA is essentially a body that looks after the clean athlete. Sport relies on athletes for its survival. Sport does not exist without athletes. These athlete groups are most important in terms of representation. There are many areas in which appropriate representation can lead to proper voices for athletes. Sport must be very aware of its athletes and must take careful steps to ensure they are engaged. The rights of the clean athlete must be protected. The voice of the clean athlete must be heard.

Entourage

The sport movement and governments must realize that, in most cases, it is not athletes acting alone who abandon everything for which they should stand. They are assisted, counseled, sometimes tricked, and occasionally forced into the downward spiral of cheating.

Coaches, trainers, medical doctors, scientists, sports administrators – even some misguided parents – all of whom ought to know better, make a mockery of their responsibilities, and trivialize the years of training and dedication of the trusting athletes whom they betray.

Again, this was addressed to a degree in the revised Code, but imposing sanctions often relies on governmental processes, not sport tribunals.

WADA can share the experience it has gained as a unique international organization for the possible formation of a body to protect the integrity of sport, with all aspects that challenge integrity to be encompassed, anti-doping being but one arm.

Sport cannot deal with issues of sport or match fixing, bribery, and corruption, or other challenges to its integrity on its own. Certainly, we have witnessed enough high-level, widespread scandals at present – the findings of WADA's independent commission come to mind – to indicate that sport is simply ill equipped to cope with its own internal problems.

Is the governance so wrong that it "encourages" or condones corruption and cannot be changed under current rules – presidents for life, money for bids, buying votes?

WADA has worked very closely with national law enforcement agencies, INTERPOL, and other investigators responsible for maintaining integrity in individual sports or sporting leagues. It is the unanimous view of all those experienced individuals that the criminal underworld responsible for trafficking steroids and other prohibited substances is also engaged in illegal betting, bribery, and corruption.

Let us not be naive either. Legal betting also attracts bribery and corruption, even if the significant risks here might be easier to deal with, relatively speaking. Legal betting is the one area where the underworld launders its dirty money, not worrying if the bet is at odds where the return is negative. There are not 2, 3, or 4 separate groups – they are all part and parcel of the same problem. Bad people do bad things.

Establishing a World Sports Integrity Agency

From a commonsense perspective, is it efficient and effective to consider a united world body formed between sport and government to tackle these intertwined issues, with engagement and involvement of others where appropriate?

A world sports integrity agency could be established with the same governance as WADA. In other words, requiring an equal sharing of governance between sport and governments. Why not have an overarching board equipped with different arms that address specific aspects – namely doping, betting, bribery, and corruption? Membership could easily be extended, if necessary. This has not been necessary in WADA's case, as memoranda of understanding have been more appropriate.

What can be gleaned from the successful WADA sport-government model? Sport cannot undertake inquiries or investigations in order to gather evidence to be used in tribunals. Sport has no real power or jurisdiction – governments do. There are already several international treaties in place for corruption, whilst others have laws to cover betting and bribery.

Funding of any new arm of this agency could be considered separately. For example, the illegal betting arm might benefit from appropriate contributions from the legal and regulated betting bodies of the world, which need to protect their business, and/or from the collection of amounts received by law enforcement in dealing with illegal betting. During the 2010 FIFA World Cup, over just a few weeks, INTERPOL discovered USD 155 million in illegal betting and seized USD 9.9 million.

The arm relating to bribery and corruption could again quite properly be funded by the funds that might be collected as a result of investigations, prosecutions, and seizures. The agencies concerned might be usefully modeled on WADA with a small management team operating internationally but engaging those who are in the field.

Why limit this challenge to match fixing and illegal betting? Expand it to include the ever-increasing aspect of corruption and bribery. They all pose challenges to the integrity and values of sport.

Purity of competition and value-led, doping-free sport are what clean athletes and the public at large desire. Clean athletes deserve fair and even competition. The public wants to see fair play in action.

We all would like to see everyone playing true. Why delay?

References

1 World Anti-Doping Agency: The Code. Montreal, WADA, https://www.wada-ama.org/en/what-we-do/the-code.
2 Jones M: Life in the Fast Lane – An Illustrated Autobiography. Boston, Grand Central Publishing, 2004.

David Howman, CNZM
Harbour Chambers
111 The Terrace
Wellington 6011 (New Zealand)
E-Mail David.Howman@legalchambers.co.nz

Author Index

Ayotte, C. 68

Bigard, X. 77
Bloodworth, A.J. 177
Bowers, L.D. 77
Brueckner, S. 160
Budgett, R. 39

Friedmann, T. 119

Gerrard, D. 55

Haas, U. 22
Holz, M. 139
Howman, D. 194

Karanikolou, A. 119
Kinahan, A. 39

Ljungqvist, A. 1
Loland, S. 153

Marclay, F. 129
Mazzoni, I. 39
McNamee, M. 177
Miller, J. 68
Murray, T.H. 186

Neuberger, E.W.I. 91
Niggli, O. 34
Norman, P. 160

Petróczi, A. 160
Pipe, A. 55
Pitsiladis, Y. 119

Reedie, C. VII
Robertson, J. 139
Robinson, N. 107

Saugy, M. 129
Schumacher, Y.O. 107
Simon, P. 91
Sottas, P.-E. 107

Thevis, M. 68

Verdouka, I. 119

Wang, G. 119

Young, R. 11

Subject Index

AAS, *see* Anabolic androgenic steroids
ABP, *see* Athlete biological passport
ADAMS, *see* Anti-Doping and Management System
Alcohol, list of prohibited substances 52
ALPHA, *see* Athlete Learning Program about Health and Anti-Doping
Anabolic androgenic steroids (AAS)
    laboratory analysis 71, 72, 79–81
    list of prohibited substances 43, 44
    out-of-competition testing 4
    prohibited list inclusion 3, 4
Anti-Doping and Management System (ADAMS) 150
Armstrong, Lance 130, 197
Athlete biological passport (ABP)
    gene doping detection 100
    hematological module
        critical challenges 112, 113
        expert evaluation 112
        markers and analytics 111, 112
    overview 107–111
    personalized medicine 116, 117
    prospects
        endocrine module 115
        omics 115, 116
        steroidal module 113–115
Athlete education
    Athlete Learning Program about Health and Anti-Doping 172–174
    challenges in anti-doping 157, 158
    ideals of education 154
    overview 153, 154
    prospects 158
    reason-based behavioral change in value-based anti-doping intervention 168–171
    sport interpretations
        human enhancement 155, 156
        human excellence 156, 157
        instrumentalism 154, 155
Athlete Learning Program about Health and Anti-Doping (ALPHA) 172–174
Autologous blood transfusion, *see* Blood doping

BALCO, *see* Bay Area Laboratory Co-Operative
Bay Area Laboratory Co-Operative (BALCO) 6, 102, 197, 198
Beta-2 agonists
    accidental consumption 75
    list of prohibited substances 45, 46
Beta-blockers, list of prohibited substances 52, 53
Black market, pharmaceuticals 198, 199
Blood doping
    laboratory analysis 72, 73, 81, 83, 121–125
    omics detection
        prospects 125–127
        rationale 119, 120
        research findings 120–125
    prohibition 48, 49
Blood sampling, historical perspective 5, 6

Cannabinoids, list of prohibited substances 51
CAS, *see* Court of Arbitration for Sport
Clenbuterol, accidental consumption 75
Court of Arbitration for Sport (CAS)
    centralization of jurisdiction 26–28
    control standard 28–30
    establishment 14

national law
- curtailing 25, 26
- remaining influence 30
- overview 15, 23
- sport environment effects 36, 37

CRISPR/Cas9, gene doping 98, 99, 103

Designer drugs
- historical perspective 6, 7
- laboratory analysis 74, 75, 86

Diuretics, list of prohibited substances 47, 48

Doping
- constructs 161, 162
- control and deterrence 164
- definitions 163
- motivations 165, 167
- performance enhancement mindset for prevention 166, 167
- pragmatic view 165, 166
- reason-based behavioral change in value-based anti-doping intervention 168–171

Education, *see* Athlete education
Ephedrine, history of use 2, 3
EPO, *see* Erythropoietin
Erythropoietin (EPO)
- gene doping 93, 95, 100
- laboratory testing 83–85, 121–125
- list of prohibited substances 44, 45

Ethics, anti-doping
- anti-doping rule violations 179, 180
- fairness and search for advantage 188–190
- gratuitous logic of sport 178, 181–183
- health and safety considerations 187, 188, 196, 197
- meanings and values in sport 190-192
- preservation of admirable qualities of sports 180, 181, 183, 184
- values and integrity in anti-doping 195, 196

Follistatin, gene doping 92, 95
Forensic intelligence
- anti-doping application 133–137
- operational intelligence 132
- overview 131
- strategic intelligence 132, 133
- structured memory 133
- tactical intelligence 131, 132

Gene doping
- historical perspective of M3 gene doping 92–94
- laboratory analysis
  - direct versus indirect detection 100
  - overview 99, 100
- small interfering RNA and transgene detection 101, 102
- transgenic proteins 100, 101
- overview 91, 92
- prohibition 48, 49
- prospects 102–104
- techniques
  - classical gene therapy 94–96
  - RNA interference 97–99
  - stem cell therapy 96, 97

Gene SMART study 125
GH, *see* Growth hormone
Glucocorticoids, list of prohibited substances 51
Growth hormone (GH)
- laboratory analysis 73, 74, 83, 84, 115
- list of prohibited substances 44, 45

IGF-I, *see* Insulin-like growth factor-I
Insulin-like growth factor-I (IGF-I)
- gene doping 92, 95
- laboratory analysis 115
- list of prohibited substances 44, 45

Intelligence gathering
- Anti-Doping and Management System 150
- financial information 145
- INTERPOL-WADA collaboration 145–148
- law enforcement 150, 151
- overview 139–143
- personal information 144, 145
- substance information 145
- World Anti-Doping Code incorporation 148–150

International Olympic Committee Medical Commission (IOC-MC) 2, 6
INTERPOL, WADA collaboration 145–148, 198
IOC-MC, *see* International Olympic Committee Medical Commission

Jensen, K.E., death during Olympics 1, 2, 155
Jones, Marion 198

Laboratory analysis
- accidental consumption 75
- accreditation of laboratories 69–71
- anabolic androgenic steroids 71, 72, 79–81
- blood doping 72, 73, 81, 83
- challenges
  - alternative matrices 86, 87
  - designer drugs 74, 75, 86
  - overview 85, 86, 197
  - population reference range and metabolism studies 86
  - reference materials 86

gene doping
    direct versus indirect detection 100
    overview 99, 100
    small interfering RNA and transgene detection 101, 102
    transgenic proteins 100, 101
growth hormone 73, 74, 83, 84
    historical perspective 68, 69
    prospects 75, 87
    research needs 77, 78
    scope of assays 71
    standardization 3, 4
List of prohibited substances and methods
    classification of substances and methods 40, 41
    historical perspective 3
    inclusion criteria 41, 42
    legal context 39, 40
    method prohibition 48, 49
    Monitoring Program 42, 43
    nomenclature 43
    publication and revision 40
    sections
        anabolic agents 43, 44
        beta-2 agonists 45, 46
        cannabinoids 51
        diuretics and masking agents 47, 48
        glucocorticoids 51
        hormone and metabolic modulators 46, 47
        narcotics 50
        non-approved substances 43
        peptide hormones and growth factors 44, 45
        stimulants 49, 50
    sport-specific prohibitions
        alcohol 52
        beta-blockers 52, 53
    therapeutic use exemption 42

Ma Huang 2
Meldonium
    list of prohibited substances 47
    Monitoring Program 43
MicroRNA, laboratory analysis 85
Monitoring Program, list of prohibited substances and methods 42, 43
Morality, see Ethics, anti-doping

Narcotics, list of prohibited substances 50

Omics
    athlete biological passport 115, 116
    blood doping detection
        prospects 125–127
        rationale 119, 120
        research findings 120–125

OOCT, see Out-of-competition testing
Out-of-competition testing (OOCT), historical perspective 4, 5

Performance enhancement mindset, doping prevention 166, 167
PPAR agonists, list of prohibited substances 47
Pseudoephedrine, Monitoring Program 42, 43

RNA interference, gene doping 93, 94, 97–99

Stimulants, list of prohibited substances 49, 50

Testosterone, see Anabolic androgenic steroids
Therapeutic use exemption (TUE)
    applications
        management 65, 66
        retroactive applications 60
        review 59, 60
        submission 58, 59
    beta-2 agonists 46
    challenges 61, 62
    committees
        appeals 60, 61
        overview 57, 58
    Expert Group 61
    historical perspective 5, 56, 57, 61
    international standard 57
    list of prohibited substances 42
    scope of processes 62–65
Trickle-down effect, doping 199, 200
TUE, see Therapeutic use exemption

WADA, see World Anti-Doping Agency
WADC, see World Anti-Doping Code
World Anti-Doping Agency (WADA)
    athlete protection 200
    code, see World Anti-Doping Code
    historical perspective 7–9, 194, 195
    INTERPOL collaboration 145–148, 198
    prohibited list, see List of prohibited substances and methods
    research funding 9
World Anti-Doping Code (WADC)
    arbitration, see Court of Arbitration for Sport
    democratic legitimating 24, 25
    historical perspective
        2003 code
            drafting process 12, 13
            substance 13–15
        2009 amendments
            drafting process 15
            substance 15–17

2015 amendments
    drafting process 17, 18
    substance 18–20
overview 8, 195
information gathering incorporation 148–150
legal environment influences
    data protection 37
    human rights 37
    national legislation evolution 37, 38
prohibited list, *see* List of prohibited substances and methods
rationale 11, 12
regulatory authority 23, 24
sport environment influences
    athletes 35, 36
    Court of Arbitration for Sport 36, 37
    current environment 35
    governance of sport 36
World sports integrity agency, establishment 200, 201

Zilpaterol, accidental consumption 75